J. P. Lintermans W. G. van Dorp

Differential Diagnosis in Pediatric Echocardiography

With 110 Figures and 20 Tables

Springer-Verlag
Berlin Heidelberg New York 1981

Dr. Jean Paul Lintermans

Université Catholique de Louvain
Cliniques Universitaires St. Luc
Cardiologie Pediatrique
B-1200 Brussels
Belgium

Dr. Willem Gerrit van Dorp

De Graafschap 118
2904 XX Capelle aan den IJssel
The Netherlands

ISBN-13:978-3-642-67517-1 e-ISBN-13:978-3-642-67515-7
DOI: 10.1007/978-3-642-67515-7

Library of Congress Cataloging in Publication Data.

Lintermans, Jean Paul 1935–. Differential diagnosis in pediatric echocardiography. Bibliography: p. Includes index. 1. Ultrasonic cardiography. 2. Pediatric cardiology. 3. Diagnosis, Differential. I. Dorp, Willem Gerrit van, 1951– joint author. II. Title. [DNLM: 1. Diagnosis, Differential – In infancy and childhood. 2. Echocardiography – In infancy and childhood. WG141.5.E2 L761d] RJ423.5.U46L56 618.92'007543 80-12801

2127/3020–543210

To the Sick Child

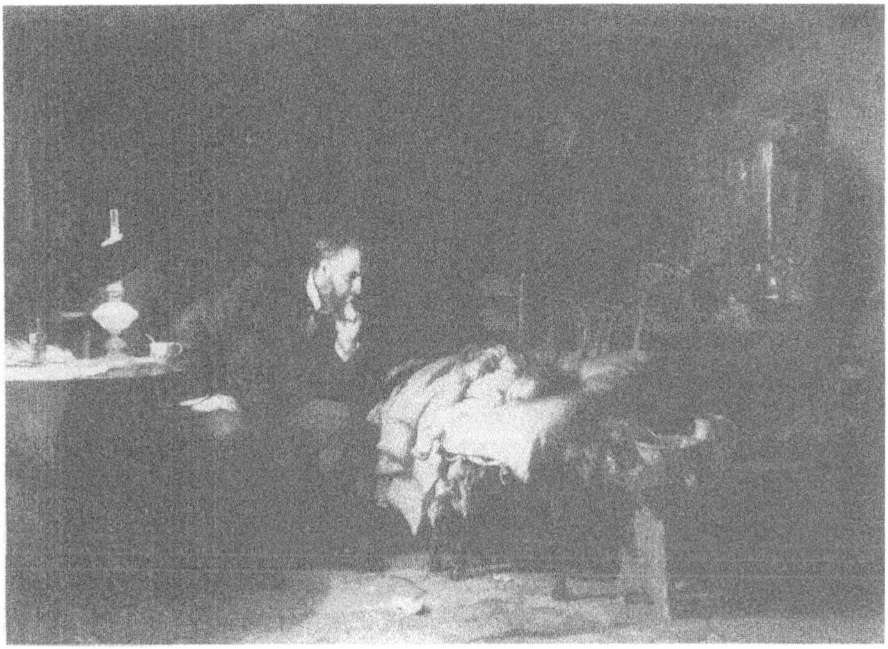

Sir Luke Fildes
The Doctor, 1891
© The Tate Gallery, London

Foreword

Dr. Jean Lintermans came to Seattle in 1962 from his general pediatric residency at the University of Iowa. He worked with us in clinical pediatric cardiology and in our animal physiology laboratory for the next three years. He was the most productive individual in the history of our training program, publishing seven papers in those three years, four clinical papers and three involving pulsed ultrasonic flowmeters and implanted ultrasonic displacement devices in animals. The work, from laboratory to publication, was always done with the utmost attention to accuracy, and was well developed conceptually. Although English was not his native language, Jean's mastery of English was not only excellent, I felt that he actually communicated better than many of our native physicians.

During the past year, I was delighted to learn that Jean was preparing a textbook on pediatric echocardiography with Dr. van Dorp, and was even more pleased to be asked to write a foreword. However, the greatest pleasure came from actually reading this book, and finding that it does indeed have a unique approach, and with the additional genuine benefit to the reader of a thorough, consistent, segmental approach to the diagnosis of congenital heart disease.

As a medical student, and as a resident physician, I have often been unhappy with being confronted with a difficult clinical problem, and when attempting to read about the significance of some clinical finding or other to find a huge number of pages that began from the position of the diagnosis, when, in fact, none was known. It seems infinitely preferable, but surprisingly rare, to find a subject such as echocardiography approached from the point of view of the individual findings, followed by a logical sequence leading toward the diagnosis, rather than requiring knowledge of the diagnosis prior to appreciating the significance of the echocardiographic findings.

As to the segmental approach to cardiac anatomy, Dr. Lintermans and Dr. van Dorp have done all of us a great service by this thorough and unambiguous approach to the diagnosis and classification of abnormalities that are subtle, difficult to describe, and even difficult to comprehend. One of the aspects of congenital heart disease that makes it exciting, but difficult, is the incredible variety of combinations of defects. The temptation to use eponyms to describe some of these complicated combinations is strong, but fortunately has been resisted, in favor of genuinely descriptive terminology. This permits a much more general approach, and causes less confusion in the diagnosis and surgical treatment of children who are unlucky enough to have, in addition to obstructive defects and septational defects, major abnormalities in the location and relationships of the heart chambers and great vessels.

In addition, sector scan echocardiography, or cross-sectional dynamic echocardiography, is an integral part of their approach, in contrast to some earlier textbooks in which the approach is primarily M-mode echocardiography, with only a hint of the usefulness of the two-dimensional approach. Further, the authors have used the cross-sectional visualizations in a flexible and exploratory manner that optimizes the echocardiographic diagnosis in complicated cases.

In addition to the careful systematic approach to the segmental relationship, the later chapters indicate an unusually thorough understanding of physiology. Almost all echocardiographic findings are related by the authors to the normal and abnormal function reflected in the dynamic anatomy. An additional excellent feature is that they make very clear when the mechanisms they propose as explanations are controversial, or whether they represent a well-documented concensus. Overall, there is a clear dedication to regarding the echocardiographic findings within a clinical picture. Common sense is regularly evident in their approach – a welcome presence.

In summary, Drs. Lintermans and van Dorp have made a very substantial contribution to the advancement of our knowledge of echocardiography, and more important, to the entire field of pediatric cardiology. I offer them my sincere congratulations.

Warren G. Guntheroth, M.D.

Professor of Pediatrics
Head, Division of Pediatric Cardiology
University of Washington School of Medicine
Seattle, Washington U.S.A.

Preface

Undoubtedly, when our book finally makes it, sceptical physicians will ask: another book on pediatric echocardiography? And seconds later they will ask: does that book offer something new?

Both questions can be answered affirmatively. Not only is this a new book, but it presents current echocardiographic data in a new way.

Since the first publication by Ultan et al. [393] of the application of ultrasound in a child, a steady stream of publications and several textbooks on the subject have been published. The approach to ultrasonic diagnosis has so far been authoritative, with little attempt at differential diagnosis. Our aim was to provide anyone interested in the art of echocardiography with a simple, schematic guidebook in which every echocardiographic feature is discussed from a diagnostic viewpoint. This was made possible through the collection of data from about 450 publications, and through the authors' experience.

The presentation of these data is, so far as we know, innovative: classically, in a textbook or article on pediatric echocardiography, a disease entity is discussed and only subsequently are the ultrasonic features of this abnormality presented. Throughout this book a more clinical sequence is followed: An echocardiographic sign or abnormality is presented, followed by a list of the conditions in which the ultrasonic feature has been reported to occur. Differentiating echocardiographic features are then discussed.

Each echocardiographic sign has a number (the chapter number followed by a serial number such as 1.1), while every disease entity listed under that ultrasonic feature has the same number followed by one additional digit (such as 1.1.1). Any pathologic condition characterized by different echocardiographic features may therefore be mentioned repeatedly in the book, at different places and under different serial numbers. However, a complete ultrasonic description of every condition is to be found at the place in the book where its most characteristic or specific sign is described. This place is indicated by an asterisk in the index to each chapter, listing the different anomalies referred to in that chapter, and in italics in the general index at the end of the book. Our book is thus intended to be a guidebook: when an abnormal feature is found on an echocardiographic tracing, the various diagnostic possibilities listed under that feature are then considered.

Finally, it should be realized that this book is a user's manual, and not a textbook on echocardiography. Indeed, an introduction to the physics of ultrasound, examination techniques, and the normal echocardiogram have been omitted intentionally.

The book is divided into three parts totalling 24 chapters. The first part, labeled Qualitative Anatomy and including the first nine chapters, deals with abnormal echocardiographic anatomy. Ultrasonically, anatomy may seem to deviate from the normal, because recorded structures are abnormally located (Chaps. 1–3), because normally expected structures cannot be recorded (Chaps. 4–7), or to the contrary, because normally absent structures are visualized (Chaps. 8 and 9).

The second part of the book is titled Quantitative Anatomy and is subdivided into two sections. In the first section, abnormal valve motion patterns are discussed (Chaps. 10–13), while in the second section (Chaps. 14–21) the echocardiographic appearance of structures is analyzed quantitatively. Cardiac chambers and great arteries may have abnormal intracavitary dimensions, while the intraventricular septum (IVS) may be abnormal in either thickness or motion.

The final part of the book is devoted to functional assessment. Chapter 22 introduces contrast echocardiography, while the last two chapters (Chaps. 23 and 24) review the clinical usefulness of various echocardiographically determined parameters.

An appendix at the end of the book lists normal age-related values for the most important echocardiographic measurements. Some of these data are from the study of Dr. P. J. Voogd, who echocardiographically studied 425 healthy school children between the ages of 4 and 17 years, and which were presented at the Third Symposium on Echocardiography at Rotterdam in June 1979. Other data pertaining to younger age groups were obtained from the literature.

Most of the conclusions in this book represent the opinions and experience not only of the authors but of the majority of echocardiographers as stated in the recent literature. Obviously, some observations await confirmation.

The echocardiograms used to illustrate this book were made at either St. Joseph's Clinic, Herent, at the Université Catholique de Louvain, Belgium, or at Sophia Kinderziekenhuis in Rotterdam, The Netherlands. Two different echocardiographic systems have been used – either a Smith Kline Ekoline apparatus, or an Echocardiovisor (Organon Teknica) including the multiscan facility. Almost without exception, extensive clinical, physiologic, angiographic, surgical, and sometimes autopsy observations were available.

It is our sincere hope that this book will benefit all children with heart disease, everywhere, by providing a better understanding of echocardiography.

Personal Acknowledgements

I am greatly indebted to Dr. V. H. de Villeneuve, head of pediatric cardiology at Sophia Kinderziekenhuis at Erasmus Universiteit, Rotterdam, The Netherlands, who for 7 months accepted me in his service and did his utmost to provide me with the necessary echocardiographic environment, and to Dr. S. Spitaels, pediatric cardiologist at Sophia, who through her constructive criticism was the first to contribute to my ultrasonic education. Similarly, I am indebted to Dr. A. Vliers, head of pediatric cardiology at the Clinique St. Joseph, Herent, Université catholique de Louvain, Belgium, for allowing me to leave his service for more than a semester.

I also wish to acknowledge my debt to the individual who contributed most to my pediatric cardiac education from 1962 to 1965. This is Dr. W. G. Guntheroth, head of pediatric cardiology at the University of Washington School of Medicine, Seattle, Washington.

Finally, it is impossible to express my debt to my wife, M. Cecilia, and our children, Solange, Christian and Thierry, for while I was writing this book, I must have been as a distant echo to them.

J. P. Lintermans

Acknowledgements

It was Dr. J. Roelandt who first introduced me to the basics of echocardiography, early during my medical studies. I am most grateful to him and to Prof. P. G. Hugenholtz, head of the department of Cardiology at the Erasmus University Hospital in Rotterdam, who not only stimulated me scientifically but made it possible for me to keep on working in the echolaboratory during most of my medical studies. At Sophia Kinderziekenhuis, headed by Prof. Visser, Dr. S. Spitaels taught me the most complex but fascinating field of pediatric cardiology. Together we spent many hours making and analyzing echocardiograms from hundreds of children. For many reasons, echocardiography would not have been possible without the active head of the department of pediatric cardiology, Dr. V. H. de Villeneuve. I am also quite grateful to Dr. Ir. N. Bom, head of the experimental ultrasound department at the Thorax Center, Rotterdam and his staff, who were always eager to help me with technical problems. Finally, I would like to thank the many workers at both the Thorax Center and at Sophia Kinderziekenhuis for their excellent collaboration.

W. G. van Dorp

*Contents**

* A more detailed survey will be found at the beginning of each chapter.

Function

Appendix

Common Echocardiographic Abbreviations

The following abbreviations are used in both their nominal and adjectival senses, i. e., "LA" stands for "left atrial" as well as "left atrium", and "LV" stands for "left ventricular" as well as "left ventricle".

Abbreviation	Translation
aCH	anterior chamber
AMVL	anterior mitral valve leaflet
Ao	aorta
AoV	aortic valve
ASD	atrial septal defect
ASH	asymmetric septal hypertrophy
ATVL	anterior tricuspid valve leaflet
AV	atrioventricular
c	cusp
CHD	congenital heart disease
CO	cardiac output
DEVM	maximal diastolic endocardial velocity
DORV	double outlet right ventricle
d-TGA	d-transposition of the great arteries
DVO	diastolic volume overload
ECG	electrocardiogram
EF	ejection fraction
endo	endocardium
F_s	fractional shortening
HOCM	hypertrophic obstructive cardiomyopathy
IAS	interatrial septum
ICT	isovolumic contraction time
IHSS	idiopathic hypertrophic subaortic stenosis
IVS	interventricular septum
LA	left atrium
LBBB	left bundle branch block
log	logarithm
LPEP	left ventricular pre-ejection period
l-TGA	l-transposition of the great arteries
LV	left ventricle
LVEDV	left ventricular end-diastolic volume
LVESV	left ventricular end-systolic volume
LVET	left ventricular ejection time

Abbreviation	Translation
LVH	left ventricular hypertrophy
LVID	left ventricular internal dimension
$LVID_d$	end-diastolic left ventricular internal dimension
$LVID_s$	end-systolic left ventricular internal dimension
LVOT	left ventricular outflow tract
LVPW	left ventricular posterior wall
MGA	malposition of the great arteries
ms	millisecond
MV	mitral valve
PA	pulmonary artery
PAEDP	pulmonary arterial end-diastolic pressure
pAoW	posterior aortic wall
PAH	pulmonary arterial hypertension
PDA	patent ductus arteriosus
PEP	pre-ejection period
peri	pericardium
PF	pericardial fluid
Pl.F	pleural fluid
pMVL	posterior mitral valve leaflet
PTVL	posterior tricuspid valve leaflet
PV	pulmonary valve
RA	right atrium
RBBB	right bundle branch block
RF	rheumatic fever
RPEP	right ventricular pre-ejection period
RV	right ventricle
RVAW	right ventricular anterior wall
RVDVO	right ventricular diastolic volume overload
RVH	right ventricular hypertrophy
RVICT	right ventricular isovolumic contraction time
RVOT	right ventricular outflow tract
SAM	systolic anterior motion
SBE	subacute bacterial endocarditis
SEVM	maximal systolic endocardial velocity
STI	systolic time intervals
SV	stroke volume
SVAS	subvalvular aortic stenosis
TAPVR	total anomalous pulmonary venous return
T/F	tetrad of Fallot
TV	tricuspid valve
Vcf	velocity of circumferential fiber shortening
VSD	ventricular septal defect
2D	two-dimensional

Qualitative Anatomy

Abnormal Location of Cardiac Segments

1 Abnormal Location of the Atria

Index

Introduction

Rather than classifying congenital abnormalities according to the total entity, a segmental approach is preferred in which the heart is divided into its three major anatomical segments: the atria, the ventricles, and the great arteries [295]. The atrial and ventricular chambers are then located, the relationship of the great arteries determined, and finally, the connections and relations of the cardiac segments to one another are defined.

As a first step it is necessary to establish the atrial situs. The normal situation, in which the anatomical right atrium lies to the right of the anatomical left atrium (LA), is called situs solitus. Two other types of atrial situs exist: situs inversus and situs ambiguous.

Although both atria have characteristic morphologic features, at present none of these features can be recognized ultrasonically. Noninvasive diagnosis of atrial situs is, therefore, routinely inferred from other features.

(1) The Visceroatrial Rule

The atrial chambers are located by noting the position of the liver on the X-ray, where the right atrium (RA) usually lies on the same side as the greater lobe of the liver [239, 361]. In general, when the liver is in its normal right-sited position (situs solitus), the atrial chambers are expected to be normally oriented. When the liver is left-sited (situs inversus), the RA is usually located to the left of the morphological LA. If the position of the liver cannot be clearly defined, as with asplenia or polysplenia syndromes, the situs is ambiguous and the visceroatrial rule does not hold [324].

(2) The Bronchial Situs

The right and left lung have three and two lobes, respectively. On a plain chest roentgenogram, this normal asymmetrical disposition can be inferred from the disposition of the tracheobronchial tree [241]. On a well-exposed chest roentgenogram, in frontal projection, the right main bronchus is noted to have a more direct course as compared to the left main bronchus, which is more horizontally oriented. If a mirror-image or symmetrical disposition of the bronchial tree is documented, atrial inversion or situs ambiguous of the atria should be strongly suspected [241].

(3) The Electrocardiographic Examination

The sense (positive or negative) of the P wave in a standard ECG should be carefully noted [367]. An upright P wave in lead I suggests that the atria (and venae cavae) are in a normal situs solitus position, whereas an inverted P wave suggests that they are inverted. Ectopic atrial rhythms, which are not uncommon in spatial abnormalities, may unfortunately complicate this diagnostic assessment.

(4) Two-Dimensional Echocardiography

Finally, echocardiographic diagnosis of atrial situs seems possible through direct visualization of the RA and inferior vena cava. As Lieppe et al. showed [207], these structures are amenable to echocardiographic recognition using a two-dimensional technique and peripheral vein injections, with the transducer in the subxyphoid area. Once the inferior vena cava has been located either to the right or to the left of the spine, the atrial situs can be inferred, since the RA is usually concordant with (on the same side as) the inferior vena cava.

1.1 Abnormally Sited Right Atrium

1.1.1 Left-Sited Right Atrium

In this condition, also called atrial inversion, the morphologic RA lies to the left of the morphologic LA. As a rule, it is encountered in mirror image dextrocardia.

As discussed before, noninvasive diagnosis of atrial inversion will rely on the visceroatrial rule, the bronchial situs, the sense of the P wave in lead I of the ECG, and the direct visualization of the inferior vena cava using two-dimensional and contrast echocardiography [207].

Quite exceptionally, isolated atrial inversion with venoatrial concordance and visceroatrial discordance may occur. This situation, which upsets the visceroatrial rule, has been described once in an infant with dextrocardia [60].

1.1.2 Situs Ambiguous of the Atria

At present, a noninvasive diagnosis of situs ambiguous of the atria is not practical.

2 Abnormal Location of the Ventricles

Index

Introduction

The next step in the echocardiographic diagnostic approach to a complex heart lesion is the study of the second major anatomical cardiac segment: the ventricular chambers. Both the right and left ventricles must be identified, their respective position noted, and their connection with both the atria and the great arteries must be determined. Concordance refers here to a normal connection, either atrioventricular or ventriculo-arterial, whereas discordance implies an abnormal connection.

The ventricular chambers are located by the echocardiographic identification of the tricuspid valve (TV) and the mitral valve (MV), which are a part of the morphological right and left ventricle respectively [361]. Based on their M mode echocardiographic patterns alone, the MV and TV cannot be distinguished from each other. However, the atrioventricular (AV) valves can be differentiated through their relationship with the semilunar valves. As a general rule, the AV valve whose anterior leaflet is continuous with the posterior margin of a semilunar valve is the MV [361]. Conversely, the AV valve whose anterior leaflet is not continuous with a posterior semilunar valve is the TV. Regardless of whether one is dealing with levocardia or dextrocardia, if the TV is found to the right of and/or anterior to the MV, there has been ventricular d-looping.

However, mitral-semilunar fibrous continuity may be absent or not always evident echocardiographically. Two more ultrasonic features may then help in the recognition of the AV valves [208]: (1) the study of AV valve closure on an M-mode tracing: normally the MV closes before the TV; and (2) the cross-sectional dynamic visualization of the two AV valves: indeed, a transverse cross section

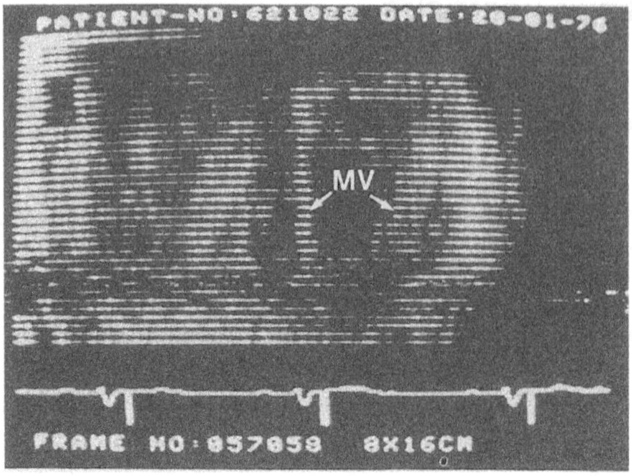

Fig. 2.1. Two-dimensional transverse cross section through the LV in mid-diastole. The MV is fully opened and the two leaflets can be recognized

through the MV clearly shows two leaflets with a characteristic opening and closing movement resembling a "fishmouth". (see Fig. 2.1).

To the contrary, a transverse cross section through the tricuspid valve – not always possible as this valve is positioned behind the sternum – reveals a three leaflet valve.

In this chapter, abnormalities in which the ventricles are abnormally positioned, relative to each other, will be reviewed briefly.

2.1 Right Ventricle Left-Sited Relative to the Left Ventricle (or Ventricular l-Loop)

The following abnormalities, which are characterized by a left-sited right ventricle (RV), have in common an abnormally positioned intraventricular septum (IVS) which is often not amenable to ultrasonic detection, as the IVS is usually oriented perpendicular to the chest wall, either vertically as in ventricular inversion (2.1.1 and 2.1.2), or horizontally as in the criss-cross heart (2.1.3).

2.1.1 Ventricular Inversion Without Ventriculo-arterial Discordance (Physiologic TGA)

Apart from clinical, roentgenographic and electrocardiographic evidence, ventricular inversion should be suspected echocardiographically if the AV valve which is not continuous with a semilunar valve is found to the left of the MV, i. e., the valve in which this continuity is documented [361]. The anatomical RV is then left sited relative to the anatomical left ventricle. This relative ventricular position is independent of the position of the heart in the thorax: a ventricular l-loop may occur in levo-, meso-, and dextrocardia.

In addition, a dynamic transverse ultrasonic cross section through the fourth intercostal space will show displaced side-by-side ventricles, with the IVS not always visualized as it now lies in a plane parallel to the incident sound wave [118]. The latter phenomenon may also be observed in M-mode, as is illustrated in Fig. 2.2.

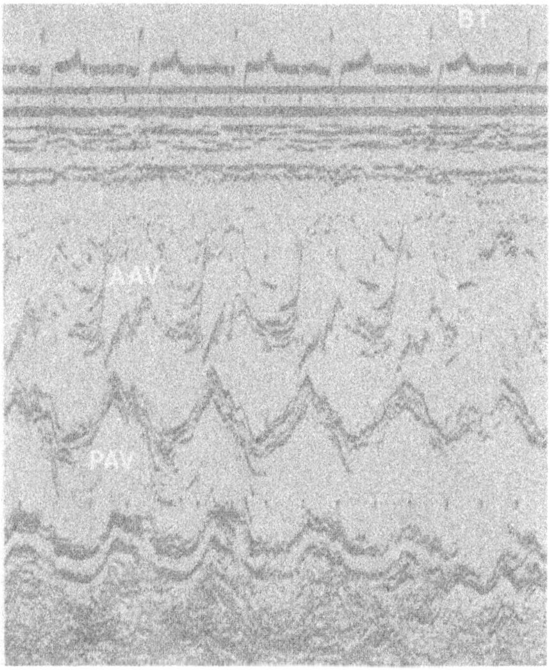

Fig. 2.2. BT: M-mode echocardiographic tracing obtained from a 7-month-old baby with angiographically documented atrioventricular discordance with ventriculo arterial concordance. Note the documentation of two AV valves without intervening septum

2.1.2 Ventricular Inversion with Ventriculo-arterial Discordance (Congenitally Corrected l-TGA) (see 3.3.2)

2.1.3 Criss-Cross Heart: Ventriculo-arterial Discordance with Misplaced Ventricles (Physiologic TGA with Misplaced Ventricles)

In some complicated forms of congenital heart disease with ventriculo-arterial discordance, the morphological RV may be left-sited and anterior relative to the morphological LV; in addition, the two ventricles may be separated from each other by a horizontally oriented IVS, with the morphologic right ventricle on top of the morphologic LV.

The abnormally positioned IVS may therefore escape ultrasonic recognition and this might lead to an erroneous diagnosis of a single ventricle with two AV valves (see Fig. 2.3a); in addition, it may be possible to record both an AV and a semilunar valve simultaneously (see Fig. 2.3b).

Once the position of the atria and the ventricles have been determined, their connections may be defined. Different possibilities exist, such as the following.

1) *A concordant connection:* The morphologic right atrium connects to the anatomical right ventricle.

2) *A discordant connection:* The morphologic right atrium connects to the anatomical LV.

3) *An absent AV connection:* (see specific entities).

4) *A double inlet heart through the absence of an inlet or posterior septum* (see 5.1.4).

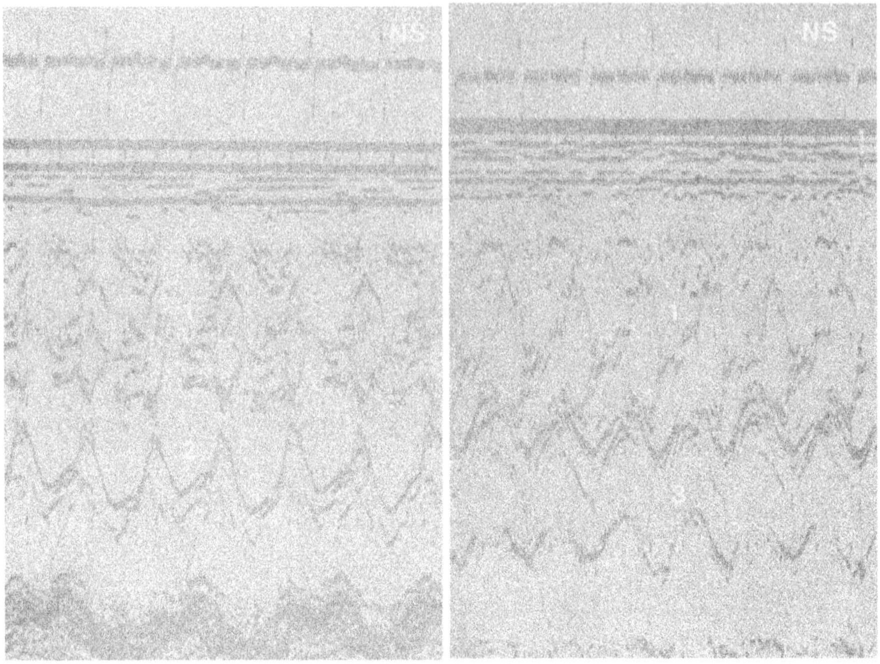

a b

Fig. 2.3 a, b. NS: Echocardiogram obtained from a 2-week-old cyanotic baby in congestive heart failure. Note in **a** the simultaneous visualization of two AV valves (labeled 1 and 2) without intervening septum. In **b**, with the transducer oriented differently, an anterior AV valve (labeled 1) is visualized simultaneously with a posteriorly oriented semilunar valve (labeled 3). The baby was found to have TGA with malpositioned ventricles, separated from each other by a horizontal septum

3 Abnormal Location of the Great Arteries

Index

Introduction

Unless cross sectional echocardiography [130] is performed ultrasonic recognition of the great arteries is difficult, as neither the aortic arch nor the pulmonary artery (PA) branches are well suited to conventional echocardiographic detection.

However, M-mode echocardiographic identification of the great arteries is possible. The following ultrasonic features will help in the identification of the great arteries.

The Loop Rule

This is a general anatomic rule stating that in a ventricular d-loop (right ventricle to the right of the morphologic left) the aortic valve is usually to the right of the pulmonary valve (PV). The opposite is true in a ventricular l-loop [361]. Unfortunately, in ventriculo-arterial discordance it is known that the anteriorly placed aorta is to the right in only 70% of cases [25]. Thus the loop rule should probably not be evoked when trying to identify the great arteries in complicated forms of transposition complexes.

The Recognition of the Spatial Relationship of the Great Arteries at Semilunar Valve Level or at Their Origin

In a normal heart, the aortic valve (AoV) lies posterior, inferior, and to the right of the PV. In classical d-TGA, the AoV remains to the right of the PV but assumes, with respect to that valve, a more anterior and superior position. In more complicated vascular derangements a number of great artery interrelationships at valvular level may be documented.

The relationship between these two semilunar valves can be approached diagnostically using conventional and, more ideally, cross sectional echocardiography.

In the normal situation the more posteriorly recorded valve should be obtained by a more rightward orientation of the transducer in M-mode. Unfortunately, the exact location of the transducer at the time of recording is not always precisely known. This difficulty can be overcome using cross sectional echocardiography: indeed, a high transverse scan will show the precise spatial relation of the great arteries. If the vessels are normally related, the aortic origin will be viewed as a posterior and right-sited circular echo-free space containing a central diastolic cusp echo. The right ventricular outflow tract (RVOT), which crosses anterior to it before turning posteriorly to its left as the main PA, will be viewed as a crescentic anterior and a left-sited echo-free space [162] (see Fig. 3.1).

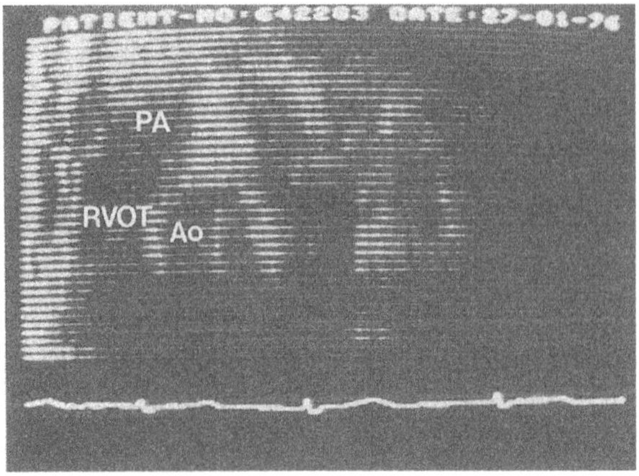

Fig. 3.1. Still frame of a dynamic cross section through the long axis of the RV outflow tract and the origin of the main PA. Note that the Ao is sectioned transversely, appearing therefore as a circular structure. Within the aorta the aortic valve is visible

To the contrary, if the vessels are transposed so as to become parallel at their origin, they will be viewed, on a high transverse scan, as two perfectly circular spaces, opposite in orientation to the echo-free spaces observed in normal subjects [160]. Indeed, the origin of the posterior vessel (the PA) is now left sited relative to the origin of the anterior vessel. Even so, in some complex heart lesions, including l-TGA, the semilunar valves may have an apparent normal right-left and anterior-posterior interrelationship, with a right valve in a posterior location. However, in this instance, the valve is the pulmonary and not the aortic as in a normal heart. Even if a normal vascular relation is found, l-TGA can be suspected, if on a high transverse cross sectional scan, two perfectly circular echo-free spaces are viewed.

The Diameters of the Great Arteries at the Level of Their Ostia

Van Meurs et al. [232] studying necropsy specimens of normal hearts from children whose ages ranged from 25 weeks of gestational age to 9 years postpartum showed that the pulmonary artery ostium was always slightly larger than the aortic ostium. The pulmonary ostium is thus larger than the aortic ostium unless there are obstructive lesions of either the right or the left heart, depending on whether or not transposition of the great arteries is present.

Time Intervals

Ventricular ejection time is another useful parameter, as it is known that the aortic ejection time is generally shorter than the pulmonic ejection time. The shortest ejection time thus points to the systemic ventricle. Exceptions exist when pulmonary resistance approaches systemic resistance, such as, for instance, in a distressed newborn infant. Conversely, the interval between onset of the QRS and ejection, the aortic pre-ejection period (LPEP), is usually longer than the pulmonic pre-ejection period. Both intervals can be measured reliably from the semilunar valve echoes and a concomitant electrocardiogram (see Chap. 23).

M-Mode Sweep

In normal subjects, a M-mode sweep upward from the aortic valve shows the upward continuation of both the anterior and posterior walls of the aorta. In patients with classical d-TGA, this upward sweep will show the upward continuation of the anterior wall of the PA, whereas the posterior wall terminates abruptly where the PA turns posteriorly [161].

All the above features or techniques are not completely reliable for the separate identification of the aorta and main pulmonary artery [161]. This identification can usually be obtained using cross sectional echocardiography

Detection of the Aortic Arch

Aortic identification is possible by noting the continuity of the ascending aorta with the aortic arch. Echocardiographic detection of the aortic arch has been described in order to detect coarctation of the aorta [428]. The transducer of a real-time cardiac imaging sector scan is placed in the suprasternal notch, and is swept from the ascending aorta to the aortic arch.

Sweeping the transducer in the opposite direction, from the aortic arch to the ascending aorta, should show that the aortic arch is in continuity with the ascending aorta. In addition, no arterial branches should originate from this ascending vessel.

Detection of the Main Pulmonary Artery

If the ascending aorta cannot be visualized adequately, it may be important to show branching of an artery, which establishes that vessel as the PA [162], at least in the absence of a surgical shunt.

In children with d-TGA, branching of the PA can be viewed with the scanner directly transverse at valvular level and tilted to carry out a headward sweep, as with M-mode echocardiography, in order to follow the course of the pulmonary artery.

Assessment of Ventriculo-arterial Connections

Once the ventricles and great arteries have been identified, their mutual connections must be defined. As the semilunar valves may have different relationships in any connection, this definition may be hard to get at echocardiographically. For instance, in TGA, the AoV is right-sited, in accordance with the loop rule, in approximately 70% of cases. Sometimes, even in TGA, a normal connective relation can be documented. Nevertheless, if mitral semilunar valve continuity is present, elucidation of the ventriculo-arterial connection should not be difficult. Barring the rare possibility of a double outlet left ventricle, there are but two possibilities: a normal (or concordant) connection, or a transposed (or discordant) connection. However, if the presence of a left ventricular conus is responsible for mitral semilunar valve discontinuity, determination of the ventriculo-arterial connection may be more difficult. Cross sectional echocardiography, because of its greater capacity to display the anatomy of the ventricular outflow tracts, the septum, and the origin of the great vessels, will often be necessary. Longitudinal scans will show the relation of the mitral valve and ventricular septum to the posterior great artery; multiple transverse scans, parallel to the outflow tracts and the semilunar valves, will permit study of the interrelations between ventricles, the IVS, and the great vessels so as to allow a spatial reconstruction of the heart, including a definition of the ventriculo-arterial connection. Alternatively, the transverse scanning plane can be tilted up and down from outflow tract to great vessel origin.

Contrast echocardiography may be of further help in defining ventriculoarterial connections in complex great vessel positional abnormalities.

Four basic patterns of ventriculo-arterial connections may be recognized.

Normal or Concordant Connection

The aorta arises from the anatomic LV and the pulmonary artery arises from the anatomic RV. A normal great artery relationship will be documented most of the time, with the AoV posterior, inferior, and to the right in relation to the pulmonary valve.

However, an abnormal great artery relationship is possible in the following entities:

1. In mirror-image dextrocardia, where atrial situs is inversed, there is a ventricular l-loop and the AoV lies posterior, inferior, and to the left of the PV.

2. "Anatomically corrected malposition" [354] indicates here an abnormal relationship between the two semilunar valves, classical transposition being excluded. In anatomically corrected malposition, the aorta is connected to the anatomical LV, and the PA to the anatomical RV. However, the relationship between the two semilunar valves is, abnormal. For instance, the aorta may be to the left and anterior with respect to the PV. Whether or not the circulation is normal will depend on the type of atrioventricular connection.

Transposition or Discordant Connection

The aorta arises from the anatomic RV and the PA from the anatomic LV: the great arteries are placed across the IVS.

Double Outlet Ventricle

Following Kirklin's et al. definition [179], a double outlet ventricle is defined as that condition in which more than one and a half great arteries arise from the same ventricular outlet chamber. This leaves out entities such as tetrad of Fallot, which is therefore defined as a "normal" connection. Both great vessels may arise either from the morphologic right (DORV) or from the morphologic left ventricle (DOLV). Entities such as single ventricle without outlet chamber may be included in this category.

The abnormal relationship between the aorta and the pulmonary artery is then referred to as "malposition" of the great arteries (MGA), and the position of the aorta relative to the pulmonary valve may be indicated [295].

Single Outlet

In this condition, a single great artery arises from the anatomic right or anatomic left ventricle, or overrides the IVS.

Persistent truncus arteriosus, single aortic trunk with pulmonary atresia, and single pulmonary trunk with aortic atresia are examples of single outlet.

One of the advantages of the segmental approach is that the position of the heart within the thorax does not interfere with the terminology and abbreviations used.

Commonly used abbreviations consist of three letters enclosed in brackets, which refer to the three main cardiac segments, the atria, the ventricles, and the great arteries. The following abbreviations are used: (1) S = situs solitus, right-sited right atrium; (2) I = situs inversus, left-sited right atrium; (3) D = dextro or right, right ventricle or aorta, right-sited; and (4) L = levo or left, right ventricle or aorta, left-sited [295 a].

Thus SDL, for example, means situs solitus of the atria, a right-sited right ventricle (ventricular d-loop), and a left-sited aorta (to the left of the PV).

Often, this three letter abbreviation is not used, save for indicating the position of the aorta, such as, (1) d-TGA, or transposition of the great arteries with the AoV to the right of the PV, or (2) l-MGA, or malposition of the great arteries with a left-sited AoV.

In this chapter, only the more commonly encountered abnormal ventriculo-arterial connections amenable to echocardiographic diagnosis will be presented. Some of the abnormalities, such as persistent truncus arteriosus, will be discussed elsewhere.

3.1 Right-Sited Aorta Connected to the Right Ventricle

3.1.1 d-Transposition of the Great Arteries

The echocardiographic diagnosis of d-TGA rests fundamentally upon the identification of (1) the ventricular chambers, and (2) the great arteries, noting their spatial orientation in relation to each other and to the ventricular chambers [208].

The Ventricular Chambers

Identification of the ventricular chambers is based primarily on the detection of mitral-semilunar valve continuity. Two other features are helpful: the study of AV valve closure, and the appearance of the mitral valve on dynamic cross-sectional examination (see Chap. 2).

The Great Arteries

Having identified the MV, its position relative to the TV can then be determined. If a normal ventricular relation is found, with the TV located to the right and anterior to the MV, ventricular d-looping has occurred [361] and, in accordance with the loop rule [296 a], dextroposition of the aorta is expected. M-mode recording of an anteriorly located vessel with rightward orientation of the transducer is, therefore, strongly suggestive of d-TGA [127].

This abnormal vascular arrangement, as seen in d-TGA, can be diagnosed more precisely using cross sectional echocardiography, which will allow a separate identification of the aorta and of the PA [327]. In all patients with d-TGA, a longitudinal scan or sagittal cross section will identify the PA by its directly posterior course immediately beyond the PV [161]. This posterior course can be surmised using M-mode echocardiography when an upward sweep from the pulmonary valve shows abrupt termination of the echoes from the posterior pulmonary artery wall coinciding with the posterior arching of the main pulmonary artery. The same longitudinal scan will identify the aorta by its retrosternal course upward before turning posteriorly above the main pulmonary artery [161]. In addition, it may be possible to note that the anterior (aortic) semilunar valve is slightly more superior than the posterior (pulmonary) semilunar valve as it now rests upon the right ventricular conus (see Fig. 3.2).

When the transducer is placed perpendicular to the long axis of the LV and more or less parallel to the right ventricular outflow tract, the precise spatial relations of the great arteries can be determined. Indeed, a high transverse scan will reveal two adjacent circular echo-free spaces, representing the two great vessels scanned perpendicular to their long axis. The anterior vessel will be seen to be more to the right as compared with the posterior vessel. This is in contrast to the normal situation, in which a sausage-shaped structure (the right ventricular outflow tract and the origin of the PA sectioned longitudinally) is displayed in front and to the left of a circular structure (the transversely sectioned aorta) [148, 217] (see Fig. 3.1).

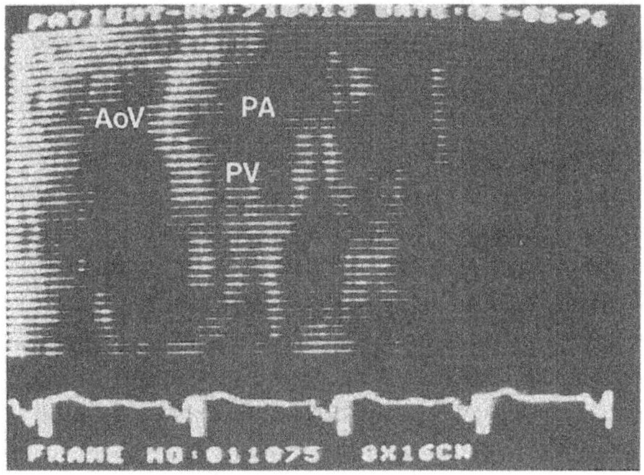

Fig. 3.2. Still frame of a dynamic cross section through the long axis of the LVOT in a 5-year-old child with d-TGA and subpulmonic obstruction after Mustard's operation. The aortic valve is seen to be positioned more anteriorly and superiorly; the PA is perhaps slightly dilated. Within the original left atrial cavity echoes of the Mustard's baffle are documented

Furthermore, tilting the transverse plane upward from the pulmonary valve may show branching of the main PA [161].

Due to the abnormal vascular arrangement seen in d-TGA, it is quite common to record both great arteries and their respective semilunar valves may, quite frequently, be recorded simultaneously on M-mode registration [208] (see Fig. 3.3).

Two other echocardiographic criteria may be important to help confirm that the anteriorly recorded vessel corresponds to the aorta.

The Diameter of the Two Vascular Trunks. At all ages, barring the possibility of subpulmonary obstruction in d-TGA, the pulmonary trunk exceeds the aortic trunk in width [232].

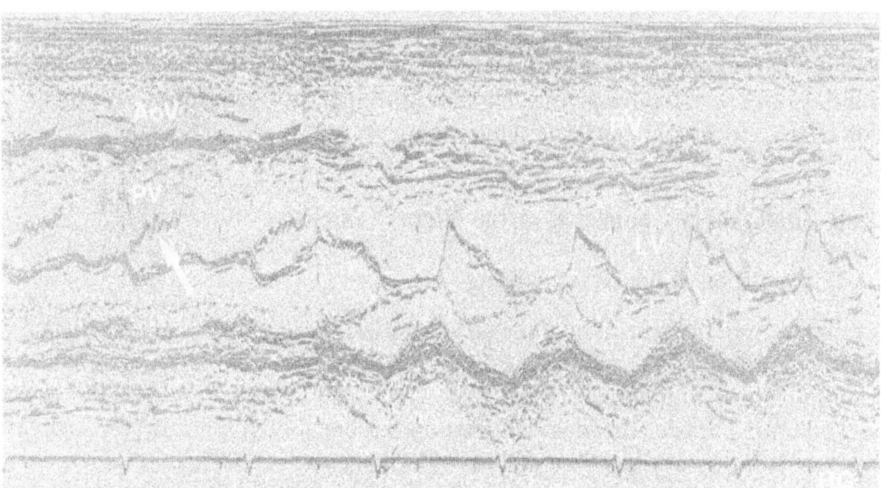

Fig. 3.3. HG: M-mode scan obtained from a 10-year-old boy with d-TGA after a Mustard's operation. Both great arteries are recorded simultaneously, the aorta being now the anterior vessel. Note the coarse fluttering of the PV due to subpulmonary obstruction (*arrow*), and the presence of disproportionate septal thickening

The Study of Ejection Times. The shortest ejection time, in the absence of increased pulmonary vascular resistance, indicates which vessel is the systemic [152]. This remains valid even in the newborn period [133], and after a Mustard's operation [152].

In addition, following echocardiographic features are often seen in d-TGA [278] (see Figs. 3.3, 13.13). (1) RV end-diastolic dimensions larger than normal, and tending to increase after a Mustard's operation; (2) LV end-diastolic dimensions often below normal preoperatively, with a further reduction postoperatively; (3) SAM of the AMVL, more often encountered postoperatively; (4) Fluttering of the AMVL in almost every patient who has undergone a Mustard's operation; and (5); Abnormal septal motion in about four out of ten patients with d-TGA.

Finally, contrast echocardiography may contribute to the diagnosis (see Chap. 22).

3.1.2 Corrected d-TGA in Situs Inversus of the Atria

In this condition [361], the anatomical RA is left-sited, and connects with the left-sited anatomical LV. Mitral-semilunar valve continuity is normal but the PA connects to the anatomic LV.

The association of atrioventricular discordance and TGA is responsible for a normal circulation, unless additional cardiac abnormalities are present.

Situs inversus of the atria should be suspected from other noninvasive techniques (Chap. 1). Position of the ventricles relative to each other can be determined echocardiographically (Chap. 2). Diagnosis of the vascular derangement is discussed in 3.1.1.

3.2 Left-Sited Aorta Connected to the Left Ventricle

3.2.1 Mirror-Image Dextrocardia

This condition is almost always associated with complete situs inversus. The heart is located in the right hemithorax and all structures show a reversed right-left relationship: the aortic valve is thus left-sited, although it remains posterior and inferior relative to a right-sited pulmonary valve.

3.3 Left-Sited Aorta Connected to the Right Ventricle

3.3.1 l-Transposition of the Great Arteries

In this rare form of transposition of the great arteries, the loop rule is at fault. The position of the atria and ventricles is the same as in d-TGA, but the AoV is now left-sited (and anterior) with respect to the PV.

This condition has been diagnosed at least once echocardiographically, through the study of systolic time intervals (STI) [361].

3.3.2 Corrected l-TGA

This condition is characterized by situs solitus of the atria with ventricular inversion (atrioventricular discordance) and transposition of the great arteries. Blood circulation thus remains normal as blood streams from the right atrium via a morphological left ventricle into a posteriorly positioned PA.

Although on a high cross sectional scan, the great vessel orientation, at valvular level, appears to be normal with the anterior semilunar valve (now the aortic) "normally" located to the left, the echocardiographic diagnosis of corrected l-TGA remains possible and is based on following criteria.

1. On a high transverse scan, at valvular level, the two vessels will appear as circular echo-free spaces, because of the parallel orientation of the great arteries. In normal subjects this scan does not show the two great arteries simultaneously as circular spaces, as discussed in Chap. 3 (see Fig. 3.1).

2. Tracing both vessels back from a high transverse scan, to their ventricles of origin, it will become apparent that the anterior leftward great artery arises from the anterior leftward portion of the left-sited ventricle and is not continuous with the left-sited AV valve [118].

3. A low transverse cross section will show displaced side-by-side ventricles and AV valves. The IVS lies in a plane parallel to the incident sound wave and will often not be visualized, except using unusual transducer locations.

4. A sagittal cross section will show the anterior vessel to have a long retrosternal sweep characteristic of the aorta in transposition anomalies [118].

5. Using M-mode echocardiography, continuity may be noted between the anterior leaflet of the anterior right-sited AV valve and the posterior wall of the posterior great artery. It can therefore be deduced that this AV valve is the mitral valve and that ventricular inversion has occurred.

6. The recording of two AV valves without intervening septal echoes (see Fig. 2.2) is due to the fact that the IVS is abnormally oriented, lying in a plane parallel to the incident sound waves. In these cases, diagnosis is still possible, as the two AV valves may be identified by studying their respective closure time, knowing that in transposition the tricuspid valve usually closes first.

3.4 Both Great Arteries Connected to One Ventricle

3.4.1 Double Outlet Right Ventricle (DORV) (see 4.2.1)

Echocardiographic data on these patients are scarce. The diagnosis will remain difficult, because many varieties of DORV exist.

Two semilunar valves, lying side-by-side and in approximately the same anterior-posterior plane may be recognized. Mitral-semilunar valve discontinuity is usually present.

3.4.2 Double Outlet Left Ventricle

Definite echocardiographic features of this entity have not been reported; cross sectional echocardiography should be helpful.

3.5 One Great Artery Arising from the Ventricles

The inability to record two semilunar valves does not necessarily indicate the existence of a single artery leaving the heart: the second semilunar valve may be inaccessible for echocardiographic detection because of stenosis or hypoplasia, etc. Echocardiographically, patients with two great arteries, albeit one hypoplastic such as in severe tetrad of Fallot, may be erroneously included in this category.

True examples of a single arterial trunk include:

3.5.1 Truncus Arteriosus Persistens (see 4.1.3 and 4.2.2)

3.5.2 Single Pulmonary Trunk with Aortic Atresia (see 17.2.1)

3.5.3 Single Aortic Trunk with Pulmonary Atresia (see 4.1.4)

Absence of Normally Present Structures

4 Discontinuity in Cardiac Structures

Index

Introduction

Although a segmental approach was advocated to arrive at a correct echocardiographic diagnosis of a complex heart lesion (Chaps. 1–3), some complicated heart abnormalities can be recognized ultrasonically, essentially through the documentation of abnormal patterns [422] such as echocardiographic discontinuity.

Normally, echocardiographic continuity exists between: (1) the IVS and a semilunar cusp (or anterior continuity); (2) the AMVL and a semilunar cusp (or posterior continuity); (3) the interatrial septum and the IVS; and (4) the interatrial septum and the mitral valve.

The IVS and a Semilunar Cusp

This reflects the continuity which is normally found between the IVS and the semilunar system including a wall of a great vessel, either the aorta in a normal heart or the PA in transposition. Echoes of both structures are recorded, on M-mode registration, as a single uninterrupted line.

The Anterior Mitral Valve Leaflet (AMVL) and a Semilunar Cusp

This is essentially an anatomic definition and corresponds to the fibrous continuity normally present between the AMVL and a semilunar cusp, either aortic or pulmonary. This normal continuity is easily detectable through both conventional (M-mode) and two-dimensional echocardiographic examination.

The Interatrial Septum and the IVS

This continuity can only be detected using cross-sectional echocardiography, when the ultrasonic beam is swept up along the IVS from the body of the left ventricle into the left atrium. Normally, an abrupt shift in septal direction occurs as the beam leaves the IVS to encounter the interatrial septum (IAS) [82], which then appears as a series of linear echoes extending from the inferior medial border of the aortic root to the junction of the posterior left and right atrial walls.

The Interatrial Septum and the Mitral Valve

On a mitral to tricuspid valve scan, MV echoes are seen to be continuous with atrial septal echoes noted posterior to the tricuspid valve echoes [26, 139]. This can be documented using M-mode (see Fig. 4.1) and cross sectional echocardiography.

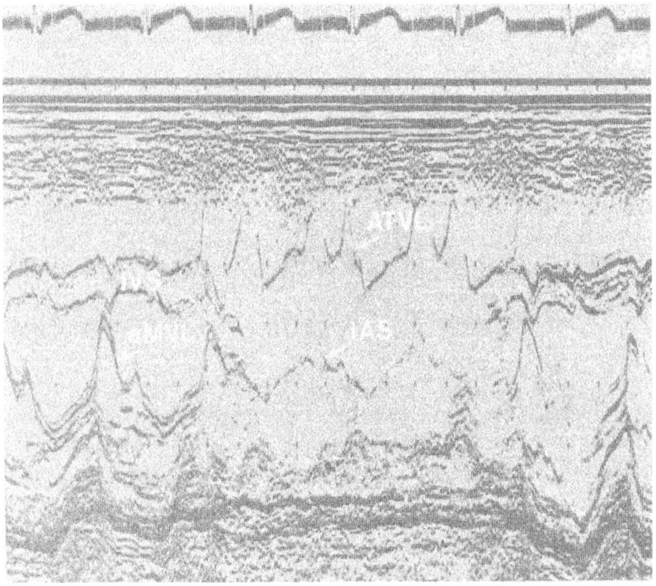

Fig. 4.1. PB: Echocardiogram from a 7-year-old child, 3 months after surgical closure of an ASD. Note the normal relationship between IVS, ATVL, IAS, and MV

Using this last technique, a horizontal section is used at the level of the membranous septum [26].

Septal-semilunar (or anterior) and/or mitral-semilunar (or posterior) continuity is absent in anomalies in which there is an abnormal spatial interrelationship between the ventricles and the great arteries.

Discontinuity between interatrial and interventricular septum and between interatrial septum and the AMVL involves anomalies in which there are defects in the lower parts of the IAS.

Abnormalities characterized by one of these echocardiographic discontinuities constitute the subject of this chapter.

4.1 Anterior Discontinuity

4.1.1 Ventricular Septal Defect (VSD) (see 15.1.2)

Septal semilunar continuity is absent, or partly missing, in the presence of a high or membranous VSD with or without overriding of a great vessel [83] (see Fig. 6.5).

However, in most cases of uncomplicated VSD this discontinuity cannot be demonstrated echocardiographically, even if the ultrasonic beam is directed to the defect. The defect usually remains totally obscured, since (1) the angle between the transducer and the septum may not be 90°, and (2) the beam width usually exceeds the diameter of the defect [118, 317].

4.1.2 Tetrad of Fallot (T/F) (see also Table 4.1)

The most characteristic finding in T/F is a discontinuity, on a M-mode trace, of the echoes from the anterior aortic wall and the IVS: this corresponds to the echocardiographic registration of the presence of a VSD and an overriding aorta [59, 125, 383] (see Fig. 4.2 a). However, this overriding may sometimes persist after surgical closure of the VSD (see Fig. 4.3). This overriding can also be visualized directly using cross sectional echocardiographic systems [83, 327] (see Fig. 4.4).

Secondary ultrasonic features of T/F include (1) thickening of the right ventricular anterior wall and of the IVS, which may sometimes lead to disproportionate septal thickening relative to the left ventricular free wall; (2) decreased width of the right ventricular outflow tract [383]; (3) aortic root dilatation [431] (see Fig. 4.2); and (4) decreased pulmonary root diameter [11, 431].

Table 4.1: Differentiating echocardiographic features in T/F and truncus arteriosus

	T/F	Truncus arteriosus
Anterior discontinuity	+	+
Posterior discontinuity	−	− (+)[a] (see 4.2.2)
Left atrium	usually small	usually large
Pulmonary valve	+ or absent	−
Diastolic fluttering	−	+

[a] (+) = sometimes

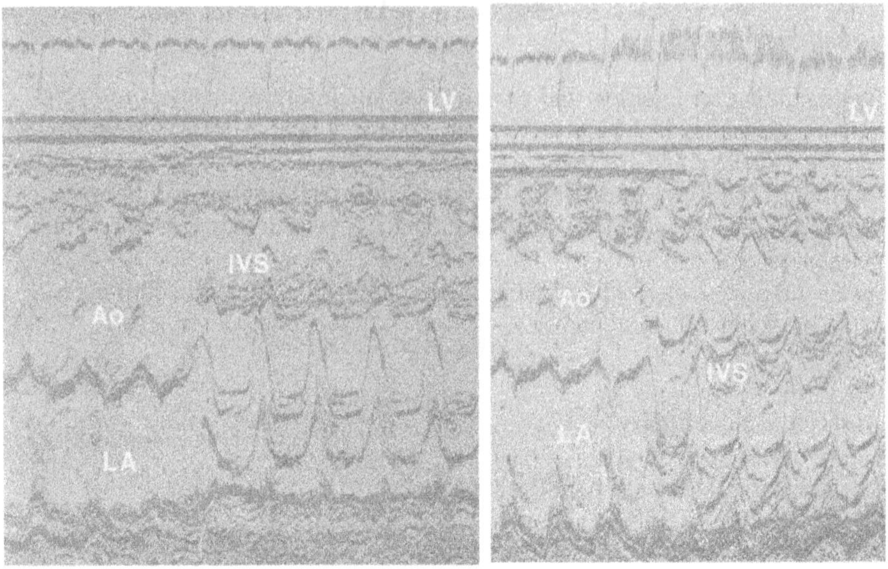

a b

Fig. 4.2 a, b. LV: M-mode echocardiogram obtained from a 2-year-old child with tetrad of Fallot and a previous Waterston operation. **a** The echocardiogram was obtained with the transducer in the standard position. It shows a dilated aorta overriding the IVS. **b** The echocardiogram was obtained with the transducer too high on the chest wall (second intercostal space), which generated the appearance of more severe degree of overriding

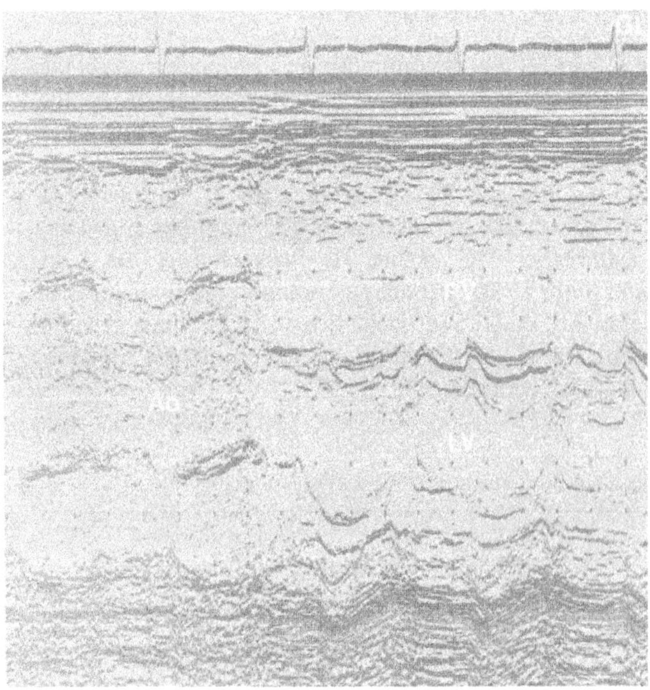

Fig. 4.3. GL: Anterior overriding is still present, also angiographically, in this 12-year-old child, 4 years after surgical repair of tetrad of Fallot with absent left PA

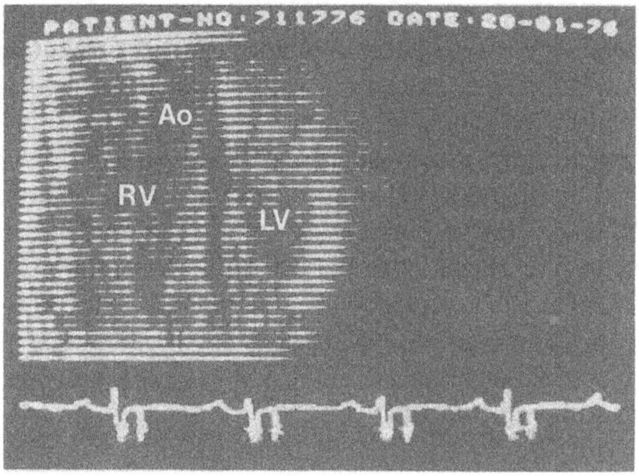

Fig. 4.4. Still frame of a dynamic cross section through the long axis of the LV obtained from a 5-year-old child with tetrad of Fallot. The aorta overrides the septum: there is no continuity between the septum and the anterior wall of the aorta. Echoes of the TV and MV are visible in their respective ventricles

4.1.3 **Truncus Arteriosus** (see also 4.2.2)

Just as in T/F, anterior discontinuity due to truncal overriding is usually present in this condition.

In both anomalies, however, it should be realized that this overriding is variable [353] and may be missed on echocardiographic examination, if, for instance, transducer placement and orientation is incorrect (see Fig. 4.2 b).

The two entities, tetrad of Fallot and truncus arteriosus, can usually be differentiated by other ultrasonic features, which are summarized in Table 4.1.

Size of the Left Atrium

Since LA size reflects the degree of pulmonary blood flow, its measurement is usually of help in the differentiation of truncus arteriosus, in which pulmonary blood flow is generally increased, and of T/F, where the opposite situation prevails. However, this ultrasonic sign is not always reliable: if pulmonary blood flow in truncus arteriosus is restricted because of either increased vascular resistance or hypoplastic pulmonary arteries, a small left atrial cavity may be recorded.

Detection of the Pulmonary Valve

In truncus arteriosus the pulmonary arteries arise from the truncus or may be totally absent: echoes from a main pulmonary artery or valve will not be recorded. To the contrary, if one can document the existence of a normally situated PA by recording a pulmonary valve leaflet, septal-semilunar discontinuity is diagnostic of T/F, and truncus arteriosus can be excluded [59]. Unfortunately, it is often technically difficult to obtain echoes from a pulmonary valve leaflet in T/F, as patients with this anomaly often have hypoplastic pulmonary arteries or even pulmonary atresia (pseudotruncus arteriosus). Thus, when a PV in anterior discontinuity is not recorded, this should be interpreted with caution.

Valvular Incompetence

Truncal valve incompetence in truncus arteriosus is fairly common: a study of a large number of patients with this abnormality has shown 20% of them to have this anomaly [41]. A previous pulmonary artery banding procedure further increases this tendency: Assad-Morell found truncal regurgitation in 60% of patients with truncus arteriosus, more than half of whom had undergone a previous banding procedure [14].

Truncal valve incompetence echocardiographically resembles aortic regurgitation: both share the following ultrasonic features: (1) fine diastolic fluttering of the AMVL and of the left endocardial surface of the IVS [48, 67, 390] (see Fig. 11.9), and (2) premature mitral valve closure, as both conditions may be associated with a rapid rise in left ventricular diastolic pressure [14, 289] (see 13.9).

As aortic regurgitation is rather uncommon in patients with T/F, the documentation of diastolic fluttering of the AMVL, in the presence of anterior discontinuity, favors truncus arteriosus.

4.1.4 Pseudotruncus Arteriosus

Pseudotruncus arteriosus, or pulmonary atresia with VSD, cannot be differentiated ultrasonically from T/F.

However, a continuous murmur in a cyanotic infant, with ultrasonic documentation of anterior overriding, should strongly suggest pulmonary atresia.

4.2 Posterior Discontinuity

Posterior discontinuity exists when conal muscle is interposed between the fibrous rings of both the mitral and semilunar valve or when both great arteries originate from the RV [83].

Echocardiographically, mitral-semilunar discontinuity is diagnosed when there is a consistent break in the echo-trace or when echoes from an intervening structure separate the echoes of the two AV valves [361] (see Fig. 4.5). This intervening structure is most often a conus, either subaortic or subpulmonic, manifested as a dense band of echoes between the semilunar and the mitral valves.

Posterior discontinuity relates primarily to the superior-inferior axis, whereas anterior discontinuity involves anterior-posterior interrelations as well.

The detection of posterior discontinuity, or of an abnormal superior-inferior interrelationship, is difficult using conventional echocardiography [118]; two-dimensional imaging, however, substantially facilitates the elucidation of this relationship [330].

Discontinuity should not be confused with mitral-semilunar valve displacement without structural separation, a condition in which the distance from the chest wall to the AMVL is different from the distance between the chest wall and the semilunar cusp or the posterior wall of a great vessel. If a displacement of less than 10 mm at end-diastole is documented, a faulty transducer position, too high on the chest wall, should be ruled out [83, 370]. True mitral-semilunar valve displacement has been described on a number of occasions [103, 371] and is well illustrated in Fig. 4.6, which is an echocardiogram obtained from a child with congestive heart failure and a dilated LV. However, this ultrasonic feature lacks specificity.

The following paragraphs deal with cardiac anomalies or disorders in which a posterior discontinuity can be demonstrated. As will be seen later, two of these

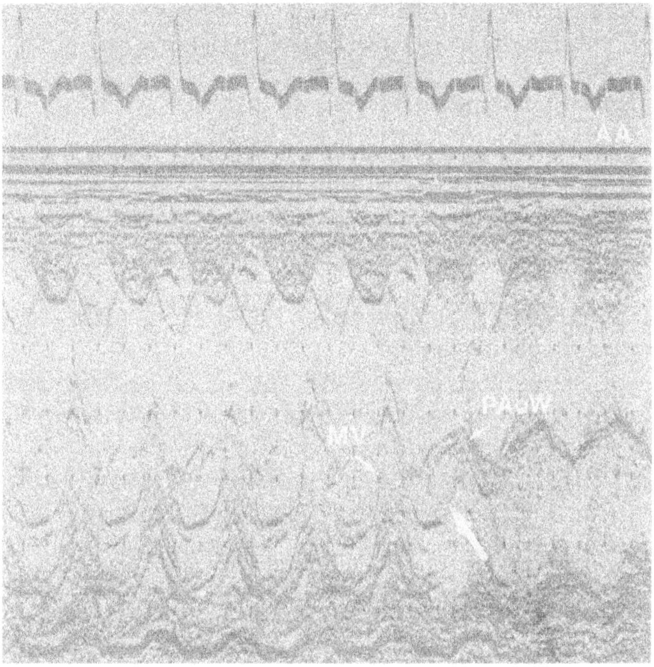

Fig. 4.5. AA: Echocardiogram obtained from a 5-year-old boy with double inlet and outlet left ventricle. The *arrow* points to the presence of true posterior discontinuity

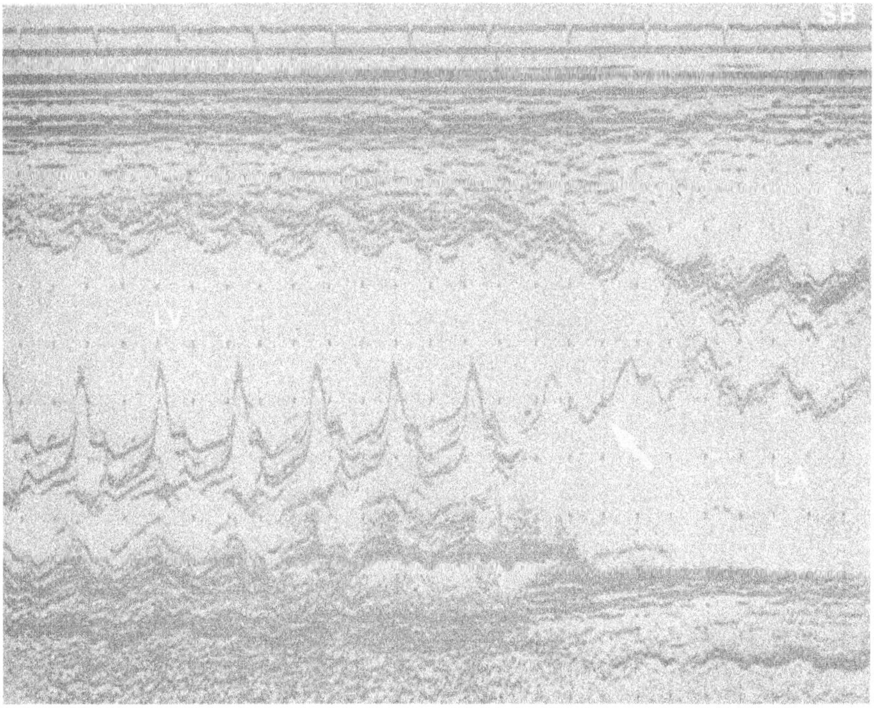

Fig. 4.6. SB: Echocardiogram obtained from a 7-year-old girl with myocarditis. Note the presence of semilunar MV displacement (*arrow*), due to severe LV dilatation

anomalies, double outlet RV and truncus arteriosus, are sometimes characterized by a double discontinuity, anterior and posterior.

4.2.1 Double Outlet Right Ventricle (DORV)

The condition in which both great arteries originate from the right ventricle has been defined differently by different workers.

For Neufeld and co-workers, the RV possesses two coni, one subaortic and one subpulmonic. Neither semilunar valve is in fibrous continuity with an AV valve [269 a].

To the contrary, for Lev et al. [198], mitral-aortic or mitral-pulmonary continuity may be present.

Finally, in some variants of DORV, an anterior overriding aorta, or PA (Taussig-Bing anomaly) can be responsible for an anterior discontinuity [103] (see Fig. 4.7).

These contradictory anatomic definitions are reflected by conflicting echocardiographic data. For some [57], a posterior discontinuity exists and enables the differentiation of DORV from T/F, in which the discontinuity is anterior [57, 58, 198]. Other centers, however, report the coexistence of both an anterior and posterior discontinuity in DORV [103]. This reported variability of echocardiographic discontinuity is not surprising, since 16 possible variations of DORV have been described with respect to interrelations of the great arteries and to location of the VSD [366].

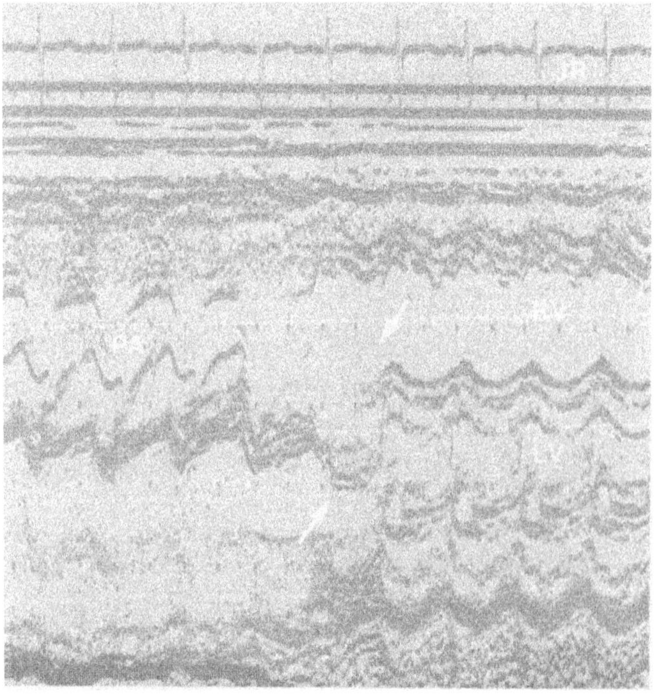

Fig. 4.7. JR: Echocardiogram from an infant with double outlet RV of the Taussig-Bing variety. Both anterior and posterior discontinuity were documented echo- and angiocardiographically (*upper* and *lower arrows*). Note the overriding of the septum by the PA

In the absence of resolution problems [317], a double discontinuity should be a fairly common finding, as the most common type of DORV consists of a side-by-side arterial relation with a subaortic VSD.

4.2.2 **Truncus Arteriosus** (see also 4.1.3)

In truncus arteriosus, the truncal vessel is usually equally associated with the two ventricles, or with the posterior ventricle primarily, resulting in anatomic continuity with the MV [296].

However, when associated principally with the anterior ventricle, both anterior and apparent posterior discontinuity can be documented both echocardiographically and angiocardiographically [48, 103].

DORV and truncus arteriosus may thus have in common the coexistence of a double discontinuity. Their differentiation rests upon other ultrasonic features.
(1) The finding of a second semilunar valve, which will exclude the possibility of truncus arteriosus [59]. However, it might be technically difficult to "visualize" two semilunar valves in DORV, as the two great vessels are usually side by side [366].
(2) With respect to the documentation of valvular regurgitation, the presence of diastolic fluttering of the AMVL and/or of the endocardial surface of the IVS is more suggestive of truncus arteriosus (see 4.1.3).
3) The caliber of the overriding vessel is also important. Bearing in mind that the truncal vessel represents the only exit of blood from the heart in truncus arteriosus, the finding of a prominent overriding vessel should certainly favor the possibility of a truncus rather than DORV [48].

4.2.3 **Single (Common) Ventricle** (see 5.1.2)

Single (or common) ventricle consists of a ventricular chamber that receives blood from two separate AV valves or from a common AV valve.

Mitral-semilunar valve continuity is most often present, as the occurrence in single ventricle of a double conus that is responsible for posterior discontinuity seems to be relatively uncommon: only eight out of 57 cases of single ventricle with two AV valves were found to present angiographic or anatomopathologic evidence for a double conus [215 a].

Echocardiographic studies have substantiated this relatively uncommon occurrence: both Felner et al. [99] and Seward et al. [348] have documented mitral-semilunar echocardiographic continuity in most of their patients.

However, with a common AV valve, valvular continuity seems to be the exception rather than the rule: Seward et al. [348] documented continuity in only one out of eight patients with a single ventricle and a common AV valve, while the overall incidence of discontinuity in all cases of single ventricle was only 13%.

4.2.4 **d-Transposition of the Great Arteries (d-TGA)** (see 3.1.1)

In the normal heart a conus is present in the RV, while there is none on the left side: this results in a fibrous continuity between the AoV and the MV [356].

In classical d-TGA, a conus leads from the right ventricle to the aorta, while no conus is present in the left ventricle. The PV and the MV are now in fibrous continuity [356]. Under unusual circumstances, complete transposition may deviate from the classical picture, in that each ventricle has a conus, the right conus leading to the aorta and the left to the pulmonary trunk. This has been documented in six out of 172 specimens from patients with complete transposition [356]. In such cases, posterior discontinuity would be expected echocardiographically and be suggestive of DORV.

4.2.5 Corrected Malposition of the Great Arteries

Most patients with anatomically corrected malposition of the great arteries exhibit bilateral coni, subaortic and subpulmonic [295 a]. Posterior discontinuity is expected in these patients.

4.2.6 Complex Heart Lesions

Other complex heart anomalies may be characterized by posterior discontinuity whenever a bilateral conus is present. This was recently described in one out of eight children with an overriding TV [191].

4.2.7 Bacterial Endocarditis

This disease can cause a large subannular ring-shaped erosion beneath the noncoronary cusp and separate the AMVL from its attachment to the aortic annulus. As a result of this erosion, the AMVL can be displaced anteriorly to the posterior aortic wall. Echocardiographically, discontinuity will be manifested as a distinct echo-free zone between the base of the anterior mitral leaflet and the posterior aortic wall. Such an occurrence has been reported in a patient with acute pneumococcal endocarditis [371].

Remarks

When assessing echocardiographically whether or not anterior or posterior (dis)continuity is present, it is essential to keep in mind that the resulting display may not always reflect true cardiac anatomy but may reflect technical factors. The "continuity-discontinuity" sign may vary according to transducer position [103] (see Fig. 4.2). Great care should be exercised in obtaining, in the third or fourth left intercostal space, a slow gentle scan from the body of the LV through the MV to the aortic root. This scan should then be repeated in the opposite direction [14]. Multiple sweeps should be observed before the echocardiogram is interpreted [14]. In certain cases, a lack of override on the echocardiogram may result from unusual transducer positions, usually too low on the chest wall [14], while override can be created or exaggerated if the transducer is placed high on the chest wall [103].

It should be acknowledged that, short of direct inspection, the precise degree of override can probably best be determined on a true lateral angiogram of the heart [103].

Despite proper echocardiographic technique, override or discontinuity may not be present in conditions expected, such as T/F or truncus arteriosus. Of Assad-Morell's 20 patients with truncus arteriosus and 28 with pulmonary atresia with

VSD, four and six, respectively, demonstrated no gross override [14]. These observations have valid anatomic explanations, namely, the well-documented variability in the degree of overriding of the aortic vessel [131, 189, 353]: in some cases the aorta will be committed primarily to the LV.

On the other hand, in the presence of chest deformities such as pectus excavatum or a straight back syndrome, echocardiographic overriding may not be real.

4.3 Discontinuity Between the Interatrial and the Interventricular Septum

4.3.1 Ostium Primum Atrial Septal Defect (see 21.1.2)

In patients with ostium primum septal defects, a loss of septal echoes occurs at the junction between the IVS and the IAS. This can be documented using cross sectional echocardiography as the ultrasonic beam is swept up along the IVS into the left atrium [82].

4.4 Discontinuity Between the Interatrial Septum and the Mitral Valve

4.4.1 Atrioventricular Canal Defects

Both in partial (see 21.1.2) and complete (see 6.1.2) AV canal defects, scanning from the MV to the TV will demonstrate continuity between the two AV valve structures with absence of atrial septal echoes posterior to the TV echoes [139] (see Fig. 6.3).

Cross sectional echocardiography along a horizontal section at the level of the membranous septum will also reveal the absence of normal continuity between the AMVL and the interatrial septum [26].

5 Simultaneous Visualization of Two AV Valves Without IVS

Index

Introduction

The simultaneous visualization of the two AV valves without an intervening ventricular septum is certainly a distinct echocardiographic pattern and suggests the possibility of a common (or single) ventricle.

However, other entities exist that have a similar echocardiographic pattern.

All these conditions will be discussed in this chapter.

5.1 Two AV Valves Without Intervening Septum

5.1.1 Large Ventricular Septal Defect (VSD) (see 15.1.2)

If the ultrasonic beam is sufficiently narrow to pass through a VSD, both AV valves will be recorded without an intervening septum; this may lead to an erroneous diagnosis of a common (or single) ventricle (see Fig. 5.1).

However, in cases of VSD, definite septal echoes will appear with inferior orientation of the transducer. In addition, it should be acknowledged that these septal echoes are in a normal plane, posterior to the diastolic echoes of the anterior leaflet of the TV.

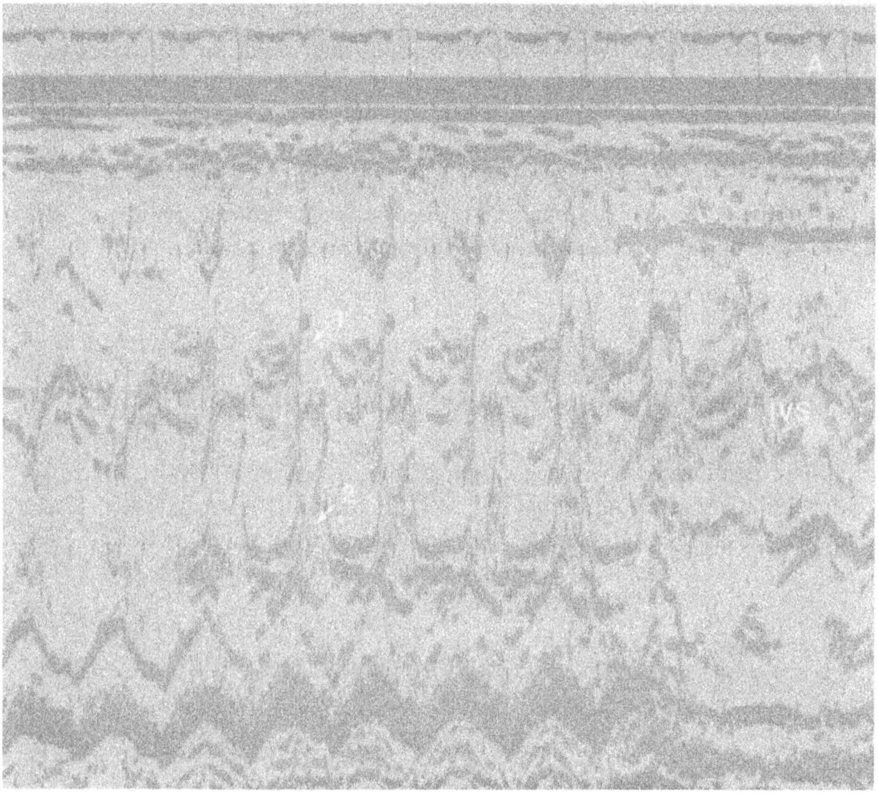

Fig. 5.1. A: Echocardiogram obtained from an infant with complete AV canal. Note on the center of the trace the simultaneous visualization of two AV valves (labeled 1 and 2) without intervening septum. IVS, however, does appear with inferior scanning of the transducer (*left side of the trace*)

Through cross sectional ultrasonic imaging of the heart [177], it is possible to demonstrate most of the larger VSD's commonly occurring in the infracristal region of the septum. Furthermore, transseptal flow directly through a VSD can be documented using pulsed Doppler echocardiography [369].

5.1.2 Single Ventricle with Two AV Valves

A single ventricle, which results from a failure of development of the posterior IVS [254, 348], consists of a large ventricular chamber which receives blood from either two separate AV valves or from a common one.

A rudimentary anteriorly positioned outflow chamber representing a persistent RVOT, and separated from the main chamber by septal remnants or a bulboventricular ridge [254], is often present and more often than not in communication with the aorta [348].

An echocardiographic diagnosis of a single ventricle with two AV valves will rest upon (1) negative, (2) positive, and (3) supportive features. In addition, contrast echocardiography will add greater diagnostic specificity to observed M-mode echocardiographic findings [349].

Negative Feature: Absence of Septal Echoes (see Fig. 5.2)

Simultaneous recording of two AV valves without intervening septal echoes, on repeated base-to-apex echocardiographic scans, [99, 348] or the demonstration of an AV valve ring or ring-like structure separating one valve from the other [27] is certainly quite suggestive of single ventricle.

However, as Beardshaw [24], Mortera [254] and their respective collaborators have shown, the echocardiographic diagnosis of a single ventricle need not rest solely on negative features but is based on positive findings as well.

Positive Findings

1) An apparently excessive posterior diastolic motion of the septal cusp of the anterior AV valve [24, 254] (see Fig. 5.3).
2) A frequent overlapping or apposition of the diastolic motions of the septal cusps of the two AV valves [24, 254].
3) A frequent demonstration of echocardiographic posterior AV valve (mitral)-posterior semilunar valve continuity [254, 349]. In addition, Beardshaw et al. [24] documented, in a high percentage of their cases with single ventricle, an

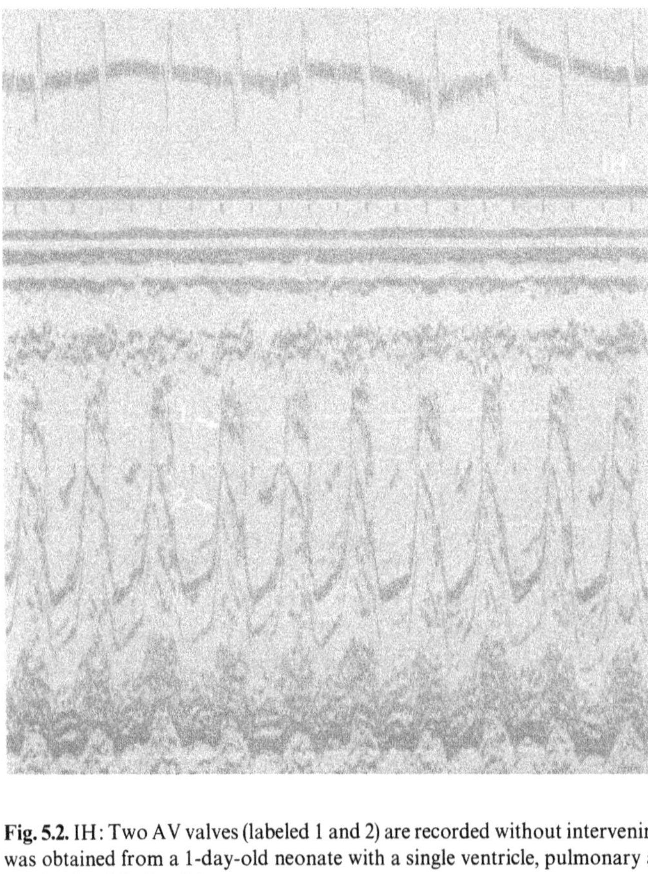

Fig. 5.2. IH: Two AV valves (labeled 1 and 2) are recorded without intervening septum. Echocardiogram was obtained from a 1-day-old neonate with a single ventricle, pulmonary atresia and PDA. The heart was in the right hemithorax

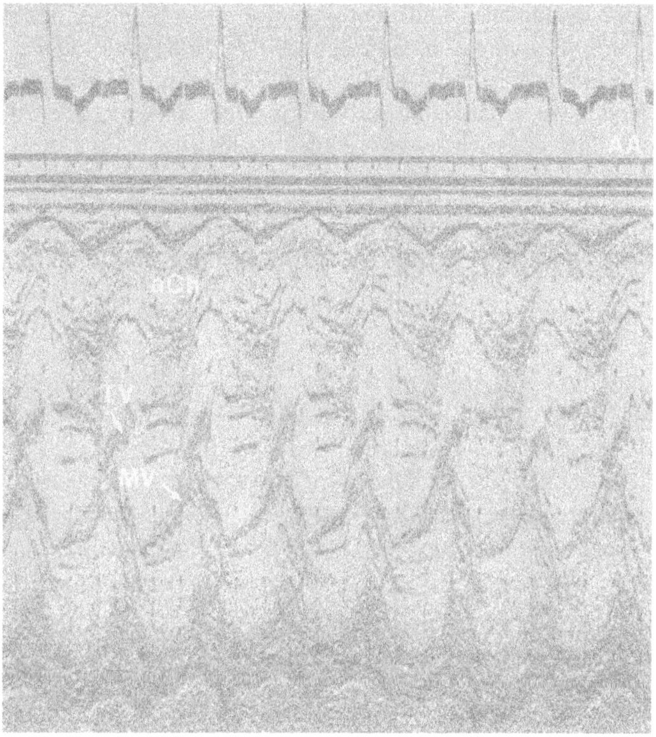

a

b

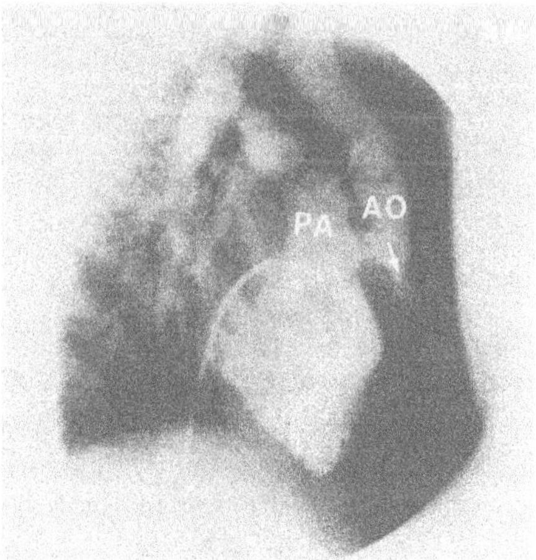

Fig. 5.3. AA: **a** Echocardiogram obtained from a 5-year-old boy with double inlet and outlet LV (same patient as in Fig. 4.5). Note the presence of a small anterior outlet chamber, aCh, shown by angiography to communicate with the main ventricular chamber through a VSD. Parts of the MV and TV leaflets are recorded simultaneously within the main chamber. Excessive motion of the septal leaflet of the TV is responsible for diastolic apposition of the AV valves. **b** Ventricular angiogram, lateral view. *Arrows* point to the presence of a small anterior outlet chamber

echocardiographic continuity between the posterior semilunar valve and both AV valves. As these authors stressed [24], there are very few other anomalies apart from single ventricle which would present the feature of both AV valves in continuity (or contiguity) with the posterior great artery in the absence of a posterior septum. Anatomically, these authors demonstrated this double continuity in 77% of necropsy specimens, with continuity of one valve and contiguity of the other in a further 14.5%.

4) The recording of a small anterior cavity with a bulboventricular ridge in cases of single ventricle with an outlet chamber. The bulboventricular ridge or septum will be recorded anterior to both AV valves [99], though, on occasion, may be straddled by one AV valve [254]. To record this abnormal echo, the transducer should be directed inferolaterally across the precordium from a relatively high position on the chest wall [349]. The outlet chamber will appear as a small echo-free space, anterior to the bulboventricular ridge (see Fig. 5.3).

Supportive Features (see Fig. 5.3)

1) A main ventricular chamber end-diastolic dimension considerably larger than normal left ventricular dimensions [56, 254].
2) Simultaneous recording of two semilunar valves, as d-TGA occurs frequently in single ventricle [80].

Contrast Echocardiography

Contrast echocardiography adds greater diagnostic specificity to observed M-mode features through the recognition of specific blood flow patterns and of anatomic features [349] (see 22.3.2).

5.1.3 Overriding Tricuspid Valve

An overriding tricuspid valve can be documented in several conditions, of which the most important are single (primitive) ventricle and d-TGA with VSD (see 6.1.1).

In the context of a single ventricle, overriding or straddling refers to an AV valve, parts of whose tension apparatus arise in the outlet chamber [254]: straddling occurs here over the bulboventricular ridge.

In the context of d-TGA, the AV valve crosses a true IVS. A commonly encountered echocardiographic pattern consists in the opening of the septal leaflet of the TV into the LV posterior to the septum [191] (see Fig. 6.1). It may be difficult to differentiate this entity from a common ventricle with two AV valves (see 6.1.1).

5.1.4 Double Inlet Left Ventricle

In this situation the TV opens entirely into the LV: this entity represents, in relation to a straddling TV, a more severe form of AV malalignment.

Echocardiography will reveal that both AV valves are located within the body of the LV, posterior to the septum (see Fig. 5.2).

Differentiation from a common ventricle with two AV valves may be quite difficult.

5.1.5 Atrioventricular Discordance with or Without TGA (see 3.3.2)

Even in the absence of a VSD, ventricular septal echoes may not be recorded adequately in "corrected" TGA (l-TGA), as the septum usually lies parallel to the ultrasound beam. A common ventricle with two AV valves can thus be diagnosed erroneously in these cases (see Fig. 2.2)

Fortunately "corrected" TGA usually has distinctive clinical, roentgenologic, and electrocardiographic features which should alert the echocardiographer. Repeated base-to-apex echocardiographic scans should then be performed from different parasternal transducer positions, including the cardiac apex. In so doing, Felner et al. [99] were able to demonstrate the IVS in four consecutive cases of l-TGA.

5.1.6 "Criss-Cross" Heart (see 2.1.3)

6 AV Valve Crossing the Interventricular Septum

Index

Introduction

This chapter deals with two disease entities: (1) Straddling tricuspid valve; and (2) AV canal.

Both of these are echocardiographically characterized by a distinct feature: echoes of an AV valve leaflet seeming to cross those of the IVS. This represents an artifact caused by the width of the ultrasonic beam, which encompasses the septal defect present in both entities. The defect itself, unless it exceeds the width of the sound beam, is not recognized ultrasonically: as a result, echoes of an AV valve leaflet, parts of which are abnormally located and/or attached to the IVS, are projected into the echoes of the septum.

In AV canal, overlapping of the septum is only apparent when, during diastole, the AMVL opens toward the septum and fuses with the septal echoes, or with the tricuspid valve as it begins to open. If the opening of the two AV valves is synchronous, an apparent confluent or single AV valve leaflet crossing the septum will then be registered [139].

The title of this chapter reflects the true anatomical situation, for the AV valve leaflet passes through the *plane* of the IVS, and of course not through the defect itself.

6.1 AV Valve Crossing the Plane of the IVS

6.1.1 Straddling Tricuspid Valve

A straddling or overriding TV is a rare cardiac defect in which the TV is positioned over the IVS and opens into both ventricles. The anomaly is associated with a ventricular septal defect of the endocardial cushion type [204]. An hypoplastic right ventricle is often encountered, as well as TGA.

Echocardiographically, the most common patterns consist in [191] (see Fig. 6.1): (1) opening of the septal leaflet of the tricuspid valve into the left ventricle, posterior to the septum, and; (2) the anterior leaflet of the tricuspid valve crossing the plane of the IVS in diastole.

Obviously, if the first pattern prevails, the two AV valves are seen without an intervening septum, which is recorded anterior to the septal leaflet of the tricuspid valve.

Ultrasonic differentiation from common ventricle with two AV valves may be difficult, especially if straddling tricuspid valve is associated with an hypoplastic RV. Septal echoes can then be mistaken for echoes of the anterior right ventricular wall.

Whenever a straddling tricuspid valve is suspected, the possibility of TGA should be investigated. (see also 5.1.3).

6.1.2 Complete Atrioventricular (AV) Canal

Common AV canal is the most severe form of the endocardial cushion defect disease spectrum, characterized by a large defect involving the lower part of the atrial septum and the adjoining proximal ventricular septum, and by gross abnormalities of the AV valves.

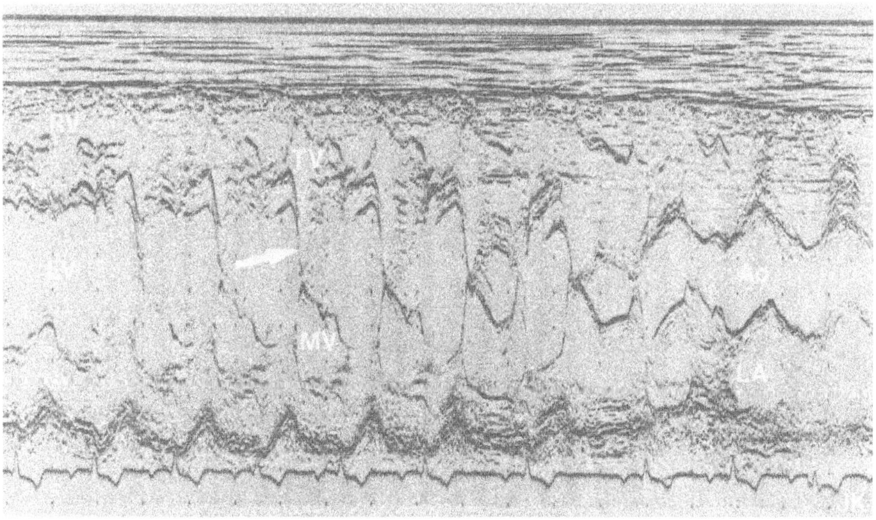

Fig. 6.1. JK: M-mode scan obtained from a 18-year-old boy with an angiographically documented overriding TV. At the level of the VSD, TV echoes are seen within the LV, actually coming into contact with MV echoes (*arrow*)

The echocardiographic diagnosis of complete AV canal is concentrated on the detection of abnormalities, in position and motion, in the mitral and tricuspid parts of the AV valve leaflets.

Position Abnormalities [139]

The mitral valve (or mitral part of the AV valve) is displaced anteriorly in the left ventricular outflow tract (LVOT), while the tricuspid valve seems to be displaced posteriorly, appearing to open in diastole from within the ventricular septal echoes (see Fig. 6.2).

An echocardiographic continuity between the two AV valve structures can be documented [22] (see Fig. 6.3). In addition, atrial septal echoes, posterior to tricuspid valve echoes and normally in continuity with echoes from the AMVL, will not be recorded (see 4.4.1).

Motion Abnormalities (see Fig. 6.4)

Abnormalities of AV valve motion are consistently found in AV canal defects. These abnormalities may consist of minimal duplication and fragmentation of systolic and diastolic valve echoes, or to the contrary, of extremely bizarre multiple and

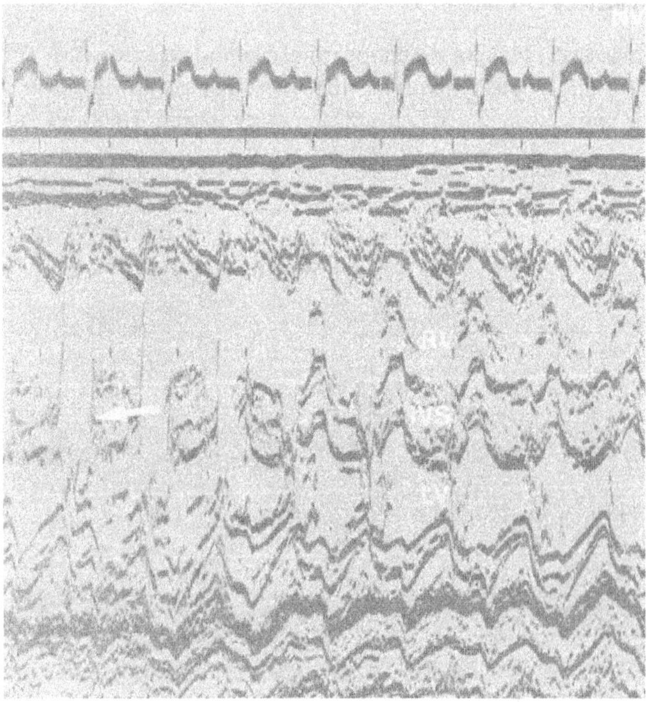

Fig. 6.2. NV: Partial left ventricular scan in a 6-week-old mongoloid child with complete AV canal and pulmonary artery hypertension (same child as in Fig. 5.1.). The transducer was directed from an area just below the AoV to the apex of the LV. Just below the AoV (*left part of the tracing*), the septal echoes drop out (*arrow*) corresponding to the VSD. With inferior scanning of the transducer (*right part of the tracing*), septal echoes reappear. Note the AV valve motion across the VSD

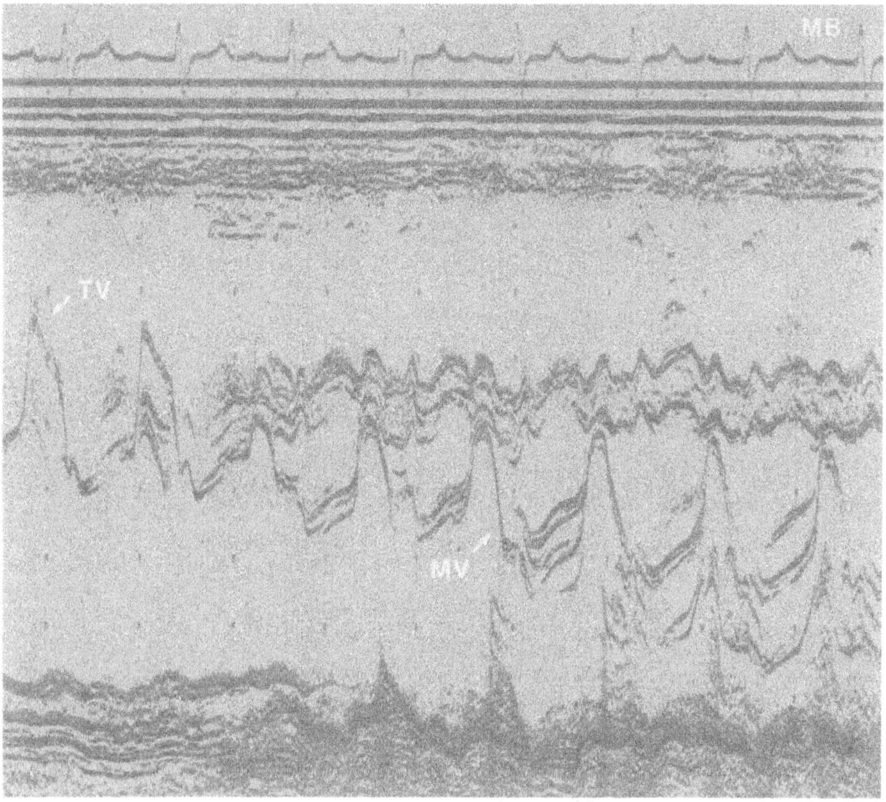

Fig. 6.3. MB: Echocardiogram from a 13-year-old child with partial AV canal. Note the confluence of MV and TV echoes

fragmented echoes of the AMVL, often with limited anterior diastolic excursion [139].

Base-to-apex scans frequently demonstrate that large segments of the ventricular septal echoes are absent, predominantly during diastole but also frequently in both systole and diastole, in the area immediately inferior to the aortic root [99, 139] (see Fig. 6.2).

Typically, at this level, the mitral valve echoes seem to move through this defect during diastole, giving the impression of a large common AV valve with excursion through an entire ventricular chamber [139, 182, 287, 328]. However, inferior scanning of the transducer will bring out the separate components of the AV valve motion, separated from each other by distinct ventricular septal echoes [139] (see Fig. 6.2).

Complete AV canal can be differentiated echocardiographically from a common ventricle with a single AV valve by (1) the appearance of ventricular septal echoes on a complete base-to-apex scan, and (2) the finding of a normal vascular relationship. Indeed, if TGA is demonstrated, complete AV canal is a less likely diagnostic possibility.

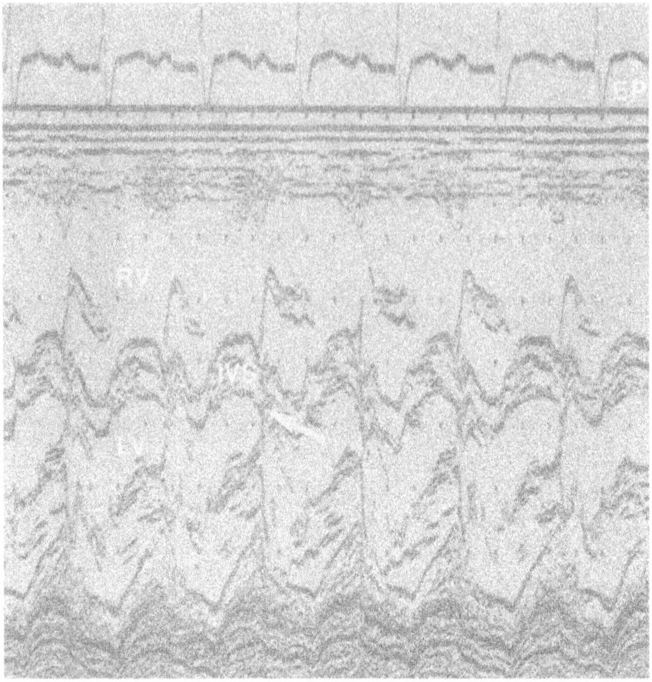

Fig. 6.4. EP: Echocardiogram from a 5-year-old girl with a large ostium primum septal defect (partial AV canal). The child had in addition a secundum ASD. Note the dilatation of the RV, the paradoxical septal motion and the bizarre systolic MV echoes, which apparently cross the IVS during diastole (*arrow*)

6.1.3 Partial Atrioventricular Canal (see 21.1.2)

Just as for complete AV canal, diagnosis of partial AV canal will rest upon the detection of abnormalities, in position and motion, in the mitral and tricuspid parts of the AV valve leaflets.

Position abnormalities [139] (see 6.1.2 and Fig. 17.6) consist of (1) anterior displacement of the mitral valve, which is responsible for a narrowed LVOT and prolonged diastolic mitral valve and ventricular septal apposition; (2) posterior displacement of the TV; (3) continuity between the two AV valves structures (see 4.4.1); and (4) absence of atrial septal echoes (see 4.4.1).

Motion abnormalities (see 6.1.2.) consist of (1) abnormal systolic and diastolic mitral valve echoes; and (2) apparent diastolic movement of a single large AV valve leaflet through the ventricular septum. (see Fig. 6.4).

Partial and complete AV canal defects share similar echocardiographic features; however, their differentiation is possible through the documentation of some features.

The Abnormal AV Valve Motion Through the Septum

This apparent motion can be observed in all types of AV canal [139].

In partial AV canal, it is usually possible to detect separate openings when recording mitral and tricuspid valve echoes [22] (see Fig. 6.4). In addition, both

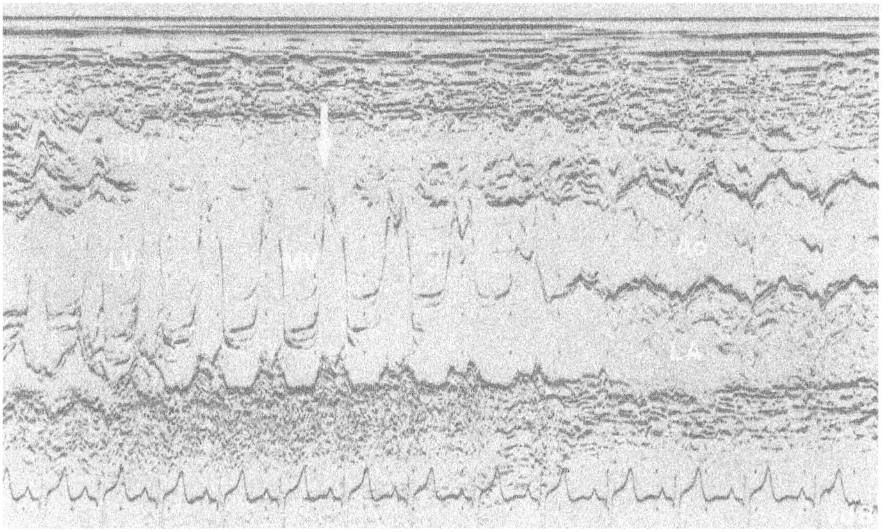

Fig. 6.5. vdB: M-mode scan obtained from a 10-year-old boy with complete AV canal. *Arrow* indicates the ventricular septal defect area, just below the AoV, where no septal echoes are recorded

components of AV valve motion usually remain separated by distinct ventricular septal echoes on a complete base-to-apex scan.

In complete AV canal, absence of large segments of ventricular septal echoes, with excursion through the defect of a large common AV valve, can usually be documented [139] (see Fig. 6.5).

Mitral-Tricuspid Valve Continuity

Continuity between the mitral and tricuspid valve is in favor of complete AV canal [22].

Abnormal Septal Motion

Abnormal (paradoxical) septal motion with right ventricular dilatation is more suggestive of partial AV canal; most patients with the complete form of AV canal defect show normal septal motion [22, 139].

Remark

One of the limitations of echocardiography consists in the fact that abnormal or unusual transducer positions on the chest wall may result in apparent aberrant structural interrelationships. A faulty transducer position, for instance, too low on the chest wall, may be the origin of an incorrect ultrasonic relation between the septum and the tricuspid valve [191]. Solinger et al [361] has stressed that the echo from the ATVL, at the onset of systole, may appear to be more posterior than the anterior wall of a large vessel, depending on the direction of the ultrasonic beam, the spatial position of the heart in the thorax, and the internal cardiac anatomy.

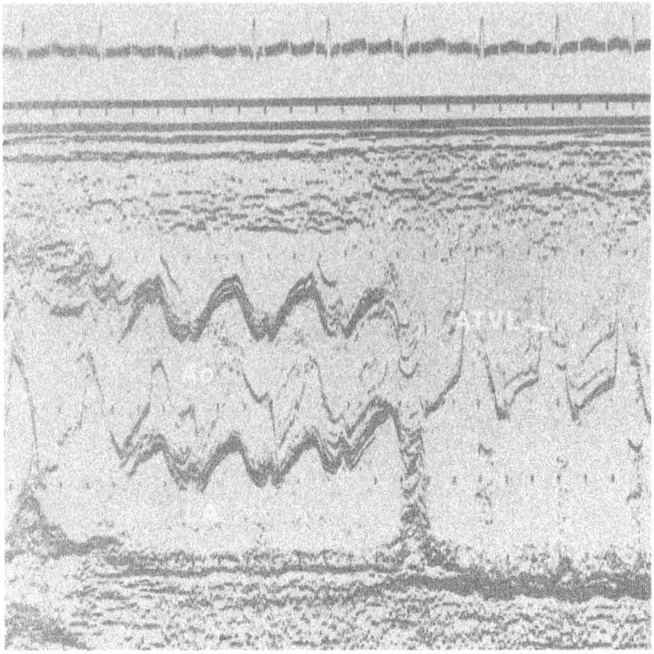

Fig. 6.6. Note the abnormal relationship between the anterior aortic wall and the ATVL, most likely resulting from a faulty transducer position on the chest wall

Figure 6.6, obtained from a child without significant heart disease, illustrates this point. It shows an abnormal relationship between the IVS and the ATVL resulting from a faulty transducer position.

7 Visualization of a Single AV Valve

Index

Introduction

Atrioventricular (AV) valves are quite mobile structures and are easy to record in the pediatric age group.

If only one AV valve can be "visualized" by an experienced echocardiographer, a complex congenital defect should be suspected.

This chapter deals with cardiac anomalies in which only one AV valve can be demonstrated.

7.1 Visualization of Only One AV Valve

7.1.1 Common Ventricle with a Single AV Valve

As stated before (5.1.2), a single or common ventricle consists in a large ventricular chamber which receives blood from two separate or from a common AV valve. A rudimentary, anteriorly positioned outflow chamber may be present.

The relative frequency reported of common ventricle with a single AV valve varies from one study to another. Seward et al. [348] found a single AV valve in eight patients out of 55 with a common ventricle. Mortera et al. [254] documented this in about half of their patients, while Bini et al. [27] reported a still higher incidence of 62%. This variability is probably attributable to the fact that in some series children with mitral or tricuspid atresia were included.

Echocardiographic features of common ventricle with a single AV valve include [254, 348, 349] (1) a single demonstrable AV valve, posteriorly located in the ventricle, with a large amplitude of diastolic excursion; (2) absence of ventricular

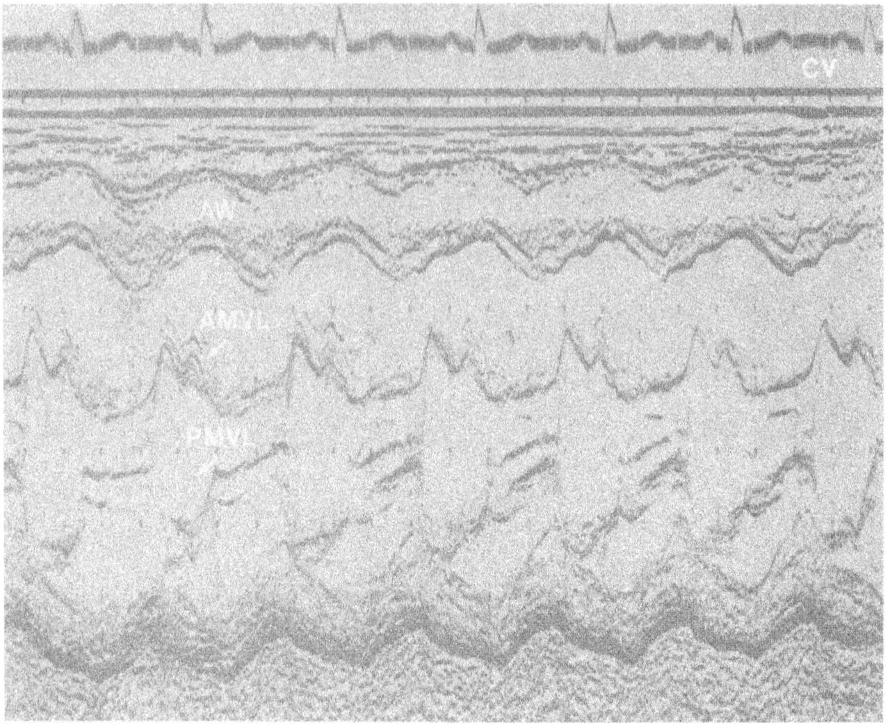

Fig. 7.1. CV: Echocardiogram obtained from a 8-year-old girl with tricuspid atresia, single ventricle and pulmonary obstruction. Exceptionally, no outlet chamber could be documented, either echo- or angiographically

septal echoes on a complete base-to-apex scan; and (3), usually posterior discontinuity.

In common ventricle with a single AV valve an outlet chamber is not usually present. However, if such a chamber is documented ultrasonically in the presence of a single recordable AV valve, tricuspid atresia would be a more likely diagnosis than single or common ventricle [349] (see 7.1.3) (see Fig. 7.1).

Contrast echocardiography is an useful adjunct to the M-mode echocardiographic diagnosis of single ventricle with a single AV valve, through the recognition of specific blood flow patterns (see 22.3.2).

7.1.2 Complete AV Canal (see 6.1.2)

In complete AV canal, at a level immediately below the aortic root, a pattern can be recognized in which a large common AV valve seems to move through the entire ventricular chamber [139, 182, 287, 328]. However, a complete base-to-apex scan will bring out separate portions of two distinct AV valves separated from each other by septal echoes (see Fig. 6.2).

7.1.3 Tricuspid Atresia

The echocardiographic recognition of tricuspid atresia rests upon the following findings, recently summarized by Seward et al. [350] (see Figs. 7.1, 7.2).

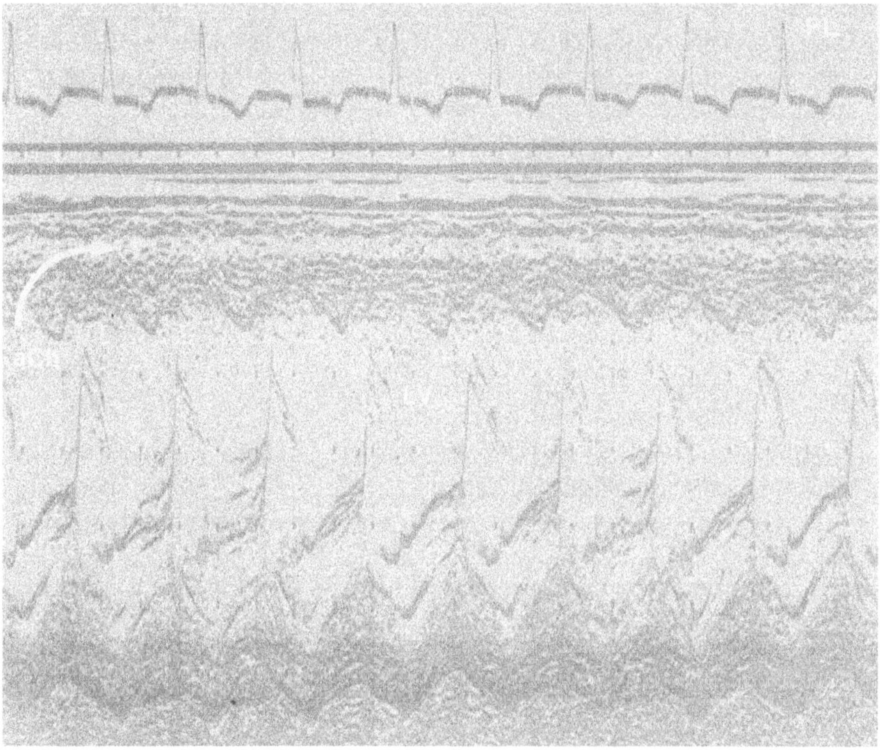

Fig. 7.2. PL: Echo trace from a 5-year-old boy with tricuspid atresia. Note the presence of a small anteriorly located right ventricular chamber (aCh)

1) Inability to record the tricuspid valve,
2) The recording of a single posteriorly positioned AV valve with large anterior excursion during diastole,
3) The frequent occurrence of MV prolapse
4) Mitral-semilunar valve continuity, aortic or pulmonary depending on whether or not the great arteries are normally oriented or transposed,
5) The presence of a small anteriorly located right ventricular chamber [257], although in more than half of the patients, right ventricular diameter is above the fifth percentile,
6) Normal septal and LV posterior wall excursion,
7) Left ventricular end-diastolic dimension at the upper limits of normal, or increased, in most patients,
8) Increased septal and left ventricular posterior wall thickness in a great majority of the patients,
9) Reduced fractional shortening of the left ventricular internal diameter,
10) Possible enlargement of the left atrium,
11) A reproducible flow pattern of contrast medium (see 22.3.2).

However, as mentioned in 7.1.1, differentiation of tricuspid atresia from single ventricle with one AV valve is not always easy echocardiographically. Two essential features should help in this differentiation: (1) in common ventricle with one AV valve, there is usually no RVOT, or anteriorly positioned chamber; and (2) in tricuspid atresia, mitral-semilunar valve continuity is invariably present, a feature rarely encountered in common ventricle with a single AV valve.

The presence of a small anterior chamber with documentation of posterior continuity is thus strongly suggestive of tricuspid atresia, if only one AV valve is found.

If tricuspid atresia is diagnosed, additional echocardiographic features may help detect associated lesions, such as: (1) the presence of TGA; (2) the presence of pulmonic stenosis; and (3) the presence of a VSD by the observation of "dropping out" of septal echoes.

7.1.4 Mitral Atresia

Mitral atresia is often associated with aortic atresia and hypoplasia of the ascending aorta, constituting the hypoplastic left heart syndrome.

In isolated MV atresia, most of the features of this syndrome will be found to some extent (see 17.2.1).

Differentiation from common (single) ventricle with one AV valve should present no problems, echocardiographically or otherwise.

Presence of Normally Absent Structures

8 Echo-Free Spaces

Index

Introduction

Echocardiography has become an extremely useful noninvasive technique in the differential diagnosis of an enlarged heart. It may show whether a large heart shadow on roentgenologic examination is due to left and/or right ventricular hypertrophy or dilatation, or if it is related to pericardial effusion [1].

In fact, echocardiography is now considered to be the most reliable and sensitive method of detecting pericardial fluid, thanks to its ability to detect soft tissues. In this respect, the most striking feature is an echo-free space between the pericardium and the epicardium of the free left ventricular posterior wall (LVPW) caused by the presence of fluid.

In addition to pericardial fluid, other abnormalities may be responsible for similar echo-free spaces, either outside or within the heart borders.

In this chapter, the most frequent causes of abnormal echo-free spaces will be reviewed; the first three subdivisions (8.1 to 8.3) will deal with echo-free spaces surrounding the heart, whereas abnormal echo-free spaces within the heart borders will be discussed in the last three subdivisions (8.4 to 8.6).

8.1 Behind the Left Ventricle

8.1.1 Pericardial Effusion (see Fig. 8.1)

As little as 15 ml of pericardial fluid is detectable by ultrasonic examination of the heart [159]. With large effusions, fluid accumulates not only behind the left ventricle but also anteriorly between the right heart border and the chest wall. Exceptionally, with effusions under high pressure, it may collect behind the left atrium [128].

Fig. 8.1. MF: Echo trace obtained from a child one week after TV replacement for an Ebstein's anomaly. Pericardial fluid (labeled PE) is present both in front of the RV and posterior to the LV

In practice, considerable skill and experience are required to diagnose pericardial effusion; indeed, the gain settings on the instruments must be appropriate, a complete scan is mandatory, and recording devices should be used optimally.

These aspects will be discussed briefly.

Appropriate Gain Settings

The damping controls of the echocardiographic instrument must be used appropriately, especially to demonstrate small efussions [159]. With gain settings that are too high, structures close to each other cannot be differentiated, so that myo-, epi-, and pericardial echoes become blurred and tend to obliterate any clear echo-free space between them. Only with proper gain settings will an echo-free space, between the epi- and pericardium, become apparent. In fact, the presence of such a space most often indicates pericardial effusion as epi- and pericardium seldom can be resolved into separate structures in the absence of intervening fluid.

The asiest if not the best way to identify the pericardium consists in progressively reducing the gain settings of the echocardiograph. Indeed, the pericardium/lung interface is the strongest reflector and therefore the last echo to disappear when returning echoes are progressively damped.

Complete Scan (see Fig. 8.2)

A continuous M-mode scan from the left ventricular apex toward the aorta or vice versa will usually allow a correct diagnosis of pericardial effusion by documenting

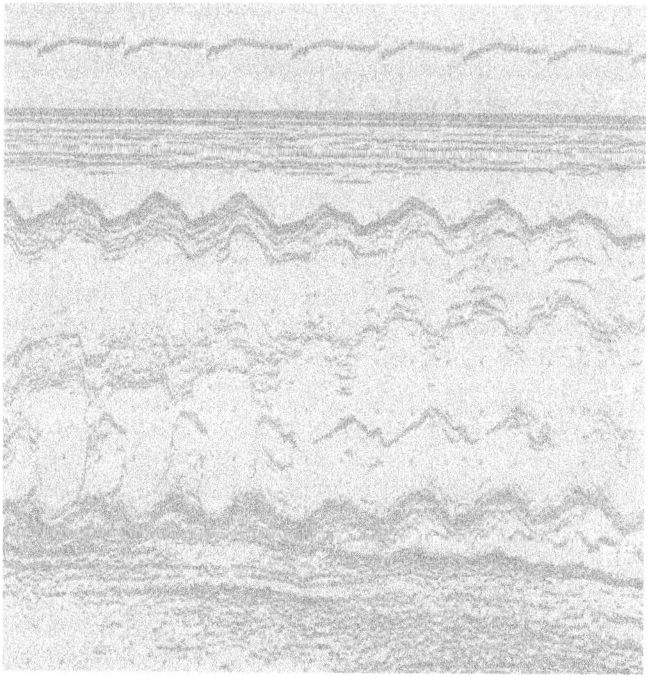

Fig. 8.2. Z: M-mode scan from subaortic region to LV. Pericardial fluid is present both in front of the RV and posterior to the LV. The posterior echo-free space progressively appears as the LV is approached

that the effusion will gradually phase out as the AV junction is approached. Indeed, unless pericardial effusion is massive, fluid rarely accumulates behind the LA, since the insertion of the pulmonary veins into the LA interrupts the continuity of the pericardial sac in this region. However, it is possible to direct the ultrasonic beam where the left atrial pericardium is free of attachment, such as at the oblique sinus of the pericardium, and to document a fluid collection at that level [266].

Recording Devices

A strip chart recording is indispensable if minimal separation between the epi- and pericardium is to be documented. A small pericardial effusion is thus more easily detected on M-mode registration than by a two-dimensional video-system apparatus. However, in the presence of a large effusion, a dynamic two-dimensional image offers the advantage of directly visualizing the extension of the echo-free space and of studying the motion of the heart within the pericardial sac.

In the presence of pericardial effusion, different patterns of epi- and pericardial movement and/or separation have been described. For Horowitz et al. [159] two patterns are considered to be abnormal on M-mode registration: (1) a flat pericardial motion with the epicardium still touching the pericardium in diastole; and (2) separation of epi- and pericardium throughout the cardiac cycle.

If such a pattern behind the LVPW cannot be documented, an anterior echo-free space in front of the right ventricle probably has no diagnostic significance [97, 159]. Indeed, any tissue interposed between the heart and the chest wall, such as fibrous and adipose tissue, or a large thymus, can generate an echo-free space. Thus anterior epi-pericardial separation alone is not sufficient evidence for the diagnosis of pericardial effusion.

The relative importance of a pericardial effusion can be estimated echocardiographically. For some the difference at end-diastole between the cubed diameters of the pericardium and epicardium (from RV to LV), indicates the volume of pericardial fluid present [159]. However, as D'Cruz et al. cautioned [75], there are some potential pitfalls in this quantitation, as the distribution of fluid within the pericardial sac is not necessarily uniform. A large effusion can be more easily defined by the finding of anterior pericardial fluid and, at least in the adult, by finding a 1 cm depth of posterior pericardial fluid. A moderate effusion can be defined by finding pericardial fluid posteriorly only and exceeding 1 cm thickness, and a small effusion can be defined by finding less than 1 cm thickness of posterior pericardial fluid [346].

If a large effusion is documented, signs of cardiac tamponade should be looked for (see 16.2.3).

Dynamic two-dimensional imaging permits studying the motion of the heart within the pericardial sac: in the presence of a large effusion, the normal contraction pattern of the heart is seen to be almost completely overshadowed by a pendular motion of the whole heart within the pericardial sac.

Abnormal valve motion patterns attributable to this swinging heart motion may be documented, such as [266] (1) prolapse patterns of mitral and tricuspid valves; (2) pseudosystolic anterior motion of the AMVL; (3) premature systolic movement toward closure of the aortic valve; and (4) midsystolic notching of the pulmonary valve.

Septal motion may also be abnormal, while aortic root motion is often attenuated.

Effusions within the pericardial sac are certainly the first cause of an echocardiographic free space. Quite often, small effusions will be documented in patients with congestive heart failure and in the immediate cardiac postoperative period. Generally, the space is entirely echo free, but rarely, scattered multiple echoes may be registered, reflecting a change in the homogeneity of the contents of the space [286]. Furthermore, in the presence of clotted blood, echocardiography can be equivocal: a pericardial clot adjacent to myocardium may fail to register a sonolucent space even though liquid blood may also be present [174].

8.1.2 Pericardial Cyst

The ultrasonic appearance of a pericardial cyst, as described by Roelandt in one adult patient [315], is similar to a localized pericardial effusion, and consists in a localized echo-free space behind the LV at the level of the MV.

8.1.3 Pseudoaneurysm of the Left Ventricle

These aneurysms, which are usually due to post-myocardial infarction and are retained by pericardial or extracardiac tissues, are in free communication with the LV cavity [316]. They may result either from cardiac rupture with localized hemopericardium or from subacute rupture with gradual and/or episodic bleeding and formation of a localized hematoma.

Obviously, this will not frequently be encountered in the pediatric age group, although viral myocarditis, endocardial fibroelastosis, or related conditions may lead to such complications.

Echocardiography alone cannot differentiate a pseudoaneurysm from a localized pericardial effusion; however, it does allow differentiation between pseudoaneurysm and a true left ventricular aneurysm [316]: in this last condition, the myocardium or its tissue replacement forms the outer wall of the aneurysm, in contrast to pseudoaneurysms whose outline is formed by the pericardium.

8.1.4 Pleural Effusion (see Fig. 8.3)

A pleural effusion may also be responsible for an echo-free space behind the LVPW. However, in this situation the echo-free space may extend upward behind the left atrium; in addition, the relation of the pericardial echo to the echo-free space will be entirely different. With pleural effusion, the pericardial echo will be in front of the echo-free space rather than behind, as with pericardial effusion.

8.1.5 Left Ventricular Diverticulum

A left ventricular diverticulum is difficult to detect using conventional echocardiography. Real-time cross sectional echocardiography may show a small, almost echo-free space, immediately behind the LVPW and changing shape during the cardiac cycle [91].

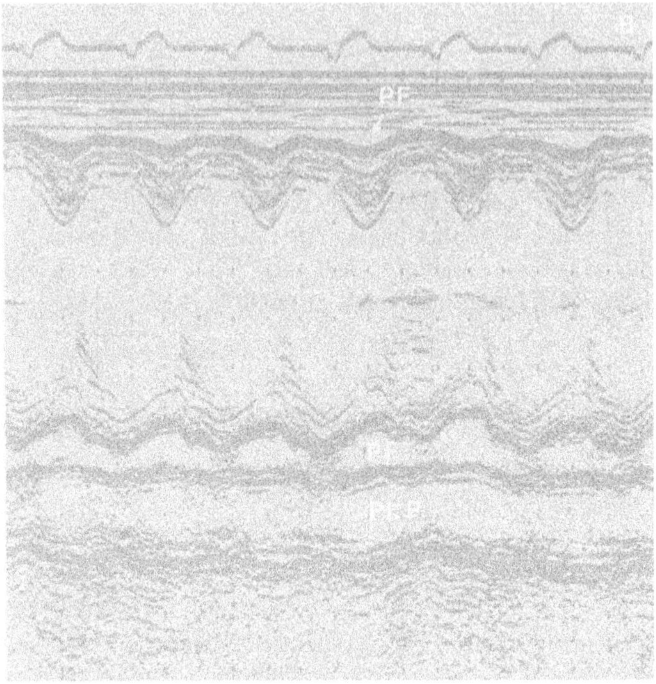

Fig. 8.3. B: Echo trace obtained from a 45-year-old male with pericardial fluid (PF) in front of the RV and posteriorly to the LV. Note an additional echo-free space behind the pericardium, compatible with a left pleural effusion (Pl.F)

8.2 In Front of the Right Ventricle

8.2.1 Pericardial Effusion

Pericardial effusion in front of the right ventricle was discussed in 8.1.1.

It suffices to remember that the finding of anterior pericardial fluid, in addition to posterior pericardial fluid, is indicative of a large effusion.

8.2.2 Pericardial Cyst (see 8.1.2)

8.2.3 Fibrous, Fatty Tissues; Thymus

8.3 Behind the Left Atrium

8.3.1 Pericardial Effusion

As discussed before (see 8.1.1) fluid rarely accumulates within the pericardium behind the left atrium, unless the effusion is under high pressure [128].

8.3.2 Pleural Effusion (see Fig. 8.3)

An echo-free space posterior to the left atrial wall is generally caused by pleural effusion. A rare pericardial effusion can be differentiated by the fact that the left atrial wall will exhibit systolic and diastolic motion, whereas with pleural effusion the left atrial wall is immobile [128] (see also 8.1.4).

8.3.3 Total Anomalous Pulmonary Venous Return (TAPVR)

No definite ultrasonic features of this anomaly have been described. However, the diagnosis is suggested if an echo-free space, dorsal to the posterior wall of the LA, is found in a cyanotic baby [277a, 380]. This space represents the common pulmonary venous channel which can be found in most cases of TAPVR (see Fig. 8.4). The posterior wall of this echo-free space should not be confused with the true left atrial wall, which may lead to an erroneous ultrasonic diagnosis of an intra-atrial membrane (cor triatriatum) [192].

Other features suggestive of TAPVR include (1) an echocardiographic pattern of RVDVO, or the association of right ventricular dilatation with paradoxic septal motion (see 21.1.4) in a cyanotic baby (see Fig. 17.4); and (2) the presence of a small left atrium [114].

Contrast echocardiography further helps in delineating the location of the pulmonary venous collector behind the left atrium [277a].

If the pulmonary venous return drains into the coronary sinus, abnormal echoes within the left atrium may be recorded (see 9.1.6).

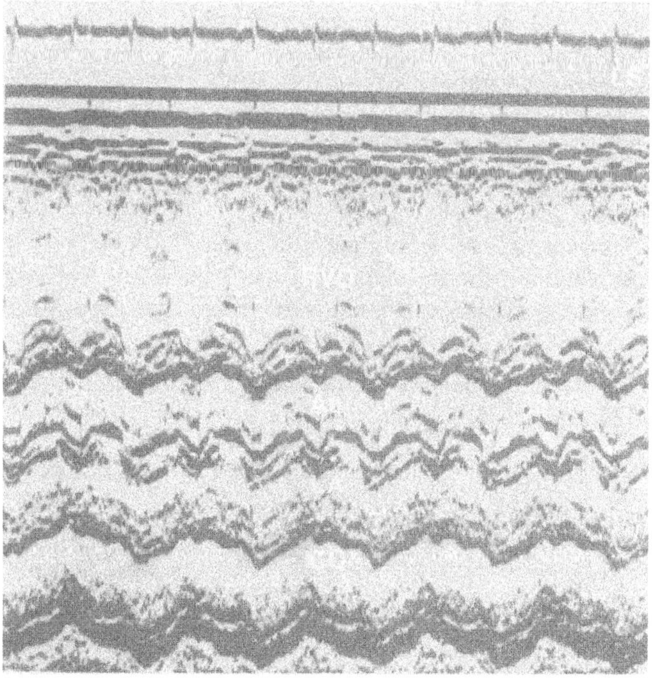

Fig. 8.4. LS: Echocardiogram obtained from an infant with total anomalous pulmonary venous return into a persistent left superior vena cava. Note the echo-free space, representing the common pulmonary venous channel, behind the left atrium

Remark

Before diagnosing an echo-free space behind the left atrium, the precise location of the left atrial wall should be ascertained. Indeed, nonstructural echoes within the left atrial cavity may be mistaken for the atrial wall, and may give the impression of an abnormal echo-free space behind these echoes.

8.4 Within the Aortic Walls (Duplication of Aortic Wall Echoes)

Demonstration of an echo-free space within the anterior or the posterior aortic wall echo, in fact, the finding of a duplication of an aortic wall echo, suggests aortic dissection [246].

However, widening or duplication of aortic wall echoes may also be seen in other unrelated conditions, with (8.4.1 to 8.4.4) or without (8.4.5 and 8.4.6) involvement of the aortic walls.

8.4.1 Dissecting Aortic Aneurysm

Aortic root dissection should be diagnosed by ultrasound, only if the patient's clinical course is consistent with this serious complication [37], and well-known echocardiographic features of aortic dissection can be documented.
These features include:
1) Widening or duplication of one or both aortic walls [37],
2) Intimal echo thinner than outer margin [37],
3) Parallel motion of the separated margins of the aortic root walls [267],
4) Aortic root dilatation [267],
5) Pronounced variation in aortic root diameter with only minor changes in transducer angulation [258],
6) The demonstration that the echo from the mitral ring diverges into two posterior wall echoes [37, 190],
7) Normal cusp echoes within the true lumen [267].

Cross sectional echocardiography is also useful in the diagnosis of dissection, as it may reveal the extension of the dissection into the supravalvular aorta [267].

8.4.2 Aneurysmal Dilatation of the Aortic Root and the Noncoronary Sinus of Valsalva [157]

This condition will more likely be encountered in elderly people.

8.4.3 Pericardial Effusion Extending into the Transverse Sinus [258]

8.4.4 Atherotic Plaques in the Aortic Walls [258]

In these conditions (8.4.2 to 8.4.4) the aortic walls are directly or indirectly involved and may seem to be widened or duplicated on echocardiographic examination.

8.4.5 Abscess or Fluid Collection in the IVS [37, 157]

8.4.6 Reflection from the Mitral Valve in Mitral Stenosis [37, 157]

In these entities (8.4.5 and 8.4.6), the aortic walls are not involved but reflections from surrounding diseased structures (either the MV or the IVS) may produce echoes which are parallel to an aortic wall echo.

Finally, it should be realized that apparent aortic wall duplication may result from artifacts. A common example of such an artifact is in the simultaneous recording of the anterior aortic wall echo with either the posterior pulmonary artery wall or with a catheter positioned into the pulmonary artery [258]. The simultaneous recording of these structures will result in an apparent duplication of the anterior aortic wall echo.

8.5 Within the IVS

8.5.1 Cystic Tumors of the Heart

Using echocardiography, Farooki et al. [96] recently diagnosed a hydatid cyst in the IVS of an 8-year-old boy with abdominal echinococcosis. This cyst corresponded to an echo-free space in the area of the septum, posteriorly delineated by a linear flat echo anterior to the MV apparatus.

8.6 Within the Heart

8.6.1 Primitive Ventricle with Outlet Chamber (see Fig. 5.3)

An outlet chamber may be present in cases of primitive ventricle with either one or two AV valves [254]. Echocardiographically, this outlet chamber is detected as an anterior echo-free space, separated from the main ventricular cavity by septal remnants or the bulboventricular septum (see also 5.1.2).

8.6.2 Calcified Mitral Annulus (see 9.2.2, Fig 8.5)

This will give an abnormal band of dense echoes within the left ventricular cavity posterior to the AMVL. These annular echoes are responsible for an additional echo-free space between these echoes anteriorly and the LVPW posteriorly [72, 74, 289].

8.6.3 Aneurysm of the Right Sinus of Valsalva

An aneurysm of the right sinus of Valsalva may extend either into the right or into the left ventricle. Figure 8.6 represents such an aneurysm protruding into the heart, between the two ventricles. An echo-free space is generated between the IVS and the anterior wall of the aneurysm. The aortic root may be dilated [431].

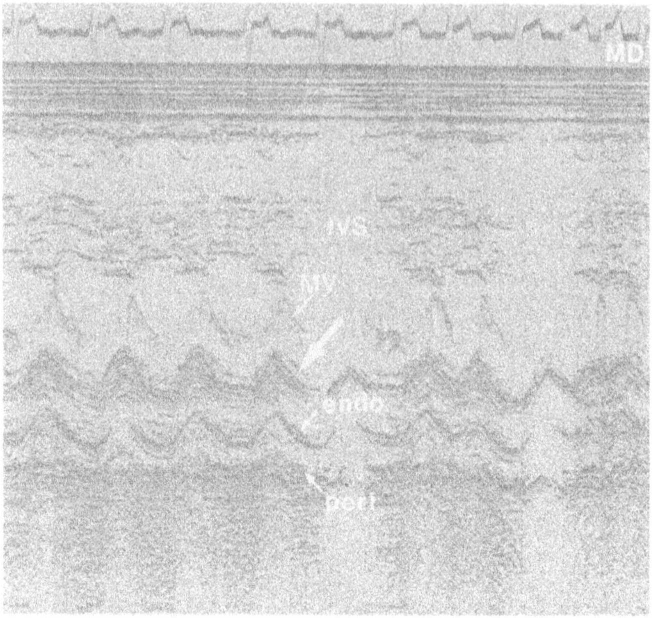

Fig. 8.5. MD: This echocardiogram might be erroneously diagnosed as showing pericardial fluid. In fact, the "echo-free space" corresponds to the LVPW. The thick band of echoes anterior to it, and indicated by an *arrow*, originate from a calcified mitral ring. This echocardiogram was obtained from a 75-year-old female

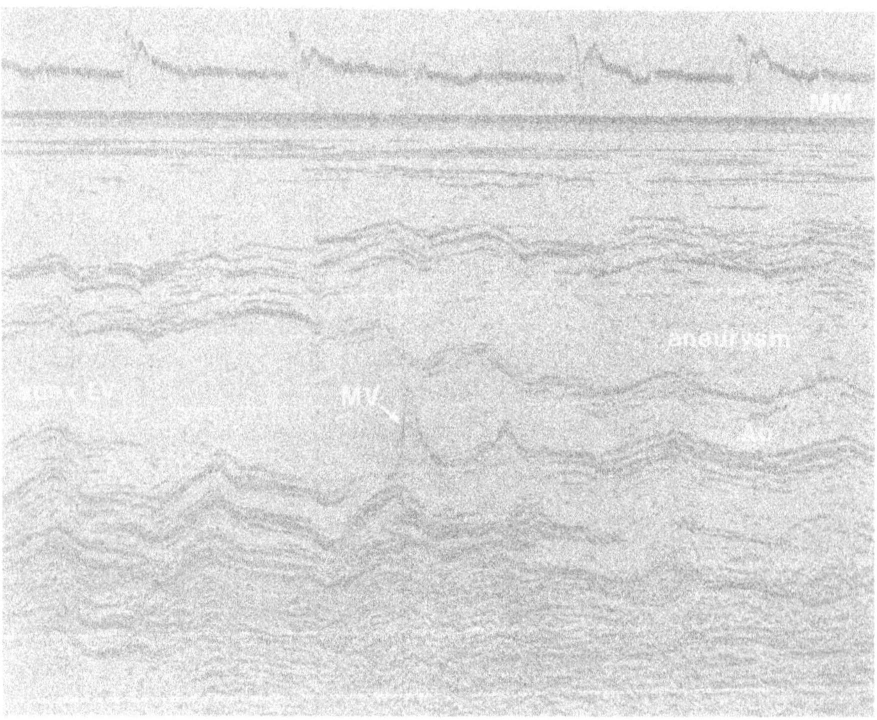

Fig. 8.6 a

b

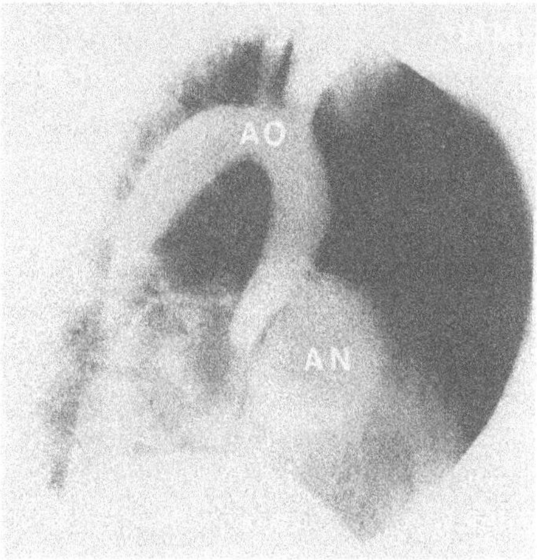

Fig. 8.6. MM: **a** Echocardiogram obtained from a 15-year-old girl with a right sinus of Valsalva aneurysm protruding into the heart. The child had, in addition, aortic regurgitation and complete AV block. The ostium of the aneurysm was closed, the AoV replaced and a pacemaker inserted. This postoperative echocardiogram shows a duplication of the anterior aortic wall, delineating the aneurysm down to the level of the MV leaflets. **b** Angiographic picture after injection of dye in the ascending aorta, preoperatively. It shows the aneurysm filling from the right sinus of Valsalva

9 Unusual, Abnormal Echoes

Index

Introduction

Abnormal echoes on an echocardiographic recording may have different causes, such as (1) intracardiac structural abnormalities as seen in some congenital heart lesions; (2) structural alterations in acquired heart diseases; (3) heart tumors; and (4) prosthetic tissues such as artificial valves, patches, conduits, etc.

However, an abnormal echo does not necessarily reflect abnormal cardiac tissue, but may be due to imperfections in presently available echo systems. Indeed, an echocardiographic M-mode recording may be confusing because of the display of spurious echoes, or echoes at a place where no corresponding structure exists. Such echoes are likely to occur with transducers having a wide acoustic beam. The disturbance on the display may also be caused by echoes picked up by the side-lobes or secondary acoustic reflections to the ultrasonic crystal.

Commonly seen examples of this distortion are parallel echoes of the MV, parts of which seem off-axis. The echoes are displayed behind each other in the form of multiple parallel echoes due to small differences in travel time [315].

Echoes from the aortic root or from laterally placed papillary muscles or chordae tendinae, with the transducer aimed at the mitral valve, represent other examples of misleading ultrasound reflections (see Fig. 13.10).

False echoes may also be produced by reverberation, a phenomenon responsible for duplication of echoes behind the true display. Reverberation can originate at transducer level or from structures within the heart. If the returning sound wave bounces back from the transducer, its reflection, which is sometimes called phantom echo, will show up at a level twice the distance to the original display.

Reflections from structures within the heart produce a mirror image posterior to the original trace. The echocardiographic appearance of a multilayered mitral valve illustrates reverberation within a calcified valve. Before diagnosing an abnormal "structural" echo, "erroneous" echoes will thus have to be ruled out.

In the following paragraphs, the most frequent causes of true "structural" echoes will be reviewed.

9.1 Abnormal Echoes Within the Left Atrium

9.1.1 Cor Triatriatum

Cor triatriatum is one of the cardiac abnormalities impeding the ventricular filling. Obstruction of blood flow is caused by the existence within the left atrial cavity of a fibrous or fibromuscular diaphragm dividing this cavity into two separate chambers. The pulmonary veins normally drain into the proximal chamber. The severity of the obstruction depends on the size of the opening(s) in that diaphragm [284]. The MV remains normal.

Echocardiographically, the diagnosis of cor triatriatum should be made with caution and only in the presence of clinical evidence. Diagnosis is suggested by the

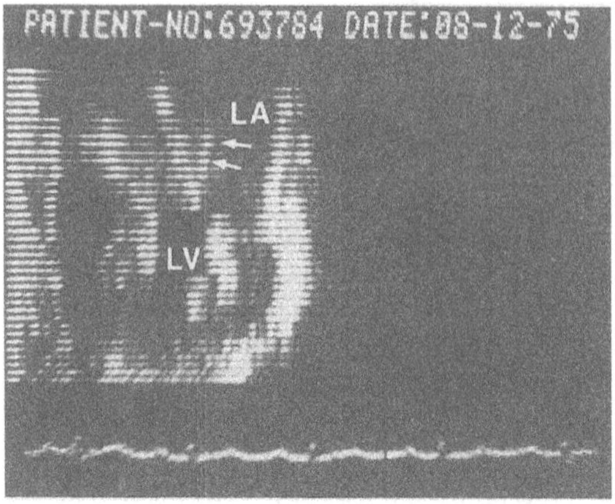

Fig. 9.1. Two-dimensional image of the heart, through the long axis of the LV, obtained from a 6-year-old girl with a supravalvular mitral membrane. *Arrows* indicate the echoes of this membrane within the LA cavity

presence of an unusual linear echo within the left atrium, either behind the posterior aortic wall or the mitral ring [15, 89, 108, 192, 250, 272] (see Fig. 9.1). This abnormal echo may move anteriorly during atrial systole [250].

As pointed out by Lacorte et al. [192], precise location of the membrane responsible for the abnormal echo depends largely on the anatomic position and motion of the membrane, as well as on transducer beam width and direction.

If a membrane is suspected echocardiographically, MV motion should be carefully studied: a normal motion is usually documented in cor triatriatum, as opposed to other obstructive left ventricular inflow anomalies such as a supravalvar mitral ring, in which MV motion may be abnormal [192, 210].

9.1.2 Left Atrial Tumors (see Fig. 9.2)

Most frequent cardiac tumors in childhood are atrial myxomas and ventricular rhabdomyomas. Up to the advent of echocardiography, detection of these tumors was a challenge requiring elaborate techniques. Today, cardiac tumors may be quite accurately diagnosed using ultrasound. Generally, one sees an organized mass of echoes that are not obliterated by low gain settings [315].

LA tumors have been repeatedly demonstrated using echocardiography [100, 213, 314, 434]. The characteristic appearance is that of a mass of echoes behind the AMVL during diastole, when the tumor prolapses through the valve [314]. The motion pattern of the AMVL is abnormal, similar to that seen in mitral stenosis, and reflects the obstruction to left atrial emptying by the tumor.

One should notice the slight delay between the time the MV opens and the time the tumor enters the mitral orifice. During systole, the tumor may move back to the LA or remain close to the AMVL, depending upon the tumor's mobility and site of attachment. In some cases the diagnosis has been sufficiently obvious to permit surgery for removal of the tumor without other diagnostic studies [269].

Sometimes a LA tumor may manifest itself by multiple, discrete linear echoes behind the MV, the anterior leaflet of which may exhibit an abrupt mid-systolic posterior movement [213].

Obviously, cross sectional echocardiography will be extremely useful in the detection of a left atrial tumor (see Fig. 9.3).

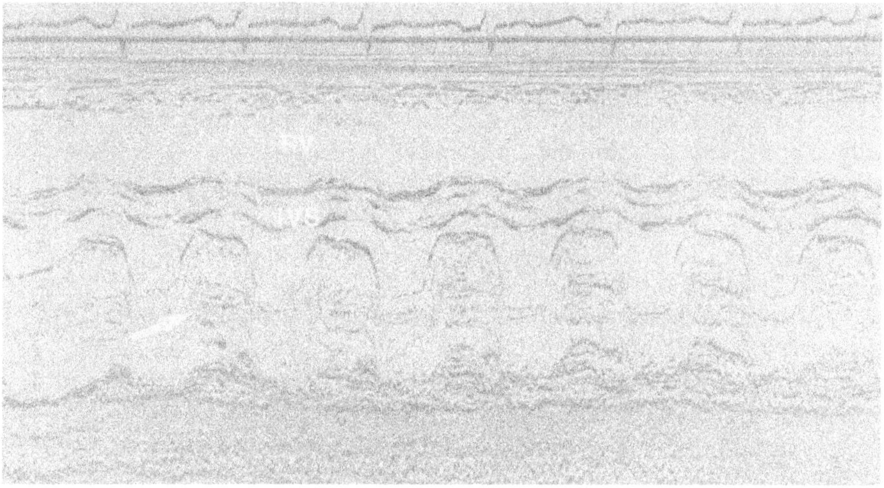

Fig. 9.2. M-mode scan obtained from a male with a documented left atrial myxoma. Echoes of the tumor are visible within the LA during systole, and in the MV region, between the two leaflets, during diastole (*arrow*). Note the abnormal motion of the MV

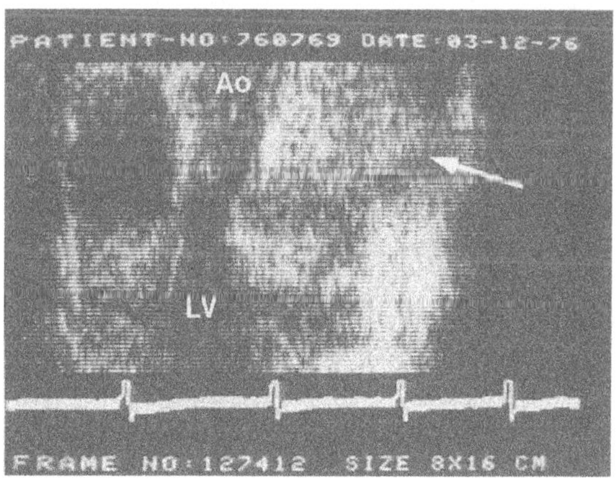

Fig. 9.3. Two-dimensional image through the long axis of the LV obtained from a male with a left atrial myxoma (same patient as in Fig. 9.2). The tumor can be seen just above the MV ring; the still frame was obtained at the onset of systole

Similar abnormal echoes within the left atrium can be found in other disease processes; these will be briefly presented in the following paragraphs (9.1.3 to 9.1.5).

9.1.3 Free Floating Left Atrial Thrombus

On occasion, abnormal echoes can be detected intermittently within the LA cavity: this may correspond to a free-floating LA thrombus passing periodically in and out of the sound beam [363].

9.1.4 Large Mural Clot

This may generate strong echoes anterior to the LA wall [363].

9.1.5 Flail Posterior Mitral Valve Leaflet (Ruptured Chordae Tendineae)

Mitral regurgitation secondary to ruptured chordae tendineae with flail mitral valve leaflets is amenable to echocardiographic diagnosis; detection rests upon several criteria recently summarized by Kotler et al. [184] and Mintz et al. [249]:
1) Multiple linear echoes within the LA chamber during systole,
2) An early systolic plunge of the leaflet to the posterior left atrial wall, followed by anterior motion, at the onset of diastole,
3) Excessive systolic motion of the left atrial wall and of the IVS [374],
4) Systolic fluttering of the mitral valve leaflets (see 13.10.2),
5) Chaotic diastolic anterior motion of the flail posterior mitral valve leaflet [39],
6) Coarse diastolic fluttering of a flail AMVL [86].

In addition, real-time two-dimensional echocardiographic studies allow identification of ruptured chordae tendineae. Here the characteristic abnormality is a rapid systolic motion of the involved leaflet beyond the line of valve closure into the atrium. The abnormal systolic motion is greatest at the tip of the leaflet, and not at its body, as it occurs in MV prolapse [249]. The normal leaflet coaptation point is lost [249].

9.1.6 Total Anomalous Pulmonary Venous Return to the Coronary Sinus (see 8.3.3)

With drainage of the pulmonary veins into the coronary sinus, it is possible to record within the left atrial cavity behind the posterior aortic wall and anterior mitral leaflet echoes, a highly mobile linear echo with a double wave form per cardiac cycle. This additional echo has been found to be related to the anterior wall of the coronary sinus [276].

9.2 Abnormal Echoes Within the Left Ventricle

9.2.1 Left Ventricular Tumors

Tumors in the LV are diagnosed by a cluster of echoes within the LV chamber [96, 202]. The left ventricle may then seem to be reduced in size.

9.2.2 Mitral Valve Annulus Calcification

Normally the mitral annulus appears as a thin discrete echo, moving in parallel with echoes recorded from the LVPW.

Distortion of the normal anatomy of the mitral apparatus by severe mitral annulus calcification results in abnormalities of MV motion and position: the mitral valve leaflets are often displaced to a relatively anterior position within the left ventricle [74]. Interposed between the thin echoes recorded from the AMVL anteriorly and the left ventricular endocardium posteriorly is an abnormal band of dense echoes representing the calcified mitral annulus [72]. These echoes should not be confused with the LVPW, lest an erroneous diagnosis of pericardial effusion be made (see Fig. 8.5 and Sect. 8.6.2)

9.2.3 Bacterial Vegetations

Bacterial vegetations may have their origin at septal level and protrude within the left ventricular cavity; this may be responsible for an abnormal tongue-like band of echoes originating from the IVS (see Fig. 9.4 a).

9.3 Abnormal Echoes Within the LVOT

9.3.1 Discrete Subvalvular Aortic Stenosis (see 11.2.1)

Two general forms of discrete subvalvar aortic stenosis exist [257]. In one, a thin subvalvar membrane or diaphragm, usually attached to the AMVL, is located under the aortic valve; in the other, there is a long fibromuscular tunnel.

The subaortic membrane has been recognized by some researchers as a thin echo within the LVOT [188, 194, 293]. However, we assume that, most of the time, recording of this membrane will be difficult because of insufficient lateral resolution of the sound beam, the membrane moving predominantly in a superior-inferior direction.

Nevertheless, if a membrane is suspected echocardiographically, more specific features of subvalvar aortic obstruction should be documented (see 11.2.1)

9.3.2 Parachute Accessory AMVL

Cooperberg et al. [65] have described an asymptomatic 9-year-old boy in whom LVOT obstruction resulted from an accessory MV leaflet attached to the base of the mitral ring. In this case, the echocardiographic findings were those of subaortic stenosis (see 11.2.1). In addition, an unusual echo moving anteriorly in systole, and separate from the AMVL echo, was found in the LVOT. Similar findings have been reported by Popp et al. [293].

9.3.3 Prolapsing Aortic Valve

9.3.4 Aortic Valve Vegetation (see Fig. 9.4 b)

Prolapsing AoV as well as aortic valve vegetation may be responsible for abnormal echoes in the LVOT [52]. These echoes will be documented during diastole only [431]. Dynamic LVOT obstruction is thus not present.

The differential diagnosis between prolapsing aortic valve and aortic valve vegetation is difficult echocardiographically: if in diastole a single, or two discrete AoV echoes are documented, eventually with fine high frequency fluttering, a floppy, prolapsing AoV is more likely than vegetative endocarditis, which is usually associated with dense diastolic echoes [52].

9.3.5 Right Sinus of Valsalva Aneurysm (see 8.6.3)

Rothbaum et al. [322], in a case report concerning a right sinus of Valsalva aneurysm, demonstrated echocardiographically that there was an abnormal structure extending from the aortic root into the left ventricular chamber adjacent to the IVS. This abnormal echo moved away from the septum during diastole and toward it during systole, and this motion appeared to correlate well with the cineangiographic filling of the aneurysm during diastole and emptying during systole. In addition, the aortic valve leaflets were found to be eccentric.

Figure 8.6 represents an aneurysm of the right sinus of Valsalva, protruding into the heart; its ostium in the right coronary sinus was closed surgically. Motion of the aneurysmal wall, represented by an abnormal echo in the LVOT, is parallel to the septal motion, as filling or emptying of the aneurysm no longer occurs.

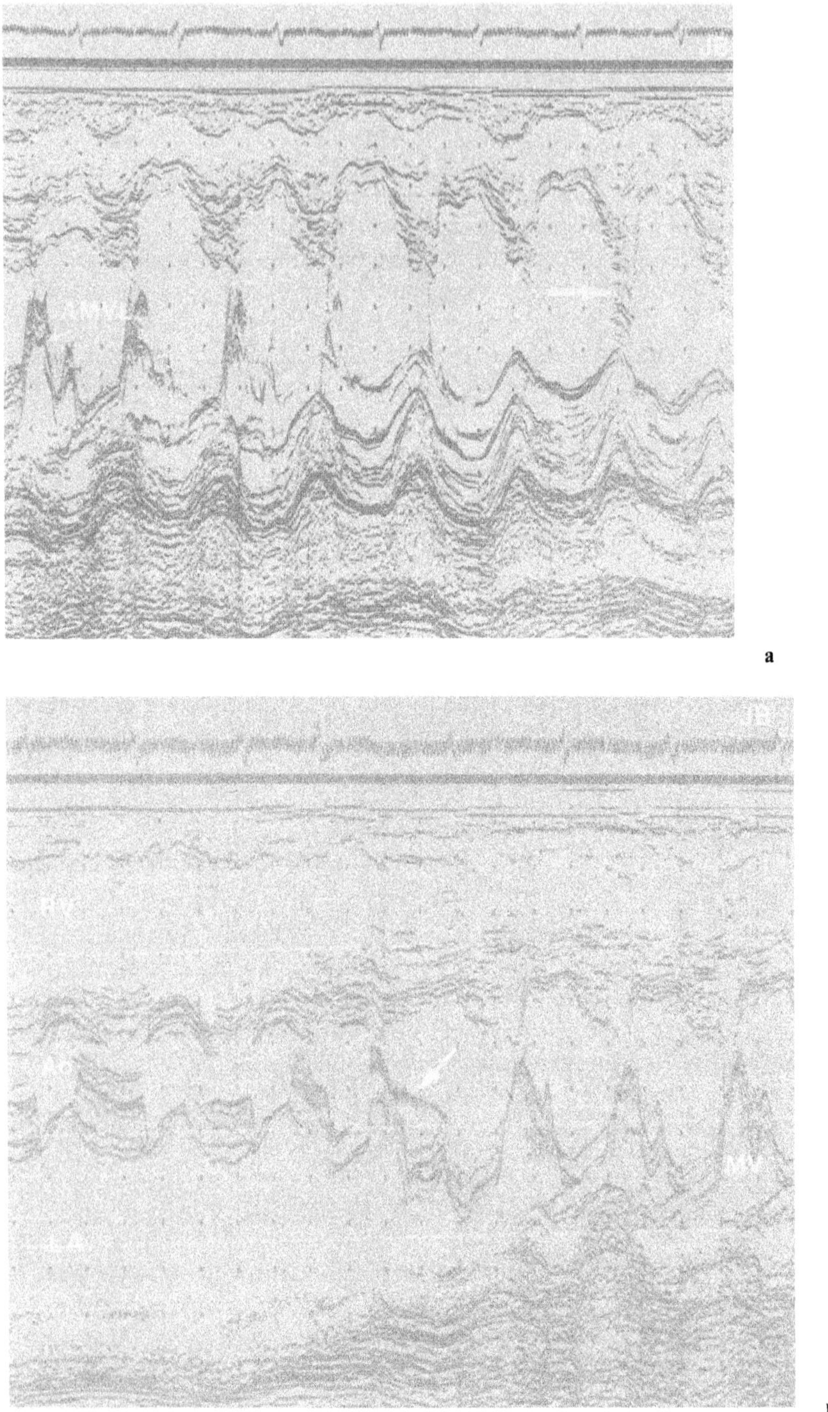

Fig. 9.4. a JB: Echocardiogram obtained from a 50-year-old man with bacterial endocarditis. Vegetations were documented at aortic, mitral and septal levels. Note the abnormal echoes distorting the MV, and deeper within the LV an abnormal mass of echoes originating from the septum and protruding into the LV (*arrow*). **b** JB: (same patient as in **a**) Scan from AoV to MV. Abnormal, irregular echoes are well demonstrated at the level of the noncoronary aortic cusp and at the AMVL. In addition, an abnormal cluster of echoes is present during diastole within the LVOT, representing a prolapsing aortic valve vegetation responsible for diastolic narrowing of the LVOT (*arrow*)

9.3.6 Aneurysm of the Membranous IVS in d-TGA

An abnormal cluster of multiple, fragmentary and posteriorly convex echoes in the LVOT, disappearing during diastole, may be seen in patients with an aneurysm of the membranous IVS in d-TGA [347].

9.3.7 Tumors in the Left Ventricle

The left ventricular cavity, including the LVOT, can be totally obliterated by a dense layer of echoes in the presence of solid left ventricular tumors [96, 202], or tumors arising from the IVS [275].

9.3.8 Calcific Deposits

Calcific deposits, either in the aortic cusps or in the region of the aortic annulus, may be responsible for a linear or bandlike echo in the LVOT region. In this situation, mitral annulus calcification is usually present [74].

9.4 Abnormal Echoes Within the Right Atrium

9.4.1 Right Atrial Tumor

A right atrial tumor is detected in the same way as a left atrial tumor: a cluster of dense echoes is documented in diastole behind the ATVL, representing the tumor as it prolapses through the valve orifice [409, 434].

It is even possible to detect echocardiographically a right atrial extension of a Wilm's tumor [93].

9.5 Abnormal Echoes Within the Right Ventricle

9.5.1 Right Ventricular Tumors

A right ventricular tumor generates a cluster of echoes within a dilated right ventricular cavity [6, 294], while a septal tumor, such as a rhabdomyoma, generates echoes in the vicinity of the IVS [92].

This cluster of dense echoes may obscure the right ventricular outflow tract throughout the cardiac cycle [53, 213], or may appear within the pulmonic valve in systole [53] (see Fig. 9.5).

Left ventricular cavity is sometimes reduced by posterior displacement of the IVS [6].

9.5.2 Abnormal Muscle Bundles

Abnormal muscle bundles within the right ventricle are sometimes responsible for a band of echoes within the right ventricular cavity (see Fig. 9.6).

9.5.3 Rupture of Right Sinus of Valsalva Aneurysm

When such an aneurysm ruptures into the right heart, unusual echoes appear in the RVOT or behind the ATVL [226, 274, 408, 420]. These echoes represent parts of

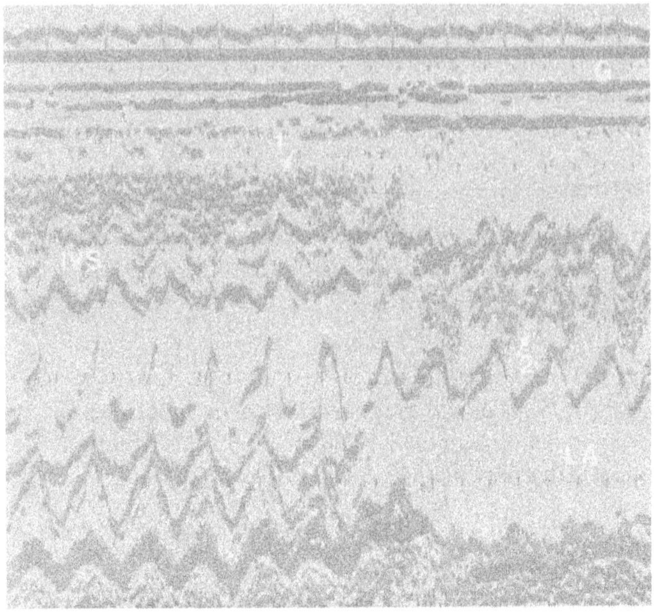

Fig. 9.5. G: Echocardiogram obtained from an infant with tuberous sclerosis. An abnormal band of dense echoes within the RV outflow tract (*arrow 1*) denotes the presence of a tumor, most probably a rhabdomyoma. Presence of a tumor mass at this location was also documented angiographically. An additional tumor mass was also visualized at the AoV area (*arrow 2*)

aortic valve tissue prolapsing into the right side of the heart. In addition, a characteristic aortic cusp motion pattern may be documented [408], i.e., early systolic closure with reopening in late systole of the right coronary cusp. Septal motion may become abnormal.

Cross sectional echocardiography can demonstrate that the aneurysm protrudes into the outflow tract of the right ventricle [274].

9.5.4 Aneurysm of the IVS

An abnormal cluster of multiple, fragmentary and anteriorly convex echoes in the RVOT, disappearing during diastole, may be seen in patients with aneurysms of the IVS and normally related great arteries [12] (see Fig. 9.7).

Aneurysms of the IVS occurring after spontaneous closure of a VSD may give similar abnormal echoes but, in general, lower within the right ventricle [338].

9.6 Abnormal Echoes in the Pericardial Region

9.6.1 Pericardial Thickening

A double band of narrowly separated intense echoes with parallel motion in the area of the pericardium is seen in most patients after heart surgery, and represents pericardial thickening [10, 289].

This is consistent with pericarditis but is not diagnostic of the functional derangement seen in the latter condition [289] (see Fig. 9.8).

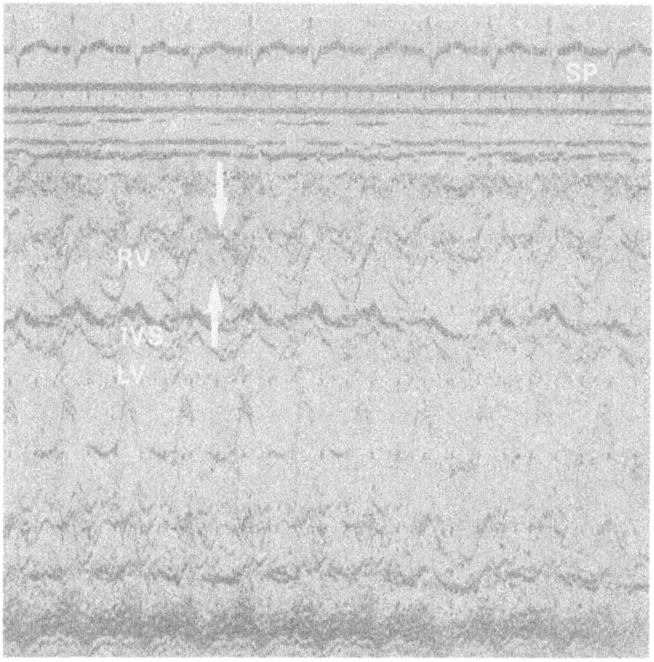

a

b

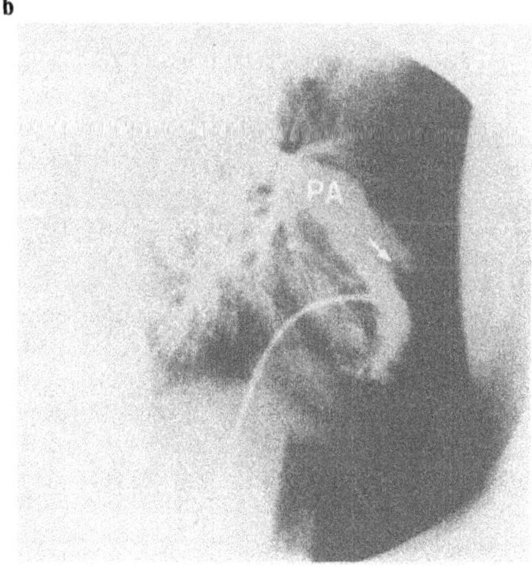

Fig 9.6. SP: **a** Echocardiogram obtained from a 2-year-old child with a left-to-right ventricular shunt, and infundibular and valvular pulmonic stenosis. Note the abnormal band of echoes in the RV, caused by the presence of an abnormal muscle bundle within this ventricular chamber (*between arrows*). **b** Right ventricular angiogram, lateral view, showing a radiolucent space (*arrow*), corresponding to an abnormal muscle bundle

9.7 Abnormal Echoes Involving the Valve Leaflets

9.7.1 Fibrosis and/or Calcification of Leaflets

Generally, it may be said that multiple intense echoes from a leaflet indicate extensive fibrosis and/or calcification [289].

An aortic valvulopathy, with cusp thickening and calcification, is suggested echocardiographically by the demonstration of multiple diastolic echoes within the aortic lumen [150] (see Fig. 11.7).

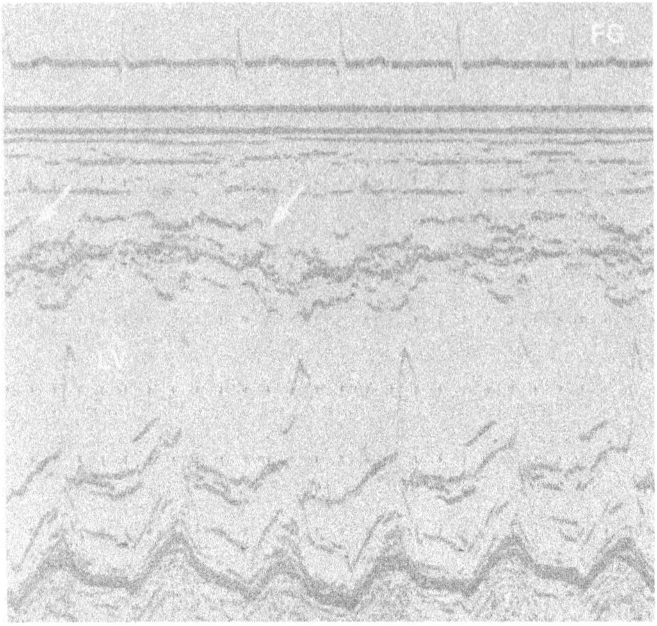

a

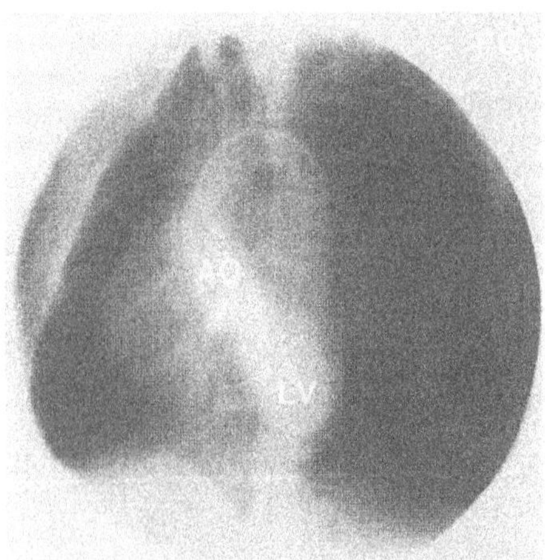

b

Fig. 9.7. FG: **a** The *arrows* point to echoes of a septal aneurysm in a 6-year-old boy after spontaneous closure of a VSD. **b** Left ventricular angiogram in a left posterior oblique position. The *arrow* points to the presence of a small membranous septal aneurysm

Similarly, multiple dense parallel $E–F_0$ (diastolic) echoes are found in patients with more than 80 mg of calcium in the MV, whereas normally, in the absence of significant calcification, or fibrosis, a single $E–F_0$ echo is inscribed [302]. It can be argued, however, that multiple systolic echoes from the AMVL are often due to the irregular nature of the valve: in general, a more redundant leaflet will occasion a greater number of echoes [289].

9.7.2 Valvular Vegetation (see Figs. 9.4 and 11.6)

Vegetative bacterial endocarditis still remains a major diagnostic problem at the onset of the disease, when prompt institution of therapy is crucial. A report on 65

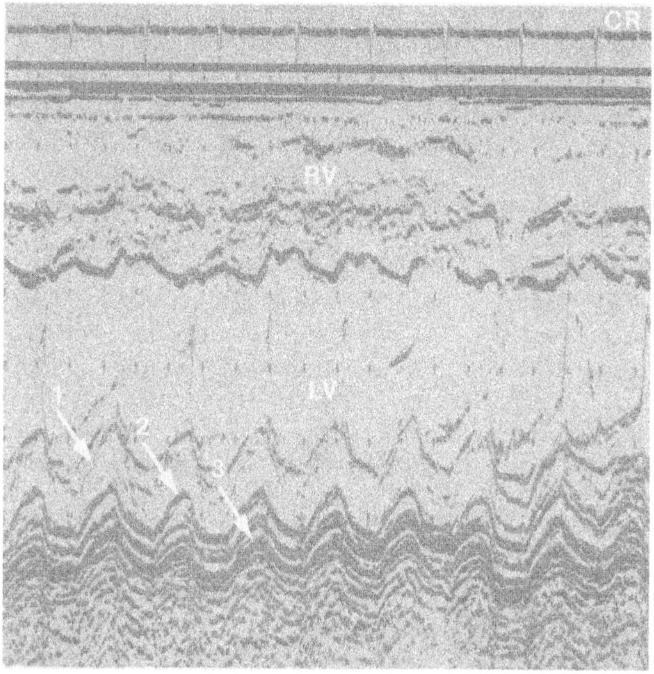

Fig. 9.8. CR: Echocardiogram obtained from a 5-year-old girl with acute rheumatoid arthritis. Pericardial irritation was present as evidenced by a pericardial friction rub. Note the parallel motion of epi- and pericardium (*arrows 2* and *3*) (*arrow 1*: endocardium of LVPW.)

patients with endocarditis [405] showed that vegetations could be visualized by ultrasound in 22 patients, or 34%. Unfortunately, echocardiographic detection of vegetation turned out to be a relatively late sign of disease, as 20 of the 22 patients either died or required cardiac operation, in contrast to those without echocardiographic evidence for vegetations. Hirschfeld and Schiller [156] showed that vegetations less than 5 mm in size could not always be detected ultrasonically.

The echocardiographic demonstration of bacterial vegetations in patients with endocarditis, initially reported in 1973, requires the presence of irregular, shaggy deposits, adherent to a valve leaflet, but not preventing its motion. Vegetations are thus more easily observed ultrasonically in diastole [79, 187, 224, 314, 405]. Calcification of vegetations, more than their size, seems to be important for their echocardiographic detection [32]. Aortic valve vegetations sometime generate abnormally dense echoes in the LVOT [52, 437] (see 9.3.4).

Fungal endocarditis presents in much the same way as bacterial endocarditis, with an even bulkier cluster of echoes filling the aortic root [122].

Unfortunately, in patients with MV prolapse, who are more liable to suffer from infectious endocarditis, echocardiography is not very helpful; indeed, thick, shaggy echoes confined to a MV leaflet may be observed in up to 40% of patients with the click-murmur syndrome [46]. At any rate, seemingly abnormal echoes attached to, or in the vicinity of a cardiac valve, are indicative of valvular vegetations only in a clinical setting of endocarditis.

Echocardiography may further help in detecting sequelae of the destructive process, such as: (1) flail aortic and MV leaflets (see 9.1.5); (2) acute aortic regurgitation, through the documentation of early MV closure [405]; and (3) a ruptured aortic valve leaflet. This is often a surgical or autopsy finding, but it is amenable to echocardiographic diagnosis, for in early to mid-diastole, a ruptured aortic valve leaflet may generate a band of fine high frequency echoes in the aortic root echogram, whereas during systole the aortic leaflet echo may consist of fine linear echoes [195, 435].

Real-time two-dimensional echocardiography, perhaps more than conventional echocardiography, may help in the diagnosis and clinical management of patients with vegetative endocarditis. Through its unique characteristics of providing spatial information concerning cardiac structures, dynamic two-dimensional echocardiography makes it possible to estimate the size of the lesion, to assess its morphology, and to document specific leaflet involvement [111]. Serially, this technique may guide the patient's management, by following destructive changes of a damaged valve [180].

Finally, dynamic cross sectional echocardiography has been shown to be useful in the differential diagnosis of aortic valve vegetations and flailing aortic valve leaflets [437], which are both complications of bacterial endocarditis, and are responsible for abnormal echo patterns in the LVOT.

9.7.3 Valvular Dysplasia

Occasionally a valve may become dysplastic as in myxomatous degeneration. This is well illustrated in Fig. 9.9, which is an echocardiogram obtained from a 6-year-old girl with Turner's syndrome and severe mitral regurgitation. Multiple abnormal echoes adherent to both leaflets, not impeding their motion, were generated by a degenerative, myxomatous MV.

9.8 Abnormal Echoes Related to Mitral Valve Leaflets

9.8.1 Supravalvar Mitral Ring

In this anomaly a fibrous shelf-like membrane or ring obstructs the inlet of the MV orifice [192].

Abnormal echoes, corresponding to the ring, are often found related to the MV leaflets, posterior to the AMVL [65, 192].

MV motion is rarely normal in these cases: either the valve is structurally altered or blood flow through it is impeded.

Cross sectional echocardiography may help to detect this anomaly (see Fig. 9.1).

9.8.2 Parachute Mitral Valve

In this anomaly MV leaflets cannot separate in diastole because of shortened tendineae chordae which insert into a single papillary muscle [45].

Parachute mitral valve is commonly associated with a supravalvar mitral ring: abnormal echoes in the vicinity of the mitral leaflets can be found in either lesion [192], and render their echocardiographic differentiation impossible.

Fig. 9.9. NA: MV echogram obtained from a 5-year-old girl with a Turner's syndrome. The MV was completely deformed by myxomatous degeneration, explaining the multiple, irregular echoes of and within both MV leaflets

As for cor triatriatum (see 9.1.1), an echocardiographic diagnosis of supravalvar mitral ring or parachute MV should be made with caution and only if there is clinical evidence of LV inflow obstruction.

9.9 Echoes of Artificial Cardiac Structures

Present surgical procedures to correct congenital or acquired heart lesions often make use of prostheses, including teflon or dacron patches and/or artificial valves. These prostheses can often be recognized ultrasonically.

9.9.1 Patches

Tetrad of Fallot

In most patients with tetrad of Fallot who are undergoing total repair, a patch is placed over the VSD and/or in the outflow region of the RV. On the echocardiogram this patch can be recognized as a relatively thin area of the septum. (see Fig. 9.10).

d-Transposition of the Great Arteries

Correction of this anomaly by a Mustard's operation is now a well-accepted procedure: the atrial septum is totally removed and a patch is placed within the atria

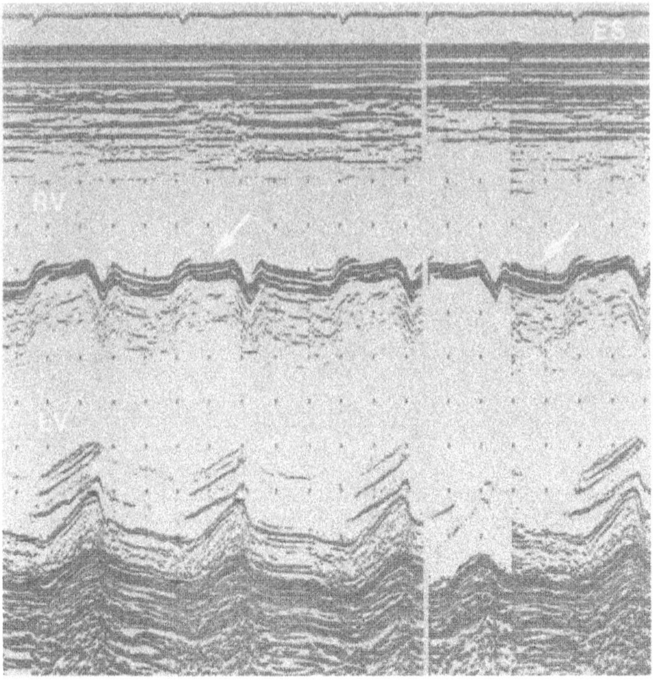

Fig. 9.10. ES: The *arrows* indicate the echoes of a ventricular septal patch inserted for correction of tetrad of Fallot in a 10-month-old baby

to connect both caval veins to the mitral orifice and to connect the pulmonary veins to the tricuspid orifice. Echoes of this patch are recognized behind the pulmonary artery as a thin, distinct line within the atrial cavity, dividing this cavity into an anterior systemic venous atrium and a posterior pulmonary venous chamber [17] (see Fig. 9.11). The motion pattern of this patch resembles the motion pattern of a stenotic MV [264]. In the presence of caval obstruction due to malposition or shrinkage of the baffle, Hunter et al. [163] found a significant difference in the echocardiographic appearance of the baffle, namely, limitation of baffle motion, thickening, and multiplicity of baffle echoes.

Correction of d-TGA using Senning's procedure, which is similar in concept and preceded Mustard's operation, results in similar echoes behind the pulmonary artery (see Fig. 9.12).

Common (Single) Ventricle

Complete surgical correction of common ventricle is possible in some cases through partitioning of the common ventricle. Seward et al. [348] echocardiographically examined eight patients in whom a dacron or teflon prosthetic septum had been inserted. This new septum gave dense echoes which moved anteriorly during systole and posteriorly during diastole.

AV Canal

Atrial septal prosthetic patches can be visualized with inferior-medial scanning of the transducer below the aortic root, in patients having undergone complete repair of AV canal defects [139].

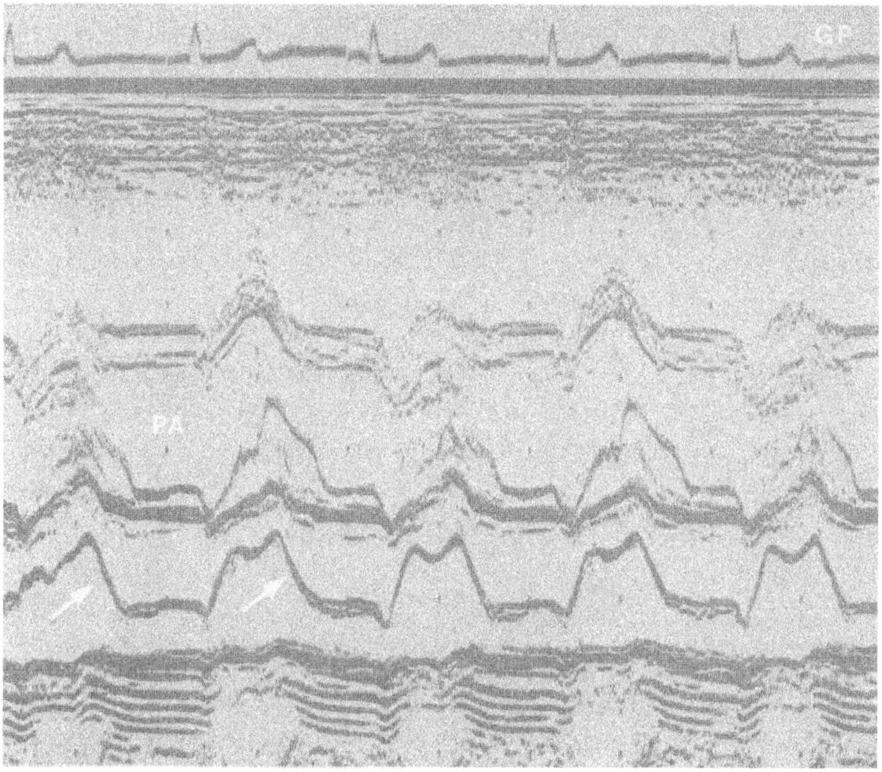

Fig. 9.11. GP: A Mustard's patch is clearly visible within the new atrial cavity (indicated by *arrows*), behind the PA, in this 5-year-old boy with surgically corrected d-TGA

9.9.2 Artificial Valves

To correct congenital or acquired valvular lesions, artificial valves may have to be inserted at any of the four locations. Most valves are constructed of plastic or metallic materials which produce extremely intense echoes and multiple reverberations of these echoes [289] (see Figs. 9.13 and 9.14). Figure 9.15 represents a porcine pulmonic valve mounted in a conduit which was inserted between the RV and the distal pulmonary arteries in a 18-month-old child with true persistent truncus arteriosus.

The potential of ultrasound in assessing prosthetic valve motion and function is now beginning to be appreciated. Information pertaining to aortic prostheses is limited; however, useful data has been obtained through echocardiographic examination of prostheses in the mitral position [314]. A baseline recording from each patient after surgery should be routine practice [290].

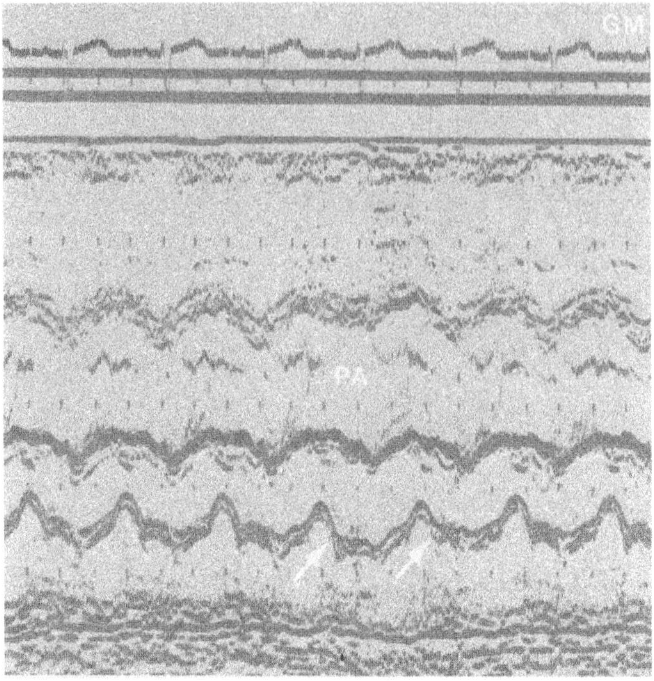

Fig. 9.12. GM: The new interatrial septum, indicated by *arrows* on the echo-trace, is clearly visible in this 6-month-old baby with d-TGA, surgically corrected with a Senning procedure

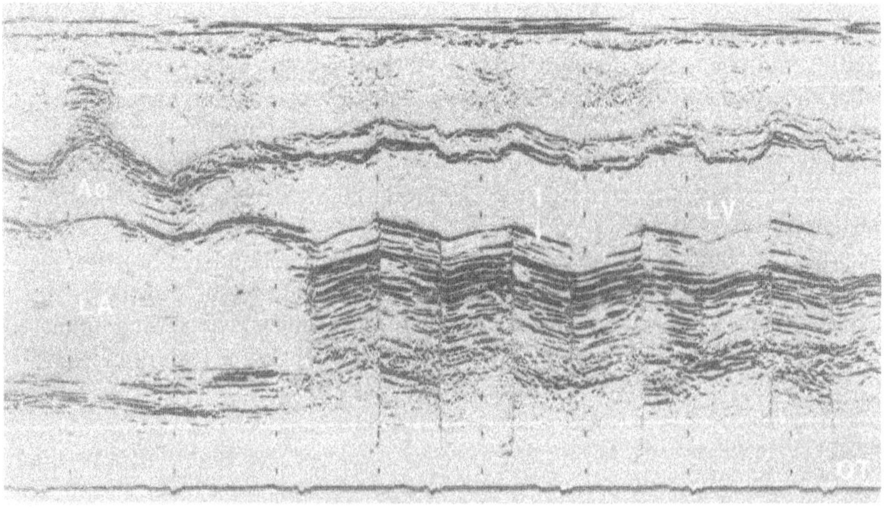

Fig. 9.13. QT: M-mode scan obtained from a 7-year-old boy with a Starr-Edwards MV prosthesis (*arrow 1*). Note the multiple echoes, mainly generated by the ball. The LA is still enlarged

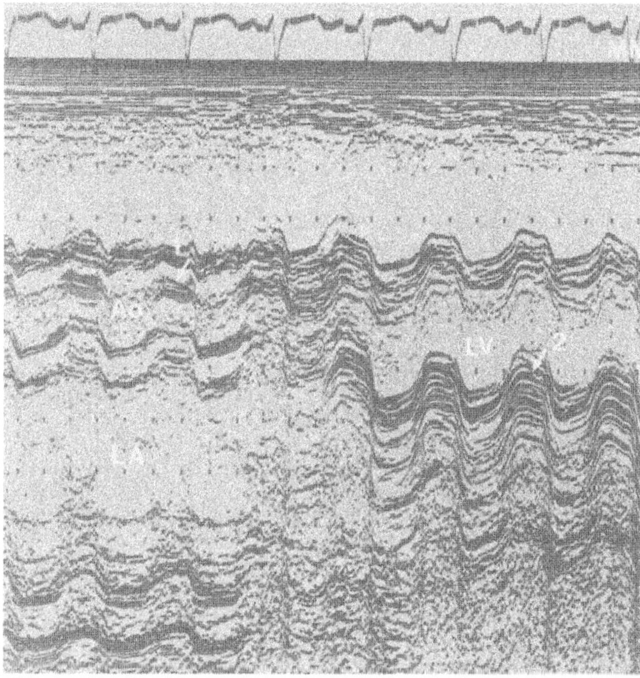

Fig. 9.14. MM: Recording of a Hancock valve prosthesis both in the aortic (*arrow 1*) and mitral (*arrow 2*) position. The valves were inserted 2 years earlier in this 10-year-old boy following valvular destruction due to acute rheumatic fever

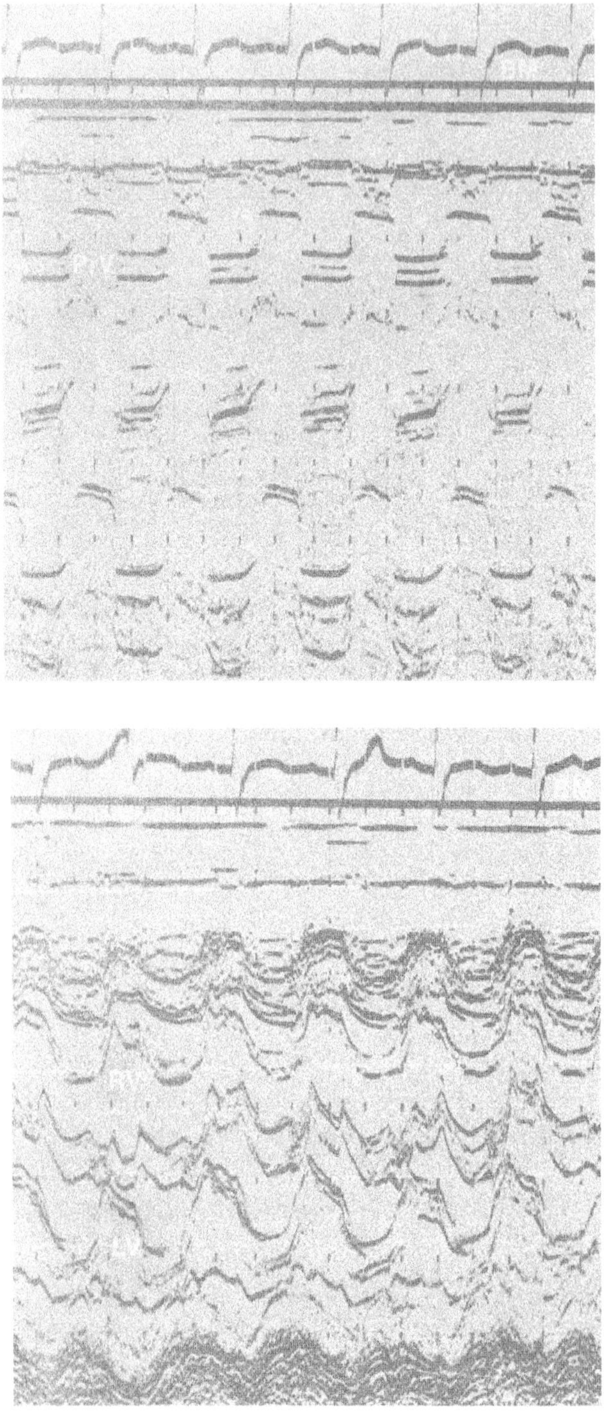

a

b

Fig. 9.15 a, b. BM: Echocardiogram obtained from a 2-year-old girl, 6 months following a Rastelli's operation for persistent truncus arteriosus. **a** Shows the external conduit with its valve; **b** Shows the two ventricles with their respective AV valves, completely separated by a reconstructed septum; note its abnormal motion (PrV: prosthetic valve)

Quantitative Anatomy

Abnormal Valve Motion

10 Abnormal Pulmonary Valve Motion

Index

Introduction

The pulmonary valve is the most difficult valve to study using ultrasound. Usually only the posterior cusp of the valve is recorded in M-mode echocardiography. Two-dimensional cardiac imaging is perhaps a more reliable method for the study of normal and abnormal pulmonary valves. Using the latter technique the entire valve can be visualized by performing a cross sectional scan through the long axis of the right ventricular outflow tract and the origin of the main pulmonary artery [426].

In this chapter, abnormal motion patterns of the pulmonary cusps, generally of the posterior cusp, as documented in M-mode recordings, will be discussed. More often than not it will become clear that an abnormal pulmonary valve echogram merely reflects an abnormal hemodynamic state: the valve itself is not necessarily diseased.

10.1 Increased a-Wave Depth

The PV normally opens at the onset of ventricular systole, when RV pressure exceeds pulmonary arterial pressure. However, the pulmonary valve may open whenever the force of RA contraction increases right ventricular end-diastolic pressure to a level equalling or exceeding simultaneous pulmonary arterial pressure [406]. This may be documented in normal people at very slow heart rates, during deep inspiration, and after premature ventricular contractions. An accentuation of this normal phenomenon – with an a-wave depth exceeding 7 mm – will be documented in the following entities.

10.1.1 Severe Valvular Pulmonic Stenosis (see Fig. 10.1)

The M-mode echocardiographic diagnosis of pulmonary stenosis is indirect and based essentially on the effects of abnormal presystolic ventricular pressure on PV motion [426]. This is reflected in an M-mode recording by a marked increase in the a-wave, or the posterior deflection of the posterior leaflet which normally occurs following atrial contraction. However, an abnormal value in a-wave depth, usually in excess of 7 mm, does not occur unless the systolic gradient across the valve is at least 50 mm Hg. Normal variations in a-wave depth resulting from respiration disappear.

RV hypertrophy, which sometimes leads to disproportionate septal thickening, further supports the diagnosis.

More reliably, an ultrasonic diagnosis of pulmonary valve stenosis can be made using cross sectional echocardiographic techniques [426] (see 10.9.1).

10.1.2 Uhl's Anomaly

The echocardiographic findings in Uhl's anomaly, or congenital hypoplasia of the right ventricular myocardium, include an increase of the depth of the a-wave.

Other features that have been reported at least once [104] are (1) delayed TV closure, 0.07 s after MV closure; (2) pansystolic prolapse of both AV valves; and (3) increased right ventricular dimensions.

10.1.3 Pulmonary Hypertension Complicated by Severe Right Ventricular Failure (see 10.5.2)

In the presence of severe pulmonary hypertension, an a-wave is usually not documented on the pulmonary valve echogram (see 10.6.1). However, when

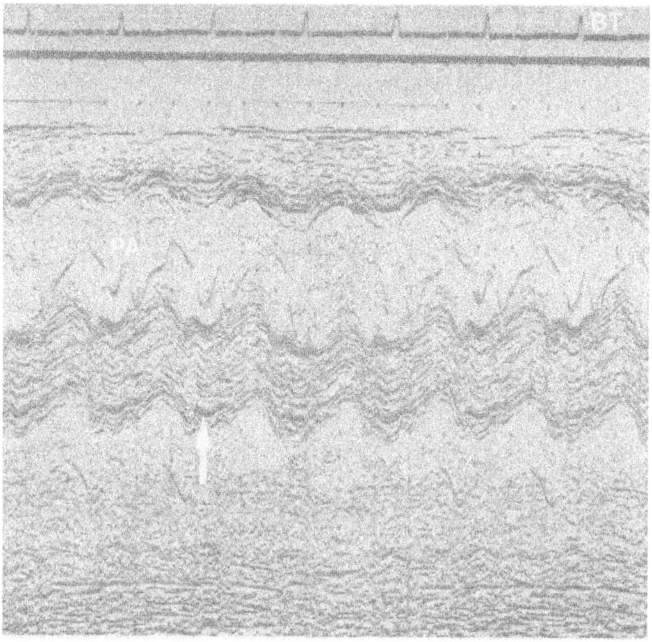

Fig. 10.1. BT: Echocardiogram obtained from a 22-year-old man with constrictive pericarditis. At operation the entire heart was covered with a fibrocalcific sheet, which also surrounded the base of the great arteries. Annular constriction of the PA was evident and probably accounts for the deep a waves of the PV echogram. The *arrow* points to the presence of dense tissues behind the PV

complicated by severe RV failure, pulmonary hypertension may be associated with increased a-wave depth [261] (see Fig. 10.2).

In all these conditions the pulmonary valve normally closes again after atrial contraction, to reopen fully with the onset of ventricular ejection.

10.2 Premature Pulmonary Valve Opening

Wann et al. [406] have shown that in the following unrelated conditions the pulmonary valve opened prematurely, so that it was already in a fully opened position at the onset of atrial systole. A rapid rise in initial RV diastolic pressure equalling or transiently exceeding pulmonary arterial diastolic pressure probably explains this phenomenon.

10.2.1 Sinus of Valsalva Rupture into the Right Atrium [420] (see also 9.5.3)

10.2.2 Constrictive Pericarditis [406] (see 21.2.5)

10.2.3 Loeffler's Endocarditis [142, 406]

10.2.4 Ebstein's Anomaly of the Tricuspid Valve (see 12.7.1)

10.2.5 Tricuspid Regurgitation (see 22.1.3)

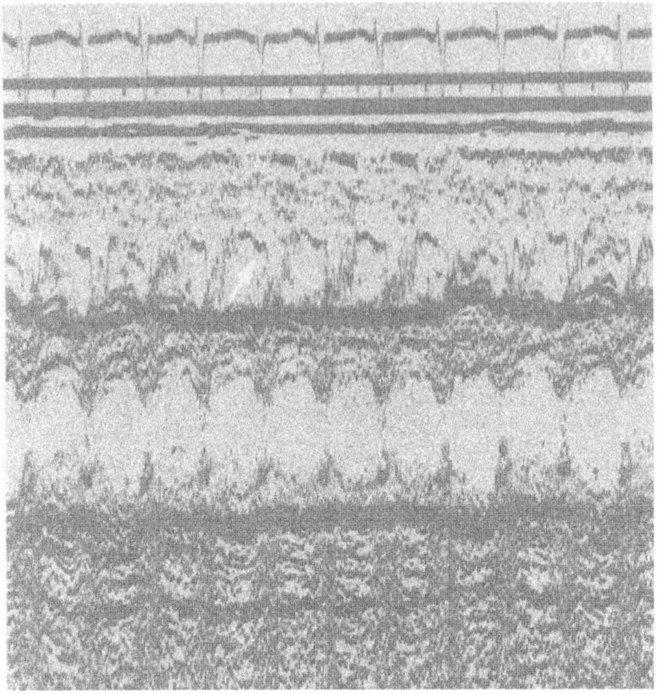

Fig. 10.2 DN: PV registration in a 2-year-old boy with PA hypertension and RV narrowing. A small a-wave is present (*arrow*). Note also the partial early closure followed by late reopening of the posterior semilunar valve with systolic fluttering

10.2.6 ASD with Pulmonary Regurgitation [406] (see 21.1.1)

In addition to the echocardiographic findings of ASD, diastolic fluttering of the ATVL or of the IVS may be documented.

10.3 Delayed Pulmonary Valve Opening

10.3.1 Pulmonary Hypertension (see 10.5.2)

In the presence of pulmonary hypertension, the RV must generate greater pressure before the pulmonary valve can open. This will have two consequences.
1) A delayed opening [196], resulting in an increased right ventricular pre-ejection period (RPEP) [261]. Mills et al. [244] showed that it is possible to infer pulmonary arterial end-diastolic pressure from the right ventricular isovolumic contraction time, or the interval from TV closure to pulmonary valve opening.
2) A greater than normal pulmonary valve opening velocity [418] (see 10.4.1).

10.4 Increased Pulmonary Valve Opening Velocity

10.4.1 Pulmonary Hypertension (see 10.5.2)

Normally, the opening velocity of the pulmonary valve does not exceed 300 mm/s. In patients with pulmonary hypertension, opening slopes of 350 mm/s or more are usually documented [261, 418] which is in keeping with a greater right ventricular dp/dt (time derivative of pressure during isovolumic ventricular contraction) [170].

10.5 Premature, Partial Pulmonary Valve Closure

10.5.1 Subpulmonic Obstruction in d-TGA (see 17.4.2)

Just as partial mid-systolic closure of the aortic valve is associated with subaortic stenosis, including IHSS, a similar closing movement of the pulmonary valve can be observed in patients with d-TGA and subpulmonic obstruction. This feature has been documented both before [265] and after Mustard's operation (see Fig. 10.3).

10.5.2 Pulmonary Hypertension (see Fig. 10.4).

Partial premature closure of the pulmonary valve in pulmonary hypertension was first described by Weyman et al. [418] and confirmed later by others [336].

This feature, though, is not pathognomonic; other ultrasonic features do exist, however and will help in the diagnosis: (1) decreased or flat pulmonary valve diastolic (E–F_0) slope (see 10.7.1); (2) absence of an a-wave (see 10.6.1); (3) delayed pulmonary valve opening (see 10.3.1); and (4) greater than normal pulmonary valve opening velocity (see 10.4.1).

In addition, secondary features are often well documented, such as:

1) Increased anterior wall and septal thickness (RVH),
2) Increased pulmonary root diameter,

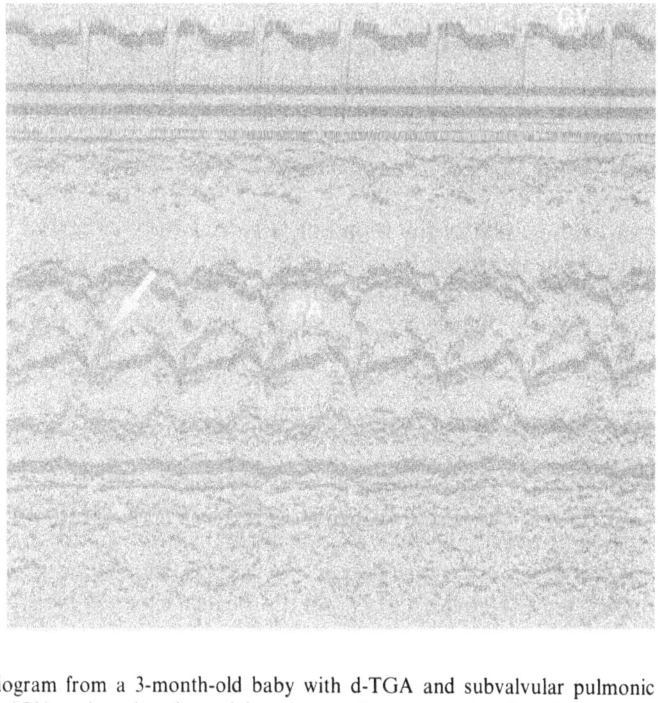

Fig. 10.3. GV: Echocardiogram from a 3-month-old baby with d-TGA and subvalvular pulmonic stenosis. Note the abnormal PV motion: there is partial premature closure (*arrow*) and marked systolic fluttering

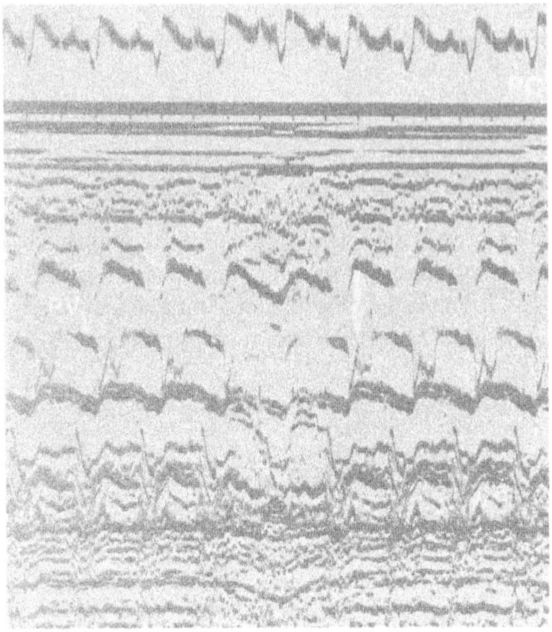

Fig. 10.4. PC: Partial mid-systolic closure of the PV (*arrow*) is documented in this recording obtained from an infant with pulmonary hypertension and total anomalous pulmonary venous return

3) Decreased mitral valve E–F_0 slope with normal motion of the PMVL (see 13.5.3),
4) Prolapse of the MV leaflets in patients with essential pulmonary hypertension (see 13.11.1),
5) Increased RPEP/RVET ratio (see 23.1.1)
6) Prolongation of isovolumic contraction time (ICT) with reduction in ejection time, resulting in an unchanged total electromechanical systole or QP_2 [71].

10.5.3 Pericardial Effusion (see 8.1.1)

Midsystolic notching of the pulmonary valve can be observed in the presence of pericardial effusion [266]. In this context, the abnormal motion pattern does not represent valvular dysfunction, but is usually a result of the exaggerated total motion of the heart. This abnormal motion pattern will disappear with the effusion.

10.6 Absence of an a-Wave

10.6.1 Pulmonary Hypertension (see 10.5.2) (see Fig. 10.4)

As discussed above, right atrial systole normally produces observable end-diastolic motion of the pulmonary valve (a-wave), because of reduced diastolic pressures on the right side of the heart [417]. To the contrary, when valve cusps are tense, as occurs in pulmonary hypertension, deflection due to atrial systole will be minimal or absent, depending on the degree of pulmonary hypertension [261, 418]. However, in evaluating pulmonary valve motion, the effect of respiration must be recognized: the a-wave may disappear entirely in normal subjects during expiration [418].

Generally, though, with a mean pulmonary arterial pressure of over 40 mm Hg [261], or a pulmonary pressure at end-diastole of at least 25 mm Hg [196], total absence of cusp motion following atrial systole is expected.

10.6.2 Severe Infundibular Pulmonary Stenosis (see also 10.8.1)

Absence of an a-wave has also been described in patients with severe infundibular pulmonary stenosis [419], a condition in which pulmonary arterial pressure is obviously very low. This apparent paradoxical finding has been explained by Weyman et al. [419] as follows: the severe obstruction below the valve prevents the relatively small pressure change caused by atrial contraction from reaching the valve with enough force to produce movements of the leaflets. Marked chaotic fluttering of the valve leaflets is then often present.

10.7 Flat Diastolic (E–F_0) Slope

10.7.1 Pulmonary Hypertension (see Fig. 10.4 and Sect. 10.5.2)

Normally, the pulmonary valve diastolic or E–F_0 slope is about 40 mm/s, although it may range as low as 6 mm/s or be virtually flat [418]. Variations in this measurement may also be due to transducer angulation [431]. A flat diastolic slope, as often described in pulmonary hypertension, is thus a poor echocardiographic criterion.

10.8 Fluttering of the Pulmonary Valve Leaflets

Although valvular fluttering is not specific and may be found in normal children, its presence on a pulmonary valve echogram has been thought to be of diagnostic interest in the following conditions.

10.8.1 Infundibular Pulmonic Stenosis (see also 10.6.2)

Weyman et al. [419] made an interesting observation regarding the duration of valvular flutter in obstructive right- and left-sided lesions: in left-sided lesions, such as in subvalvular membranous aortic stenosis [73], valvular vibration is limited to the period of systolic ejection and terminates with valve closure. In right-sided obstruction, as in infundibular pulmonic stenosis, the fluttering appears to extend well beyond the expected end of ventricular ejection, suggesting some diastolic flow in this condition.

10.8.2 Subpulmonic VSD

Glasser et al. [116] reported fluttering of the pulmonary valve in three patients with subpulmonic VSD. A turbulent stream of blood striking the pulmonary valve was thought to be the underlying mechanism.

10.8.3 Pulmonary Hypertension (see 10.5.2)

See Figs. 10.2 and 10.4 for illustrative echocardiograms.

10.8.4 Subpulmonic Obstruction in d-TGA (see 17.4.2)

Aziz et al. [18], echocardiographically assessing the LVOT in patients with d-TGA, observed a high frequency flutter of the pulmonary valve leaflets in the presence of fixed subpulmonic obstruction, whereas low, coarse flutter, along with premature closure, was noted with dynamic obstruction (see Fig. 10.3).

10.9 Systolic Inward Curvature of Pulmonary Valve Leaflets

10.9.1 Valvular Pulmonary Stenosis (see 10.1.1)

Weyman et al. [426] examined 22 patients with pulmonary stenosis by means of a mechanical sector scanner and made the following observations. (1) during systole, pulmonary valve leaflets are not parallel to the margins of the pulmonary artery as in normals, but curve inwards toward the midportion of the pulmonary artery; (2) the distal tips of the leaflets remain close together, whereas the more proximal parts of the valve leaflets make a wide arc ("doming"); and (3) in some patients, the valve is fully opened or domed after atrial systole.

11 Abnormal Aortic Valve Motion

Index

Introduction

In a normal heart, the aorta (Ao) represents a stable intracardiac landmark, halfway between the right ventricular outflow tract anteriorly and the left atrium posteriorly.

With proper transducer orientation, the aortic root containing the aortic cusps may be identified on echocardiographic examination.

The aortic root, at valve level, is visualized as two dense parallel echoes separated by an echo-free space whose width varies with age [431] (see Appendix). Within this space, two of the three leaflets of the aortic valve (AoV) may usually be recorded. As the opening and closing movements of the AoV are usually abrupt, the cusps show a box-like configuration during systole. Both the left ventricular pre-ejection period (LPEP) and ejection time (LVET) can thus be determined accurately from the echocardiogram and a concomitant ECG (see Fig. 11.1). The study of these intervals has many applications (see Chaps. 23 and 24).

In this chapter, abnormal patterns of AoV echograms will be reviewed, as these patterns may give valuable anatomical and functional information.

11.1 Premature Aortic Valve Opening

Usually the AoV opens at an average of 112 ms after the onset of electrical depolarization. Onset of opening almost coincident with the R-wave of the ECG, or premature AoV opening, may occur in rheumatic aortic regurgitation and annulo-aortic ectasia [16].

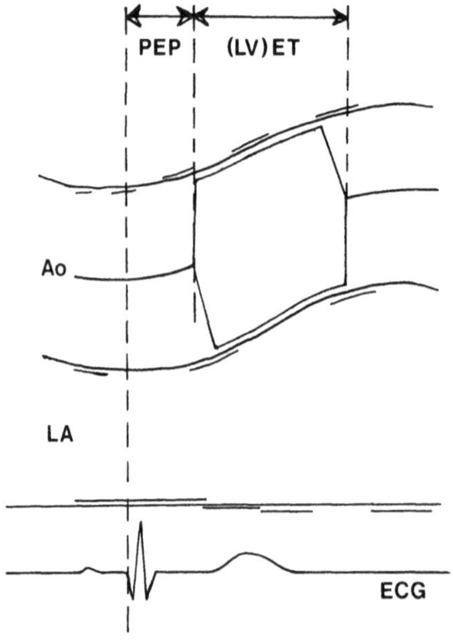

Fig. 11.1. PEP and VET (LVET) as measured from the echocardiogram and a concomitant electrocardiogram

11.1.1 Aortic Regurgitation (see 11.8.2)

Mid-diastolic opening of the AoV may be one of the echocardiographic features of aortic regurgitation [410].

11.1.2 Annulo-Aortic Ectasia

This anomaly, which consists of a dilatation of the annulus of the aortic valve and of a fusiform aneurysm of the ascending aorta up to the origin of the innominate artery, has distinct echocardiographic features [16]: (1) premature AoV opening; (2) dilatation of the aortic root; (3) abrupt premature partial closure of the AoV; and (4) abnormal backward systolic motion of the posterior wall of the aorta.

11.2 Partial Systolic Preclosure of the Aortic Valve

Early or mid-systolic partial closure of the AoV, which reflects the way blood is expelled from the left ventricle, is a well-described echocardiographic feature in subvalvar aortic stenosis (11.2.1 to 11.2.3).

However, more and more anomalies are now being recognized in which this ultrasonic feature is occasionally documented (11.2.4 to 11.2.11).

There are three types of systolic preclosure [151]: (1) an early systolic rapid closing movement; (2) an abrupt mid-systolic closing movement; and (3) a gradual systolic cusp prolapse.

The first two patterns are more specific for subvalvar aortic stenosis, whereas the last pattern is more often described in other anomalies.

11.2.1 Membranous Subvalvar Aortic Stenosis (or Discrete Subvalvar Aortic Stenosis)

As discussed in 9.3.1, it is perhaps possible to recognize the subvalvar membrane as a thin echo in the LVOT [188, 194, 293]. Nevertheless, if a membrane is suspected, more definite echocardiographic features of subaortic obstruction should be documented (see Fig. 11.2):

1) An early systolic partial closure of the AoV leaflets, a typical finding for subvalvar aortic stenosis, including IHSS [73, 431],
2) A diffusely narrowed LVOT [293],
3) A concentric hypertrophy of the left ventricle,
4) Coarse systolic fluttering of the leaflets in a semiclosed position during the latter part of systole,
5) High frequency fluttering of the MV leaflets in cases of associated aortic valve regurgitation,
6) Sometimes, abnormalities of left vertricular function [245] such as (a) SAM and delayed opening of the MV; (b) disproportionate septal thickening; (c) prolonged left ventricular filling period; and (d) asynchronous onset of contraction similar to that occurring in hypertrophic cardiomyopathies.

Cross sectional echocardiography, through its ability to improve visualization of the LVOT, makes it possible to differentiate between a subvalvular membrane and a more extensive area of subvalvular narrowing [424].

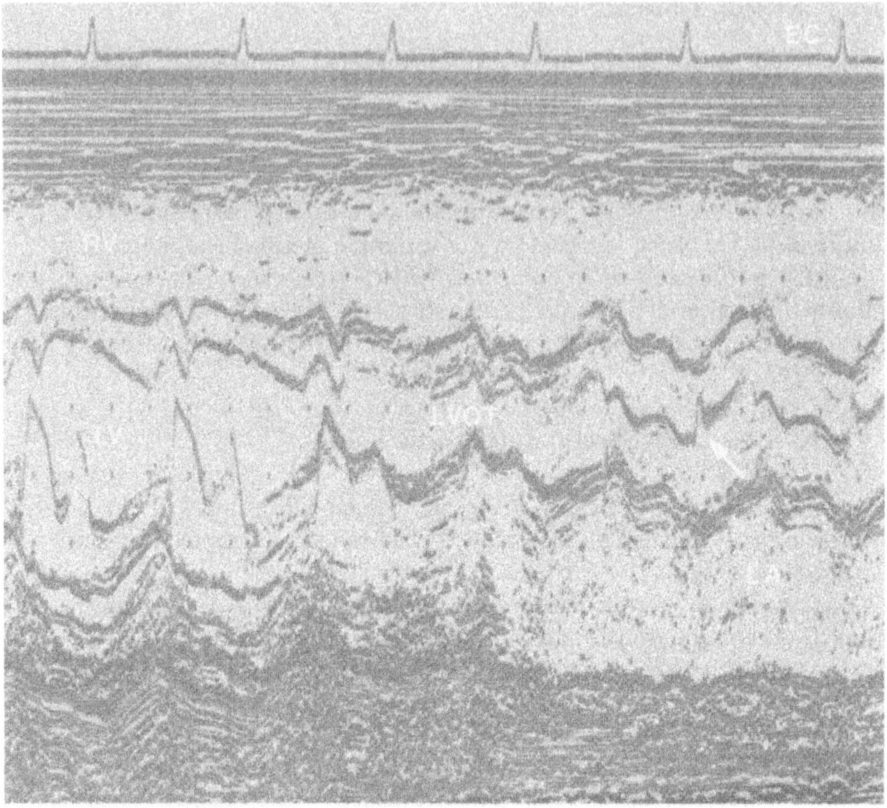

Fig. 11.2. EC: Echocardiogram obtained from a child with subvalvular aortic stenosis due to a subvalvular membrane. Note the premature systolic closure of the AoV (*arrow*) with abnormal fluttering of the leaflet during the remainder of systole. The LVOT is narrowed

In some patients, discrete subvalvular aortic stenosis may merge with more diffuse types of muscular left ventricular obstruction, including IHSS. As with IHSS, an echocardiographic examination should be made routine in relatives of patients with a subvalvular diaphragm; indeed, up to 13% of immediate family members may have left ventricular obstructive lesions [172 b].

11.2.2 Idiopathic Hypertrophic Subaortic Stenosis (IHSS)

An abrupt premature closing movement in systole is usually documented; often, this is followed by renewed opening of the valve during the later phases of ejection. Coarse fluttering of the leaflets may also occur (see also 20.1.1).

Note: The time of occurrence of early systolic closure allows the differentiation of patients with IHSS from patients with discrete subvalvular aortic stenosis [186]. A time interval can be measured from the opening point of the AoV to the point of early systolic closure (the O-ESC interval). In IHSS, this interval measures 0.14 ± 0.04 ms, whereas in discrete subvalvular aortic stenosis the O-ESC interval is shorter: 0.05 ± 0.01 ms [186].

11.2.3 LVOT Obstruction of Other Etiologies

Early systolic closure of at least one cusp, usually the noncoronary cusp, has also been described in other forms of LVOT obstruction, such as when the obstruction is caused by an accessory AMVL [65].

In the absence of subvalvar aortic stenosis, systolic preclosure of the aortic valve has been documented in several unrelated conditions.

11.2.4 Ruptured [408] and Unruptured [168] Coronary Sinus of Valsalva Aneurysm into the Right Heart (see 9.3.5)

11.2.5 "Floppy" or Redundant Aortic Valve Leaflets [51]

11.2.6 Annulo-Aortic Ectasia [16] (see 11.1.2)

11.2.7 Left Ventricular Leaks

In some cases of mitral regurgitation with reduced cardiac output, or VSD with a left-to-right shunt, AoV cusps may gradually drift toward closure and flutter during the remainder of systole [150].

11.2.8 Congestive Cardiomyopathies [151] (see 13.2.3)

11.2.9 Tetrad of Fallot [151] (see 4.1.2, Fig. 11.3)

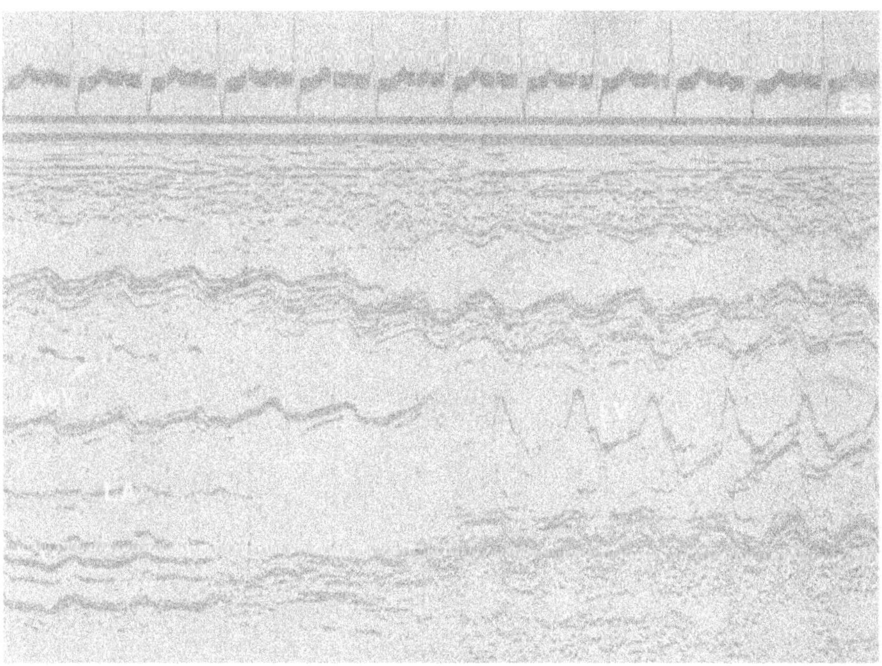

Fig. 11.3. ES: M-mode scan obtained from a 10-month-old baby with surgically corrected tetrad of Fallot. Note the premature partial systolic closure of the AoV (*arrow*), a rather uncommon finding in such patients

11.2.10 Tricuspid Atresia [151] (see 7.1.3)

11.2.11 Pericardial Effusion (see 8.1.1)

Early systolic movement toward closure of the AoV can be observed in the presence of pericardial effusion [266]. Thus this pattern does not represent, then, valvular dysfunction and will disappear with the effusion.

11.3 Eccentricity of the Aortic Cusps

11.3.1 Bicuspid Aortic Valve

Eccentricity of the diastolic line of the aortic cusps may point to bicuspid aortic valves with one small and one large cusp [260] (see Fig. 11.4).

Radford et al. [299] demonstrated that an eccentricity index (EI) of 1.3 or more, in the absence of an associated VSD, was diagnostic of bicuspid aortic valves, and could be found in approximately 75% of the patients with this abnormality. The EI is calculated as one-half the width of the aortic lumen divided by the distance of one cusp to the nearest aortic margin, as measured at the onset of diastole. Scovil et al. [342] confirmed the reliability of the EI in the diagnosis of bicuspid aortic valves, even with lesions distorting the valve, such as vegetations, myxomatous degeneration, etc.

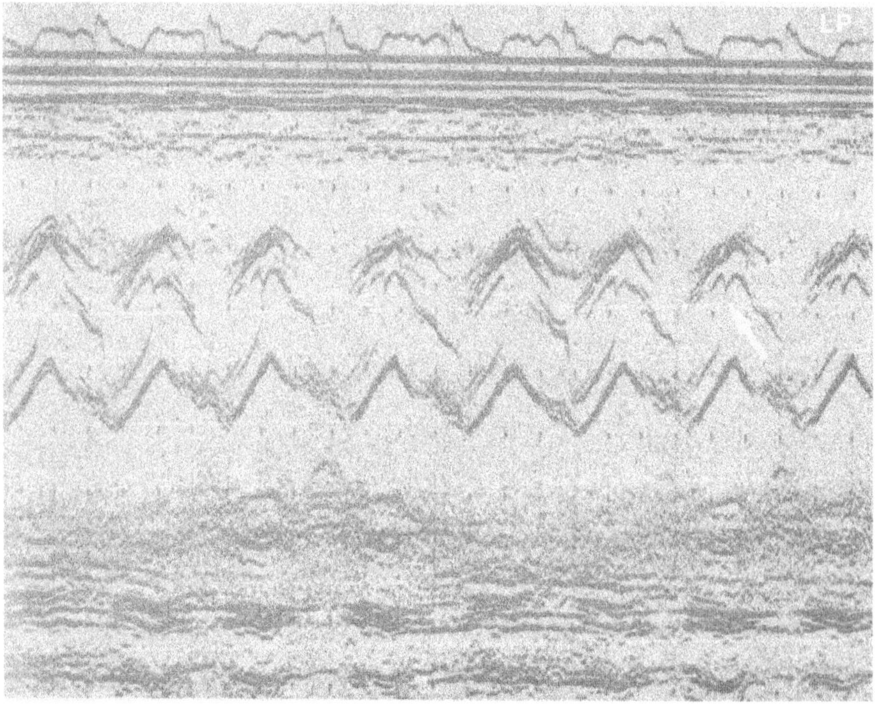

Fig. 11.4. LP: Echocardiogram obtained from a 6-year-old child with mitral stenosis and bicuspid aortic valves. Note the eccentricity of the aortic diastolic echoes (*arrow*)

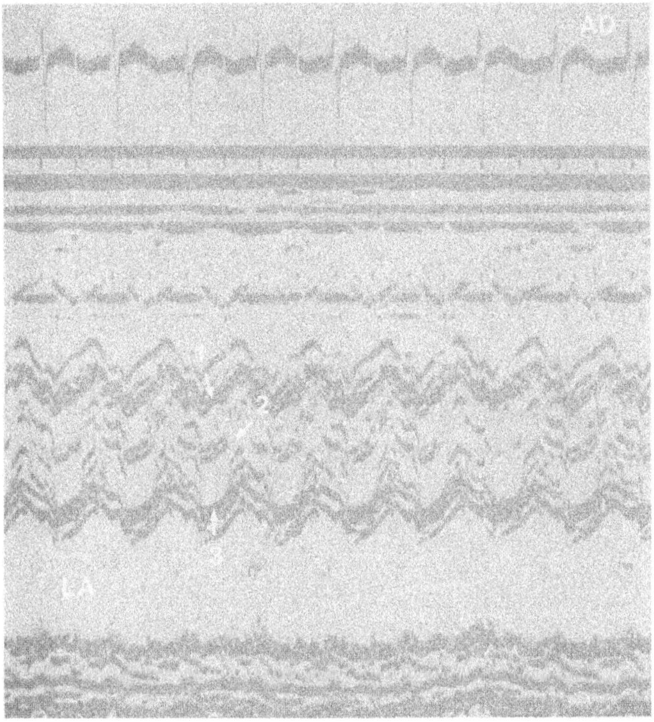

Fig. 11.5. AD: Echocardiogram from a 3-week-old infant with a severely stenotic bicuspid AoV. Although multiple eccentric diastolic echoes were suggestive of a bicuspid aortic valve, a three-cusp valve was diagnosed preoperatively because of the apparent presence of three-cusp echoes (*arrows 1, 2, 3*), during systole

However, this echocardiographic pattern lacks specificity, as it can be observed with a diseased tricuspid AoV, or even sometimes with entirely normal valves, depending on the orientation of the ultrasonic beam [83].

In addition to eccentricity, a bicuspid AoV is suggested if multiple diastolic echoes are documented within the aortic root [83, 184, 342]. These diastolic echoes may vary from beat to beat depending on the position of the transducer.

The apparent echo representation of a three-cusp valve does not exclude a bicuspid valve (see Fig. 11.5).

Patients with coarctation of the aorta often have bicuspid aortic valves. In a recent echocardiographic survey, bicuspid aortic valves, as documented by a diastolic EI over 1.5, were documented in 53% of the patients [343].

11.3.2 Cusp Dominance (?) in Anomalous Origin of the Left Coronary Artery

The ultrasonic pattern of eccentricity has been attributed by some to cusp dominance: in an echocardiographic study of four patients with anomalous origin of the left coronary artery, Glaser et al. [115] found the right coronary cusp to be dominant as if it was occupying a larger space within the aortic lumen, "pushing" the other cusps in a posterior direction. However, this finding awaits confirmation.

11.4 Shaggy or Chaotic Echoes

11.4.1 Vegetative Aortic Endocarditis (see 9.7.2)

In the clinical setting of endocarditis, unusual, shaggy, or chaotic echoes adherent to an aortic cusp either in systole or diastole, should suggest aortic endocarditis (see Fig. 11.6).

11.5 Thick Aortic Cusps Echoes

11.5.1 Severe Valvular Aortic Stenosis (see 24.3.3)

Thick, multilayered echoes within the aortic root, during systole or diastole, are suggestive of excessive calcification or fibrosis of the aortic valves [3] (see Fig. 11.7). These echoes do not necessarily imply critical stenosis [184], unless reduced systolic separation of the aortic cusps dependent on the state of the aortic commissures, is also documented.

Fig. 11.6. JB: Echocardiogram obtained from a 50-year-old man with vegetative endocarditis involving both the AoV and MV (same patient as in Fig. 9.4). Multiple, irregular fuzzy echoes, closely related to the AoV, are quite apparent during diastole

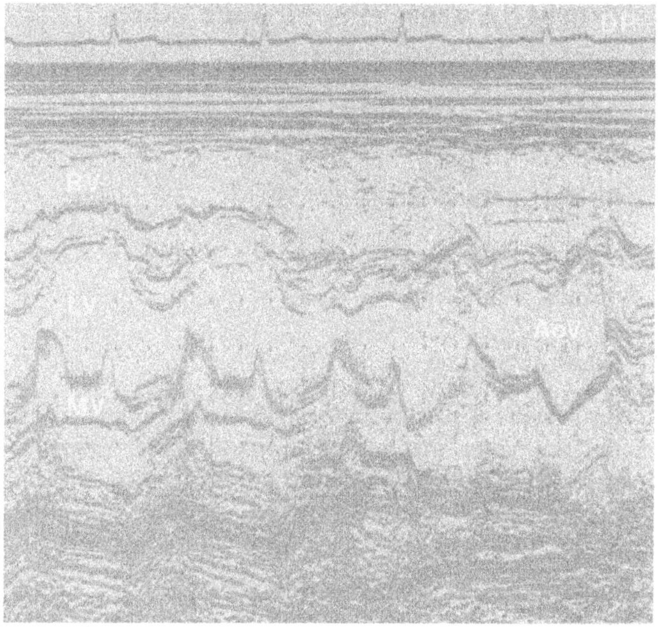

Fig. 11.7. DP: M-mode scan from an adolescent with severe valvular aortic stenosis. Multiple diastolic echoes of the AoV are present, as well as diastolic fluttering of the MV indicative of aortic regurgitation. The patient was found to have a thick, fibrotic bicuspid valve

In congenital aortic stenosis, however, thick AoV echoes are usually not encountered, as the aortic leaflets remain supple. For this reason, the AoV orifice does not correlate well with the severity of the obstruction.

11.6 Reduced Systolic Aortic Cusp Separation

The documentation of reduced aortic cusp separation should bring to mind essentially two conditions, namely, low output cardiac states and aortic stenosis.

11.6.1 Low Cardiac Output States

Reduced systolic separation of the aortic cusps, in the absence of clinical and/or echocardiographic signs of AoV disease, may be indicative of low cardiac output, for instance, secondary to impaired left ventricular function.

11.6.2 Aortic Stenosis (see 11.5.1)

The observation of reduced systolic aortic cusp separation, in addition to multiple echoes at the level of the AoV, is highly suggestive of valvular aortic stenosis.

However, in M-mode echocardiography, this reduced systolic cusp separation can be missed if there is doming of a congenitally narrowed aortic valve, as the sound beam may be directed through freely-moving parts of the AoV leaflets.

11.7 Diastolic Separation of Aortic Valve Echoes

This nonspecific echocardiographic feature may be documented in:

11.7.1 Aortic Regurgitation (see 11.8.2)

11.7.2 Bicuspid Aortic Valve (see 11.3.1)

11.8 Valvular Fluttering

11.8.1 Subaortic Stenosis (see 11.2.1)

In subaortic stenosis it is not uncommon to document a coarse type of systolic leaflet fluttering; sometimes only one cusp will vibrate depending on the direction of the eccentric jet of blood striking the aortic valve (see Fig. 11.8).

11.8.2 Aortic Regurgitation

Severe aortic regurgitation can be diagnosed echocardiographically: detection is based on the presence of definite, highly suggestive, and supportive features.

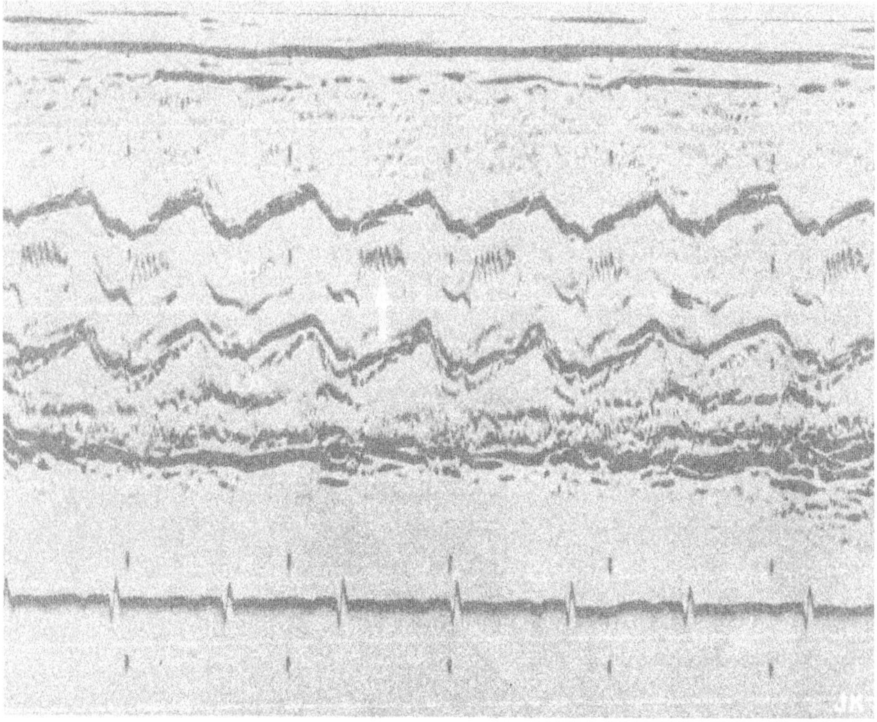

Fig. 11.8. JK: Coarse systolic fluttering of the AoV (*arrow*) is documented in this 4-month-old baby with severe subvalvular aortic stenosis

Definite Features

High frequency *diastolic* vibration of the aortic cusps is generally abnormal and considered to be the only reliable echocardiographic sign of aortic regurgitation when recording the AoV [289].

Suggestive Features

1) Suggestive features include the following:
A high frequency diastolic vibration of the AMVL [289, 315] and/or of the IVS [67], a feature which seems to be more related to the direction than to the importance of the regurgitant jet (see Fig. 11.9),
2) Premature mitral valve closure [29, 289], secondary to high diastolic left ventricular pressure,
3) Delayed MV opening (see 13.8.3),
4) Premature AoV opening (see 11.1.1),
5) Premature closure of the AoV (Premature opening and closure of aortic valve leaflets is probably related to sudden volume and pressure overload of the left ventricle) [376, 410],
6) Separate echo trace of the AoV during diastole (see Fig. 11.10).

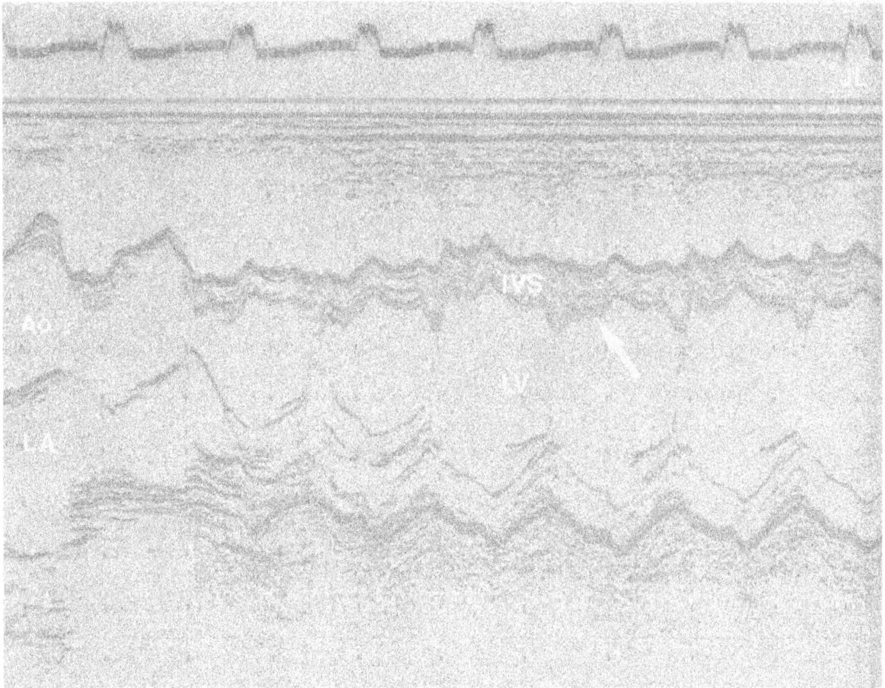

Fig. 11.9. JL: Echocardiogram obtained from a 5-year-old boy, 2 years after surgical closure of a VSD and pulmonary valvulotomy. Fluttering of the left side of the IVS is quite apparent (*arrow*) and resulted from aortic regurgitation secondary to AoV destruction following endocarditis. An AoV prosthesis was inserted

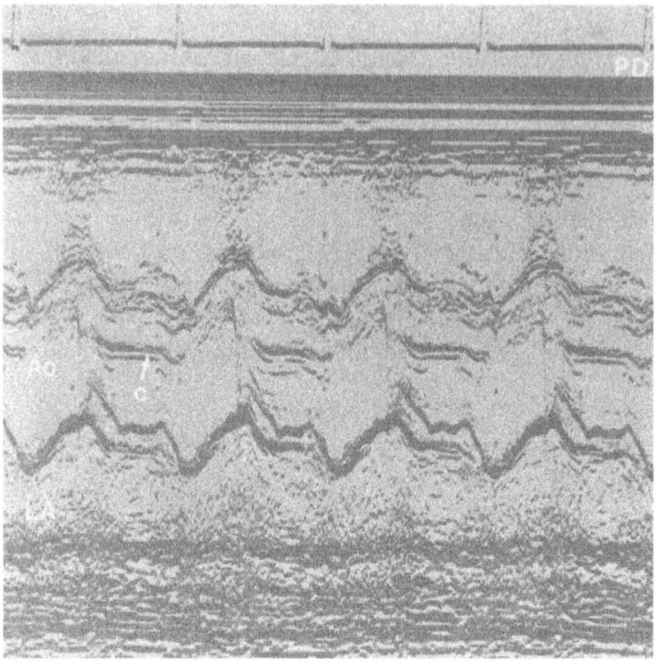

Fig. 11.10. PD: Double diastolic AoV echoes (labeled c) in aortic regurgitation

Supportive Features

Supportive features include (1) aortic root dilatation; (2) left ventricular dilatation; and (3) large amplitude of left ventricular wall motion.

12 Abnormal Tricuspid Valve Motion

Index

Introduction

Although the tricuspid valve can be identified in almost all patients, it is in general difficult to obtain a complete registration of the TV leaflets. Most often, only the anterior tricuspid valve leaflet (ATVL) is seen in systole and early diastole.

In patients with marked dilatation of the RV, the ATVL can often be followed throughout the cardiac cycle and parts of the septal leaflet may become visible as it opens toward the IVS (see Fig. 12.1).

In newborns, the TV is more readily accessible to ultrasound; at least some parts of the valve should be visualized in any distressed infant in order to rule out tricuspid atresia.

Since the ATVL is crossed somewhat tangentially by the ultrasound beam [431], its opening amplitude, in early diastole, will vary with the direction of the sound beam. In practice, the largest recorded excursion is used for diagnostic purposes. In several disease states this amplitude deviates from normal; TV motion may also be altered in other ways.

In this chapter, abnormalities in TV motion patterns will be reviewed and their diagnostic implications presented.

12.1 Increased Amplitude of the ATVL

12.1.1 Ebstein's Anomaly (see 12.7.1)

12.1.2 Atrial Septal Defect (see 21.1.1)

Right ventricular dilatation and increased flow through the tricuspid valve probably contribute, in this anomaly, to the increased excursion of the ATVL.

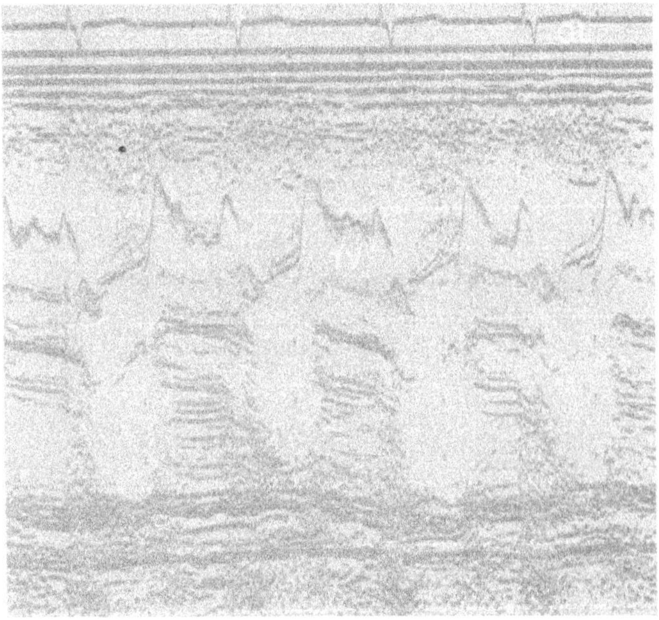

Fig. 12.1. GL: Both the anterior and septal TV leaflets are well registered in this patient, operated upon for tetrad of Fallot. RV dilatation persisted

12.1.3 d-Transposition of the Great Arteries (see 3.1.1)

Increased amplitude of motion of the ATVL may be observed in patients with d-TGA, even after a Mustard's operation and normalization of flow through the TV. This is probably related to RV dilatation and a better accessibility of the TV to ultrasound in d-TGA.

12.2 Decreased Amplitude of the ATVL

12.2.1 Tricuspid Valve Stenosis

12.2.2 Hypoplastic Tricuspid Valve

Both of these entities are associated with decreased ATVL excursion, and reduced $E-F_0$ slope (see 12.4.1). A hypoplastic TV usually accompanies pulmonary atresia with intact IVS.

12.3 Increased $E-F_0$ Slope of the ATVL

12.3.1 Atrial Septal Defect (ASD) (see 21.1.1)

The tricuspid valve $E-F_0$ slope is usually increased in ASD or in any condition characterized by diastolic volume overloading of the RV.

12.4 Reduced $E-F_0$ Slope of the ATVL

12.4.1 Tricuspid Valve Stenosis

Tricuspid stenosis is a rare congenital anomaly. As in mitral stenosis, the echocardiographic pattern consists in a marked reduction of the $E-F_0$ slope, which does not exceed 30 mm/s [171].

If tricuspid stenosis is suspected, a complete echocardiographic examination should be performed, as congenital tricuspid stenosis rarely exists as a single lesion.

Other ultrasonic features of tricuspid stenosis should be looked for, i.e., reduced opening amplitude (see 12.2); thick, dense echoes of the ATVL; or an unrecordable septal leaflet.

12.4.2 Ebstein's Anomaly [431] (see 12.7.1)

12.4.3 Right Ventricular Dysfunction [431] (see 12.7.2)

12.5 Delayed Tricuspid Valve Opening

12.5.1 Ebstein's Anomaly (see 12.7.1)

Normally, TV opening occurs slightly before or sometimes soon after MV opening [306]. In most patients with an Ebstein's anomaly, the TV usually opens after the MV [94, 211].

This feature, however, is not reliable diagnostically because of great individual differences between patients with this anomaly.

12.5.2 d-Transposition of the Great Arteries (see 3.1.1)

Delayed opening of the TV, occurring after MV opening, can be documented in patients with d-TGA.

12.6 Premature Closure of the Tricuspid Valve

12.6.1 Truncus Arteriosus with Valvular Regurgitation (see 4.1.3)

In this situation, premature closure of the TV can be documented when the regurgitant flow of blood is directed predominantly into the right ventricular chamber [14].

12.6.2 d-Transposition of the Great Arteries (see 3.1.1)

Generally, the TV closes after the MV with an average delay of 20 ms. Patients with d-TGA show a striking difference from normals in that the TV closes earlier, before the MV, irrespective of age or associated lesions [247].

12.7 Delayed Closure of the Tricuspid Valve

12.7.1 Ebstein's Anomaly

Ebstein's anomaly presents several different pathological presentations. Three of these features are relatively constant [83, 94], e.g., (1) redundancy of valvular tissue; (2) adherence of varying portions of the grossly abnormal septal and posterior cusps of the TV to the RV wall, resulting in "atrialization" of a portion of the RV; and (3) a normally attached, large anterior TV leaflet.

Although Ebstein's anomaly is often suspected clinically, radiologically, and electrocardiographically, a definite diagnosis of this malformation must be based upon invasive investigations such as cardiac catheterization and angiocardiography. These procedures are at best hazardous in patients with Ebstein's anomaly, because of the frequent occurrence of rhythm disturbances.

The introduction of echocardiography as a noninvasive diagnostic tool has proved invaluable in confirming diagnoses of Ebstein's disease, thanks to a specific finding: delayed closure of the TV (see Fig. 12.2). Normally, TV closure follows MV closure by an interval not exceeding 0.03 s [94]. Late closure of the tricuspid valve, over 0.065 s after MV closure, has been considered to be a specific finding of Ebstein's disease [94, 247, 382]; in fact, out of 19 suggested parameters, it has been found to be the only specific feature of the disease [94].

Echocardiography by revealing delayed TV closure, allows rapid dismissal of clinical entities resembling Ebstein's anomaly, such as: pericardial effusion, endomyocardial fibrosis, or anomalous muscle bundles within the right ventricle [209].

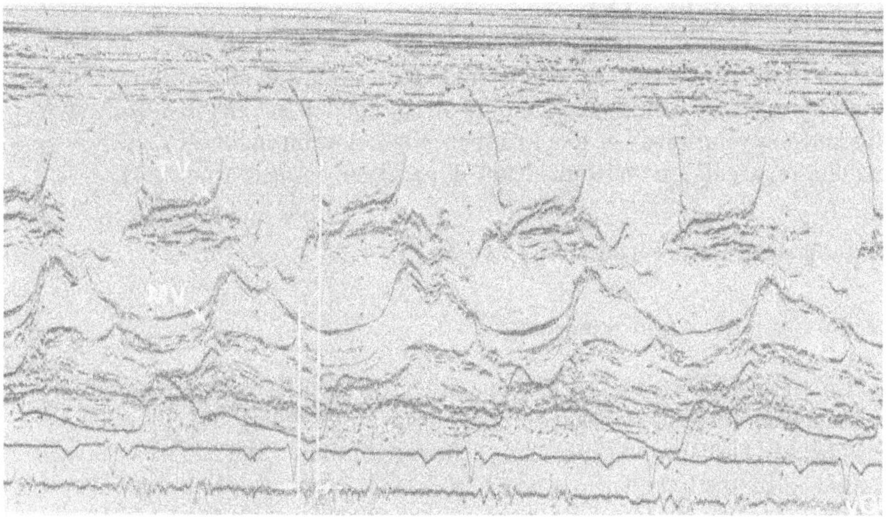

Fig. 12.2. vG: Echocardiogram with simultaneous phonocardiogram obtained from a 14-year-old boy with an Ebstein's anomaly of the TV. The large excursion of the ATVL can be well appreciated. Quite specific for the anomaly is the delayed closure of the TV (*vertical lines*)

Other, though less specific echocardiographic features may suggest a diagnosis of Ebstein's disease [94, 211, 257]. These include (1) variable diastolic closure slopes of the ATVL, depending on whether the TV is functionally competent, incompetent, or stenosed; (2) the recording of the ATVL to the left of the mid-clavicular line, the transducer being directed inferiorly and to the left; (3) the simultaneous recording of the anterior leaflets of both AV valves; (4) delayed TV opening (see 12.5.1); and (5) TV excursion exceeding mitral excursion.

The abnormal anatomy of an Ebstein's anomaly lends itself well to two-dimensional echocardiography. Not only can the large sail-like motion of the ATVL be easily followed, but it is also possible to visualize the functional RV, the large atrialized RV, and the abnormal origin of the septal tricuspid valve leaflet [227]. The severity of the displacement of the TV into the right RV can be clearly assessed using the apex four chamber view [294 a, 357].

12.7.2 Uhl's Anomaly

Abnormal delay in TV closure, 0.065 s or more after MV closure, may be a general sign of right ventricular myocardial dysfunction; indeed, in addition to Ebstein's disease, this feature has been reported in Uhl's anomaly, or congenital hypoplasia of the right ventricular myocardium [104].

12.7.3 Complete Right Bundle Branch Block (see 21.3.6)

TV closure may also be retarded in patients with complete right bundle branch block [382]. In these cases, though, the delay never exceeds 0.065 s [94].

12.8 Fluttering of the ATVL

Fluttering of the ATVL may have different causes: it may be related to increased flow through the TV, such as in secundum atrial septal defect and in d-TGA after atrial septostomy, or it may be due to a regurgitant flow hitting the TV, such as in pulmonary regurgitation and some cases of persistent truncus arteriosus.

12.8.1 Secundum Atrial Septal Defect (see 21.1.1)

12.8.2 d-TGA, After Atrial Septostomy

In ASD, fluttering of the ATVL may be due either to a rapid flow of blood across the TV, or to the existence of associated pulmonary regurgitation [205]. TV diastolic fluttering in ASD usually indicates a large left-to-right shunt [259, 300]. This is well substantiated by the fact that it is noted in d-TGA, especially following balloon septostomy or a Blalock-Hanlon procedure, when flow across the valve suddenly becomes increased [263].

12.8.3 Left Ventricular-Right Atrial Communication

A congenital left ventricular-right atrial communication can be recognized echocardiographically. In two patients with this anomaly, Nanda et al. [263] found a high frequency, low amplitude flutter on the TV echogram, during systole only. This feature, which has recently been confirmed by others [244], is assumed to be caused by the passage of a left ventricular jet of blood into the RA through a defect in the TV.

12.8.4 Pulmonary Regurgitation

Pulmonary regurgitation may be flow related, as in congenital absence of the pulmonary valve and in idiopathic dilatation of the pulmonary artery [205], or it may be secondary to increased pulmonary vascular resistance [421].

In both situations, high frequency fluttering of the ATVL may occur. In the presence of increased pulmonary vascular resistance, more specific echocardiographic features on the pulmonary valve echogram will be documented (see 10.5.2).

Finding high frequency diastolic fluttering of the ATVL may conceivably help in the differential diagnosis of a patient with a high frequency diastolic murmur at the base of the heart: if present, pulmonary regurgitation becomes more likely than aortic regurgitation in which, in addition to other echocardiographic signs, high frequency fluttering of the AMVL is expected.

12.8.5 Truncus Arteriosus with Valvular Regurgitation (see 4.1.3)

Fluttering of the tricuspid and/or MV leaflets has been documented in patients with truncal valve incompetence [14]. If regurgitant flow is important, gross curtailment of diastolic filling time of both the mitral and tricuspid valves may be recorded [14].

12.9 Systolic Posterior Motion of the Tricuspid Valve

12.9.1 Tricuspid Valve Prolapse

This is a rare condition. A small posterior displacement in mid to late systole is a normal observation and should not be confused with true prolapse. However, if a mid-systolic posterior buckling of the TV is recorded, TV prolapse should be suspected.

TV prolapse is often associated with MV prolapse.

A TV prolapse pattern may be observed in the presence of pericardial effusion [266], and of TV endocarditis [180].

12.10 Posterior Displacement of the Tricuspid Valve

12.10.1 Partial AV Canal (see 21.1.2)

12.10.2 Complete AV Canal (see 6.1.2)

12.10.3 Overriding Tricuspid Valve (see 6.1.1)

12.11 Anterior Displacement of the Tricuspid Valve During Diastole

12.11.1 Tricuspid Valve Stenosis (see 12.4.1)

12.11.2 Reduced Right Ventricular Compliance

12.11.3 Ebstein's Anomaly (see 12.7.1)

Whenever egression of blood from the right atrium to the RV is impeded, the $E–F_0$ slope is reduced and the ATVL is abnormally positioned, anteriorly, within the RV (see Fig. 12.3).

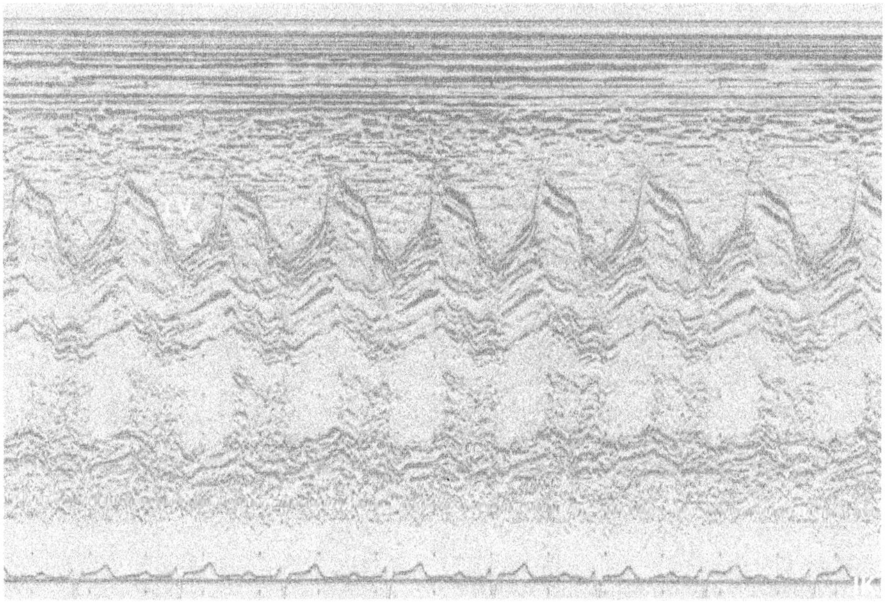

Fig. 12.3. JK: Postoperative echocardiogram of patient shown in Fig. 6.1 with an overriding TV. Though there were no clinical signs to suggest TV stenosis, the TV looks stenotic on this echocardiogram: there is no a wave, diastolic closure velocity is decreased, and there is a slight anterior diastolic motion of the septal tricuspid valve leaflet

13 Abnormal Mitral Valve Motion

Index

Introduction

Of the four cardiac valves, the MV has been the most extensively studied by echocardiography, for not only is it a relatively easily detectable intracardiac landmark, but its motion pattern has allowed, to some extent, a noninvasive assessment of LV function. Indeed, MV motion patterns result from a combination of MV flow and the interplay between left atrial and ventricular pressure [314].

Recognition of abnormal MV motion patterns therefore allows some cardiovascular abnormalities to be suspected or diagnosed. This constitutes the subject of this chapter.

13.1 Increased Excursion of the AMVL

The greatest excursion of the AMVL which appears on scanning from the aortic root to the LV apex should be selected for measurement [431]. Increased excursion is likely to be encountered in the following conditions.

13.1.1 Mitral Valve Prolapse (see 13.11.1)

13.1.2 Mitral Valve Regurgitation (see Fig. 13.1)

Specific echocardiographic features of mitral regurgitation do not exist. However, if ultrasonic examination reveals the following features, mitral regurgitation should be suspected.

1) Increased excursion of the AMVL,
2) Increased diastolic closure rate (E-F_0 slope),
3) Increased septal and LVPW excursion,
4) Left atrial and ventricular dilatation,
5) Increased left atrial filling rate [279],
6) Increased displacement of the left atrial wall [279],
7) Systolic anterior motion of the aortic root starting significantly earlier than in normal subjects [5],
8) Increased amplitude of aortic root motion [5].

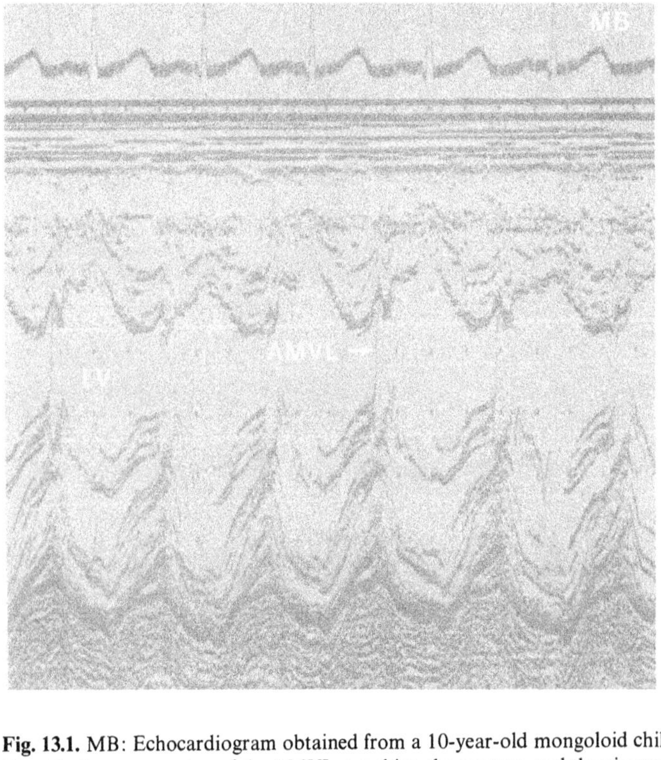

Fig. 13.1. MB: Echocardiogram obtained from a 10-year-old mongoloid child with MV regurgitation. Note the large excursion of the AMVL, touching the septum, and the vigorous contractions of the IVS and LVPW

In addition, echocardiographic examination may hint at the cause of the regurgitation, which may be, e.g., (1) MV prolapse; (2) flailing MV leaflets; (3) vegetative endocarditis, etc.

A directional range-gated pulsed Doppler technique may prove useful in the quantitative estimation of mitral flow in regurgitation [169].

Finally, significant mitral regurgitation in patients with rheumatic MV disease can be detected directly through qualitative analysis of the MV ring using short axis cross sectional echocardiography [407].

13.1.3 **Tricuspid Atresia** (see 7.1.3)

In tricuspid atresia there is only one recordable, posteriorly positioned AV valve: the MV. This valve exhibits a large anterior excursion during diastole, which often exceeds the 95th percentile (see Fig. 7.1).

13.1.4 **Single Ventricle with One AV Valve** (see 7.1.1)

As in tricuspid atresia, excursion of the single AV valve often results in a greater than normal amplitude.

13.2 Reduced Excursion of the AMVL

MV excursion (D-E amplitude), which is normally at least 20 mm [314], is a good indicator of the mobility and pliability of the valve.

Decreased AMVL opening excursion can be documented in the following anomalies.

13.2.1 **Mitral Stenosis** (see 13.7.1)

AMVL excursion not exceeding 12 mm may indicate a fibrotic, relatively immobile valve [85].

13.2.2 **Atrial Septal Defect** (see 21.1.2)

In this situation, reduced excursion has been attributed to diminished cardiac output [172]. In general, the TV leaflet exceeds the MV leaflet in atrial septal defect.

13.2.3 **Congestive Cardiomyopathy** (see 21.4.2)

Congestive cardiomyopathies are characterized by a severely dilated LV cavity and outflow tract, with generalized hypokinesis [2, 68, 314] (see Figs. 13.2 and 4.6).

On M-mode recording, low motion amplitude of both mitral leaflets is striking and sometimes there is an abnormal step formation at the middle or higher level on the descending limb of the presystolic peak [273].

13.2.4 **Idiopathic Hypertrophic Subaortic Stenosis** (see 20.1.1)

13.2.5 **Aortic Regurgitation** (see 11.8.2)

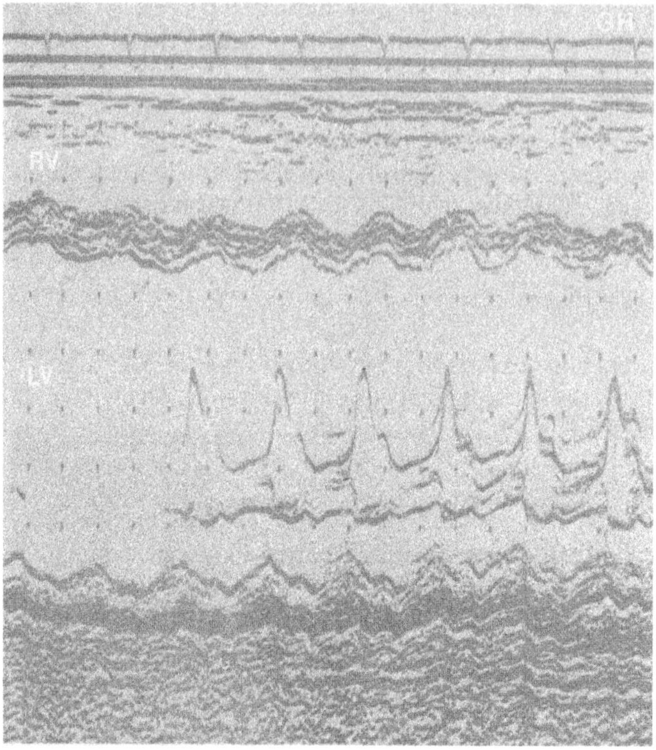

Fig. 13.2. GH: Echocardiogram obtained from a child with congestive cardiomyopathy. Note the large LV (60 mm) and the markedly reduced motion of the septum and the LVPW

13.2.6 Cardiac Tamponade (see 16.2.3)

In the presence of pericardial effusion, reduction in both MV opening excursion and E-F_0 slope (see 13.5.1) is diagnostic of cardiac tamponade. A further reduction in these parameters is often documented during inspiration [346].

13.3 Reduced D-E Slope

13.3.1 Congestive Heart Failure

D-E slope, or the rate at which the MV opens, may seem to be diminished in the presence of a high left ventricular initial diastolic pressure [98, 183]. This is usually seen in conditions with increased end-systolic volume and congestive failure which are thought to be related to decreased blood flow into an incompletely emptied LV [98].

The a-wave may then become large, indicating that a higher percentage of blood is being delivered to the ventricle during active atrial contraction [98].

The LV cavity is usually dilated, and wall motion is decreased.

13.4 Increased E-F_0 Slope

The E-F_0 slope or early diastolic closure rate represents the rate of left atrial emptying. It is thus an important indicator of MV function. The slope normally varies depending on respiration and heart rate, which reflects changes in cardiac output. E-F_0 slope is likely to be increased whenever mitral flow is increased in volume or velocity.

13.4.1 Hyperkinetic States in Normals

13.4.2 Left Ventricular Diastolic Volume Overload (DVO) States

Left ventricular DVO states include (1) aortic regurgitation [289] (see 11.8.2); (2) mitral regurgitation [289] (see 13.1.2); (3) large left-to-right shunts with increased flow through the mitral valve [11], such as in ventricular septal defects, patent ductus arteriosus, etc.; and (4) congestive cardiomyopathy [431] (see 21.4.2).

However, because several factors are involved, the E-F_0 slope may not be consistently increased in these conditions [11, 289].

13.4.3 Ventricular Septal Rupture

In ventricular septal rupture complicating acute myocardial infarction, an unusual pattern of MV motion may be documented, i.e., complete closure of the MV after its initial opening followed by almost complete reopening of the valve [49].

13.5 Reduced E-F_0 Slope

13.5.1 Impaired Left Ventricular Filling

A significantly reduced E-F_0 slope, resulting in the replacement of the typical M-shaped motion pattern of the AMVL by a square wave pattern, is a well-accepted echocardiographic criterion of MV stenosis.

However, reduction of the E-F_0 slope alone is a notoriously poor criterion of mitral stenosis [66] (see 13.7.1); indeed, anything which impairs LV filling may be associated with a reduced E-F_0 slope. Examples of this are (1) mitral stenosis (see 13.7.1); (2) supravalvar mitral ring [431] (see 9.8.1); (3) parachute mitral valve [431] (see 9.8.2); (4) left atrial myxoma [431] (see 9.1.2); and (5) cardiac tamponade (see 16.2.3).

In the presence of pericardial effusion, reduction of the AMVL E-F_0 slope is diagnostic of cardiac tamponade (see Fig. 13.3). A further reduction in the slope can be documented during inspiration; some patients may show a rounded E-F_0 slope in both phases of respiration [346] (see also 13.2.6).

13.5.2 Decreased Left Ventricular Compliance

A decreased E-F_0 slope can also be documented if LV compliance is diminished [201, 298] Examples include (1) severe valvular aortic stenosis [270] (see 24.3.3); (2) IHSS [118, 291] (see 20.1.1); (3) restrictive myocardial disease [431]; and (4) congestive heart failure [118] (see 13.3.1).

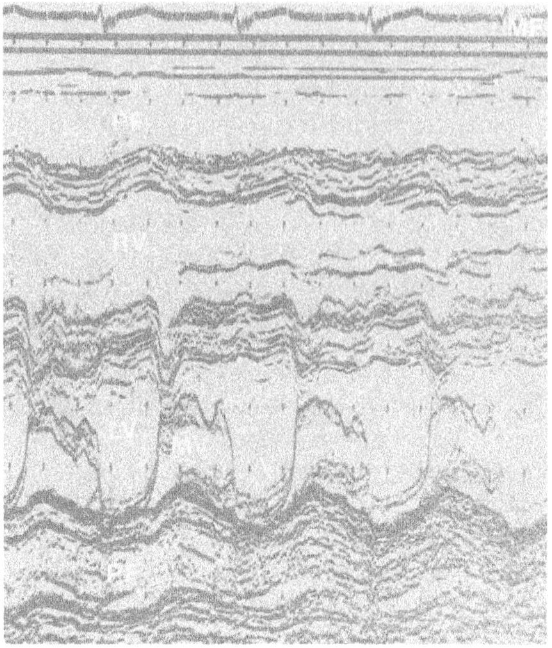

Fig. 13.3. MF: Same patient as in Fig. 8.1. Pericardial fluid is present. MV is abnormal with a reduced E-F_0 slope; a prolapse-like picture of the MV is also documented (*arrow*)

In these conditions the a-wave is always preserved and the valve is not thickened. In addition, the reciprocal posterior motion of the PMVL is preserved, thereby ruling out true mitral stenosis.

The determination of the rate of diastolic posterior motion of the AMVL may help in the quantitative assessment of the severity of some of the anomalies responsible for a MV stenosis pattern. In valvular aortic stenosis, for instance, an E-F_0 slope of greater than 55 mm/s has been found to be unlikely in the presence of critical obstruction [270]; to the contrary, a significant decrease in E-F_0 slope, down to 35 mm/s, was found whenever the AoV index fell below 0.5 cm^2, or whenever the peak systolic gradient exceeded 50 mm Hg [270].

13.5.3 Diminished Mitral Flow

Finally, the E-F_0 slope may be reduced when mitral flow is diminished. This can be documented in entities such as atrial septal defects [118] (see 21.1.2) and pulmonary hypertension [231, 431] (see 10.5.2).

As demonstrated by Vignola et al. [400], the E-F_0 slope depends greatly on the pressure-volume relationship in the LV in early diastole: in general, greater increases in the E-F_0 slope are associated with a greater downward shift of the early diastolic pressure-volume curves [401].

13.6 Decreased A-C Slope

13.6.1 Congestive Cardiomyopathy (see 21.4.2)

In patients with poor LV compliance, closure of the MV following atrial systole is abnormal: the A-point begins slightly earlier than normal, and the C-point is slightly delayed [98]. Between these two points there may be a plateau, interrupting the ordinary smooth closure [98]. This plateau or notch in mitral motion, immediately before the valve closure point, is thought to indicate a high LV end-diastolic pressure [277 b].

This pattern has been documented in congestive cardiomyopathies [273].

13.7 Anterior Motion of the PMVL

The posterior leaflet of the MV normally moves posteriorly during diastole, its direction being a mirror image of the anterior mitral leaflet motion.

Absence of this normal posterior motion should suggest an obstructive lesion to the inflow of the LV. Essentially two entities are to be considered, i. e., mitral stenosis and supravalvar mitral ring.

13.7.1 Mitral Stenosis

Echocardiographic diagnosis of mitral stenosis is based on following suggestive features.

Anterior Motion of the PMVL

An anterior diastolic motion of the PMVL is characteristic of mitral stenosis [98]. However, this abnormal motion cannot always be detected [355]. A more sensitive echocardiographic criterion is a late diastolic anterior motion of the PMVL, with the onset of atrial systole, even if the early diastolic movement of the PMVL is posterior or biphasic [355]. This feature helps to further differentiate true from pseudo-mitral valve echo patterns of mitral stenosis with reduced E-F_0 slopes (see 13.5.2).

In the only child with true congenital mitral stenosis that we were able to study ultrasonically, the PMVL remained essentially motionless throughout diastole (see Fig. 13.4)

Thickening of the Valve Cusps

Thick, multiple echoes are documented in severe mitral stenosis, rather than a single thin echo characteristic of a normal MV.

Reduced D-E Amplitude (see 13.2.1)

Increased Opening (D-E) and Closure (A-C) Slopes

As long as the MV leaflets remain pliable, their opening and closure rates will be increased as a result of elevated LA pressure.

Reduced or Absent a-Wave in the Presence of a Normal Sinus Rhythm

Distinct Deviation from Normal of Aortic Root Motion Patterns

During early diastole the normal rapid posterior movement of the posterior aortic wall is replaced by a slower motion continuing throughout the length of diastole: the plateau normally found in late diastole is thus missing [5].

The mean amplitude of posterior aortic wall motion is also significantly reduced.

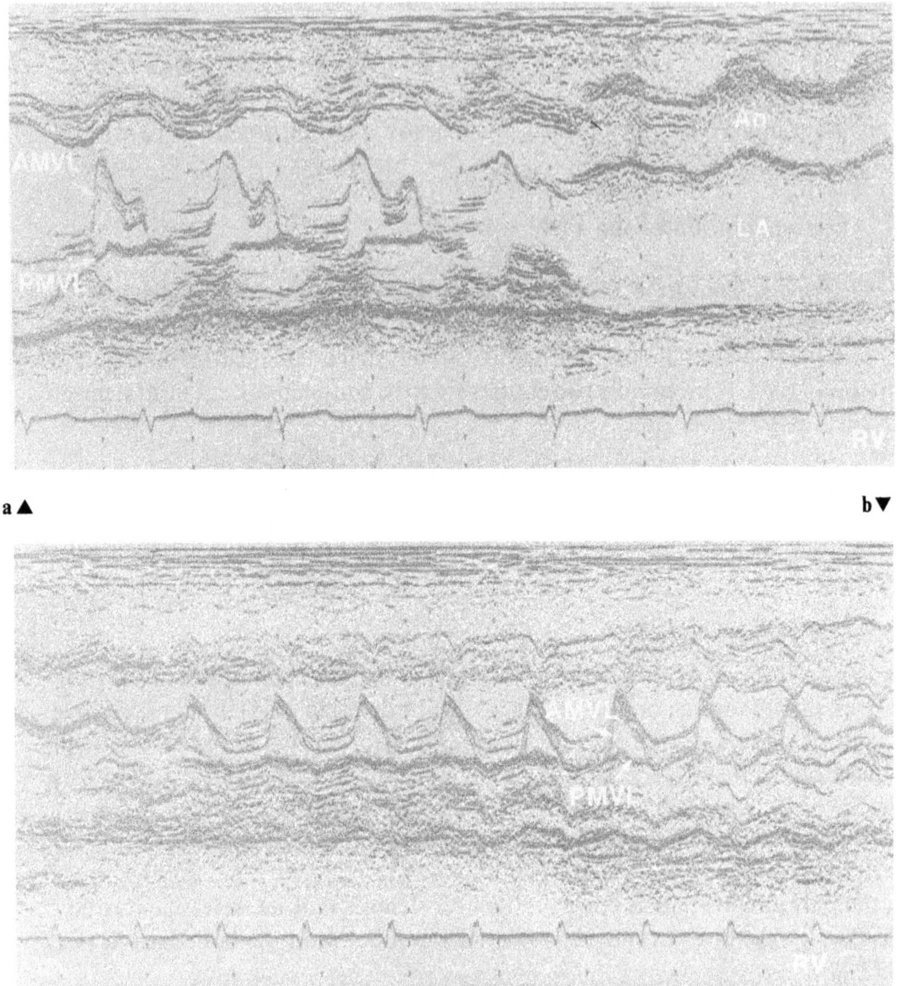

Fig. 13.4 a, b. RV: M-mode echocardiogram obtained from a 15-year-old boy with congenital mitral stenosis, due to an abnormal MV. **a** Is the preoperative echocardiogram. It shows a tickened PMVL with reduced amplitude of motion; the LA is enlarged. **b** Shows the valve after a Carpentier procedure: the thick echo posterior to the MV is generated by the metal ring. Note that the motion of the PMVL has a more normal appearance

Delayed Closure of the Mitral Valve

Akgün and Layton [5] found a Q-mitral closure interval (Q-MC) of 76 $\pm$ 4 ms in patients with mitral stenosis, whereas in normals the Q-MC was 58 $\pm$ 2 ms.

In addition, the following secondary echocardiographic features may be documented: (1) left atrial enlargement; and (2) absent a-waves on the pulmonary valve echogram if pulmonary hypertension is present.

In the presence of these criteria, objective echocardiographic confirmation of mitral stenosis can usually be made with an accuracy approaching 100% [277 b, 314].

Rough estimates of the severity of the mitral obstruction can be made based on the rate of diastolic posterior motion of the AMVL (E-F_0 slope) [314]. Normally, this slope should exceed 80 mm/s. In significant mitral stenosis it is less than 40 mm/s, and in extreme cases the slope may be under 10 mm/s [314].

The severity of mitral obstruction is, of course, most accurately assessed through determination of the MV area. This can be defined noninvasively using planimetry, directly from videotape pictures, recorded from real-time cross sectional images [271].

If congenital mitral stenosis is diagnosed, a complete echocardiographic examination should be performed accurately, as the overall frequency of associated significant cardiovascular abnormalities, such as left- or right-sided obstructive lesions, approaches 75%.

13.7.2 Supravalvar Mitral Ring (see 9.8.1, Fig. 13.5)

In a small number of patients, anterior motion of the PMVL will not result from intrinsic MV disease, but from the presence of a supravalvar mitral ring.

We have seen one patient with a crescent-like supravalvar mitral ring, located just above the PMVL. Probably due to flow changes, the PMVL showed an anterior motion in early diastole. After resection, MV motion returned to normal.

13.8 Delayed Opening of the Mitral Valve

MV opening is normally synchronous with minimal LV dimensions; when opening is delayed, abnormal relaxation is probably present [391].

Delayed MV opening has been documented in:

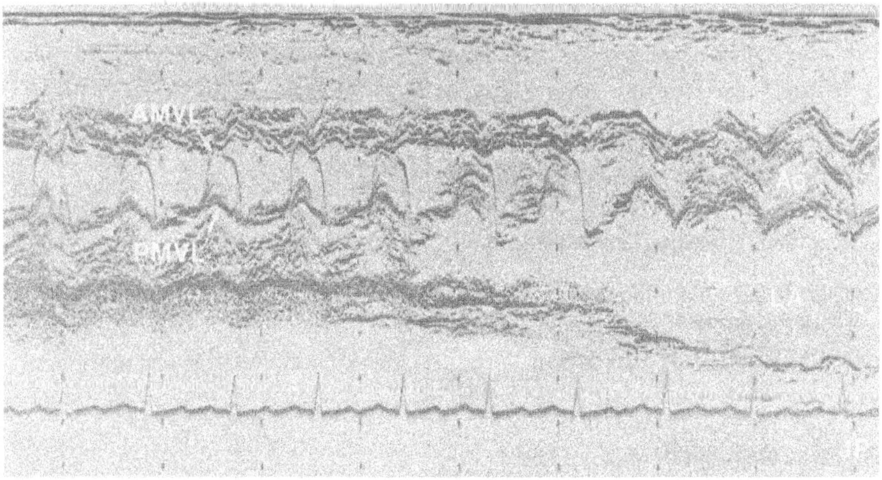

Fig. 13.5. JP: M-mode scan obtained from a 3-year-old girl with a supravalvular mitral membrane. The membrane had a semilunar aspect and was located just above the PMVL. Although the membrane itself is not well visualized on this echocardiogram, the diagnosis was suspected preoperatively by to the presence of an enlarged LA and by the abnormal anterior diastolic motion of the PMVL. Fine fluttering of this leaflet is also documented, finding which would be unusual in valvular mitral stenosis

13.8.1 **Hypertrophic Cardiomyopathy** [391] (see 20.1.1)

13.8.2 **Discrete Subaortic Stenosis** [245] (see 11.2.1)

13.8.3 **Aortic Regurgitation** (see 11.8.2)

In patients with aortic regurgitation, opening of the MV is delayed significantly: it has been found to occur 84 ms after AoV closure as compared to 61 ms after AoV closure in normal persons [5].

13.9 Premature Closure of the Mitral Valve

Valvar closure starts prior to completion of the QRS complex in most patients [29, 289], at the time of the first heart sound.

Premature MV closure, well before the subsequent QRS complex, occurs in conditions associated with a rapid rise in LV diastolic pressure. This may be observed in the following:

13.9.1 **Acute Aortic Regurgitation** [29, 289] (see 11.8.2)

13.9.2 **Truncus Arteriosus with Valvular Regurgitation** [14] (see 4.1.3, and 4.2.2)

13.10 Mitral Valve Leaflet Fluttering

Significant fluttering of the MV leaflets may be documented either in systole (13.10.1, 13.10.2) or in diastole (13.10.3 to 13.10.11).

Diastolic fluttering can be attributed to (1) a regurgitant jet of blood (13.10.3 to 13.10.7); (2) a right-to-left intracardiac shunt (13.10.8 to 13.10.10); or (3) turbulence from other causes (13.10.11).

13.10.1 Mitral Valve Prolapse After Subacute Bacterial Endocarditis

Patients with mitral regurgitation due to this association of lesions may have systolic fluttering of the MV leaflets [263].

13.10.2 **Ruptured Chordae Tendineae** (see 9.1.5)

Fine systolic fluttering of the AMVL can be seen in patients with ruptured chordae tendineae and severe mitral regurgitation.

This finding is ascribed to the action of a high velocity jet on a loose leaflet margin [233].

13.10.3 **Aortic Regurgitation** (see 11.8.2)

If aortic regurgitation directs the regurgitant jet against the AMVL, high frequency vibration of this leaflet may be recorded [289] (see Fig. 13.6).

This feature seems more related to the direction rather than the importance of the regurgitant jet.

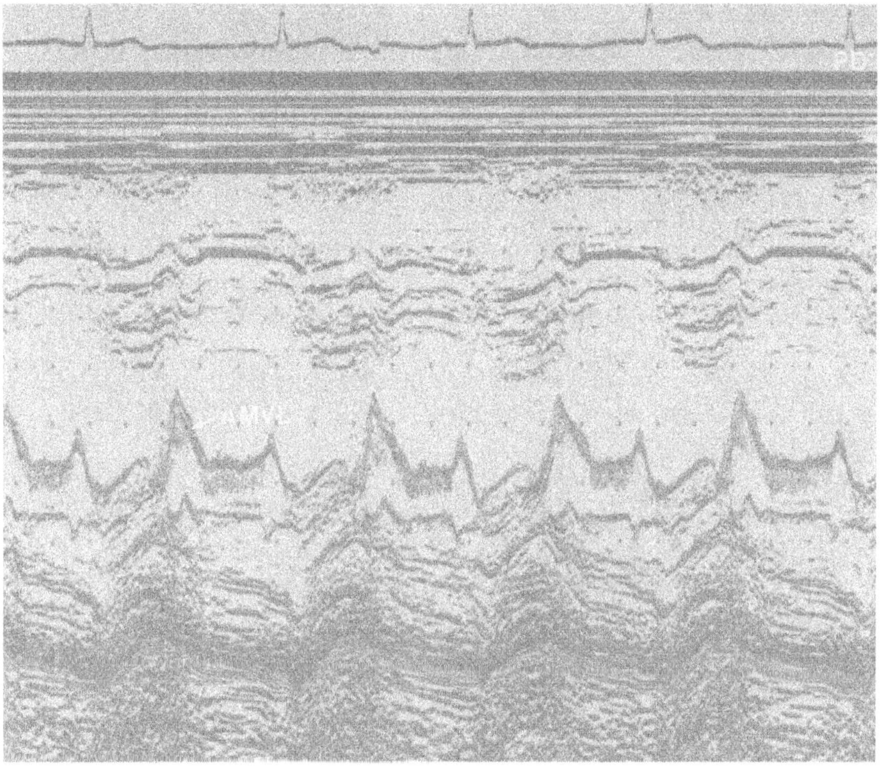

Fig. 13.6. PD: Echocardiogram obtained from a 10-year-old girl with AoV regurgitation. Note the presence of diastolic fluttering of both MV leaflets

13.10.4 Discrete Subvalvular Aortic Stenosis (see 11.2.1)

13.10.5 Bicuspid Aortic Valve (see 11.3.1)

13.10.6 Bacterial Endocarditis with Secondary Valvular Destruction (see 9.7.2)

The last three entities may be characterized by an abnormal and/or altered AoV with aortic regurgitation that is responsible for high frequency diastolic fluttering of the AMVL.

13.10.7 Truncus Arteriosus (see 4.1.3)

In patients with truncus arteriosus, fine diastolic fluttering of the AMVL and/or of the left endocardial surface of the IVS may be related to truncal valve incompetence [14].

13.10.8 Tetrad of Fallot (see 4.1.2)

13.10.9 Ventricular Septal Defect with Right Ventricular Outflow Tract Obstruction

13.10.10 Isolated Ventricular Septal Defect (see 15.1.2)

Meyer et al. [238] observed diastolic fluttering of the AMVL in 71% of patients with tetralogy of Fallot, 80% of patients with VSD and RVOT obstruction, and in 35% of patients with isolated VSD. This fluttering was assumed to be related to the passage of blood from the right to the left ventricle, striking the AMVL during diastole.

13.10.11 d-Transposition of the Great Arteries (see 3.1.1)

Fine to coarse fibrillatory movement of the MV is a frequent finding in d-TGA; this fluttering becomes even more important after a Mustard's operation [17, 141, 278] (see Fig. 13.7), and has been attributed to the relatively low level of compliance of the systemic venous atrium and high velocity of systemic venous flow through the MV [17]. An alternative explanation is that both fluttering and SAM of the MV are related to bulging of the IVS into the LV cavity with consequent distortion of the MV apparatus [278].

13.11 Systolic Posterior Motion of the Mitral Valve

13.11.1 Mitral Valve Prolapse

Since the original documentation by Barlow et al. [21] that the "systolic click-late systolic murmur syndrome" was associated with mitral leaflet prolapse, numerous

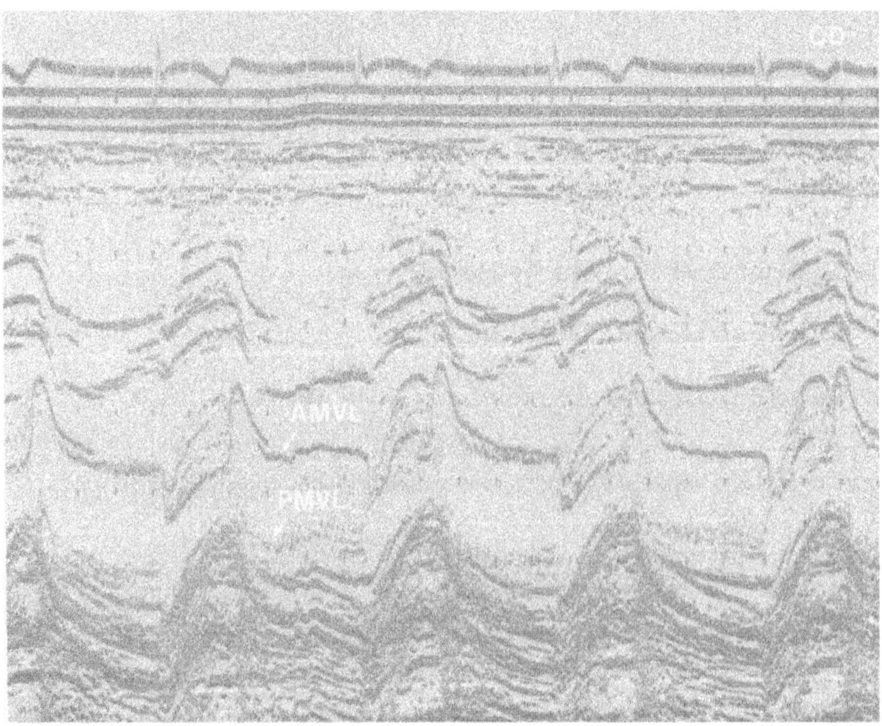

Fig. 13.7. CD: Coarse fluttering of the MV leaflets in patients after a Mustard's operation to correct d-TGA is commonly seen. This echocardiogram was obtained from a 5-year-old child. It shows, in addition, SAM of the AMVL and an abnormal septal motion

studies have described the clinical characteristics of this distinctive valvular lesion. Echocardiography has provided a better understanding of this syndrome by allowing dynamic visualization of the mitral leaflets. Mathey et al. [225] showed that the timing of prolapse, click, and murmur is governed by maneuvers affecting LV shape, thereby enhancing or reducing the disproportion between leaflet-chordal length and LV dimensions [77]: physical and pharmacologic interventions which reduce ventricular volumes will enhance leaflet redundancy, hasten prolapse, and move click and murmur earlier in systole [77]. Prolapse will thus become more significant in the standing position, after a Valsalva maneuver, and in the presence of tachycardia. Conversely, prolapse will become less apparent with squatting, bradycardia, and following the administration of vasopressors and beta-receptor inhibitors (propanolol), all of which increase LV dimensions [77].

The echocardiographic demonstration of a prolapsing MV is not difficult. However, pseudo-prolapse patterns are not uncommon ultrasonically, so that a diagnosis of true prolapse should be made only after exclusion of (1) a faulty technique or interpretation; (2) the presence of pericardial effusion (see infra 13.11.2) and/or of cardiac tamponade (13.11.3); and (3) premature ventricular activation (see infra: 13.11.4).

Indeed, if the transducer is placed too high on the chest wall, false-positive motion patterns suggesting MV prolapse may be obtained [215 b, 413]. Conversely, if the transducer is at or around the cardiac apex, a net motion toward the transducer may be registered even in the presence of documented prolapse [289].

Incomplete echocardiographic scanning of the MV may be another cause of a "false-negative" study, while a normal mitral echogram might reflect physiologic variability in patients with known prolapse. In addition, up to 10% of patients with the clinical syndrome may not have echocardiographic demonstration of prolapse [289].

Though cross sectional echocardiography is more reliable than conventional or M-mode echocardiography in diagnosing MV prolapse [110, 331], overdiagnosis is still possible by using the former technique. Gilbert et al. [110], using a phased array imaging system, noted that if the transducer was angled medially and tangentially across the mitral orifice, false posterior coaptation and minor superior arching of the AMVL could be documented in normals.

Finally, prolapse should not be diagnosed erroneously on the basis of normal posterior leaflet motion during the first 50 ms of systole [77].

M-Mode Features of MV Prolapse

A definite feature of MV prolapse is a systolic posterior motion of the MV leaflets (see Fig. 13.8).

Normally, the MV leaflets inscribe on the echocardiogram a slow continuous anterior motion during mid and late systole.

A holo or late systolic prolapse of one or both leaflets can be visualized directly by echocardiography as a posterior buckling interrupting the normal anterior motion in early or late systole. Sahn et al. [331, 335] showed that the entire spectrum of M-mode abnormalities, from late to holosystolic prolapse, could be identified in the same patient, depending on ultrasonic beam direction. This would tend to make irrelevant the differentiation between a late systolic buckling, supposedly more indicative of prolapse, and a pansystolic, hammock-like posterior motion of the valve.

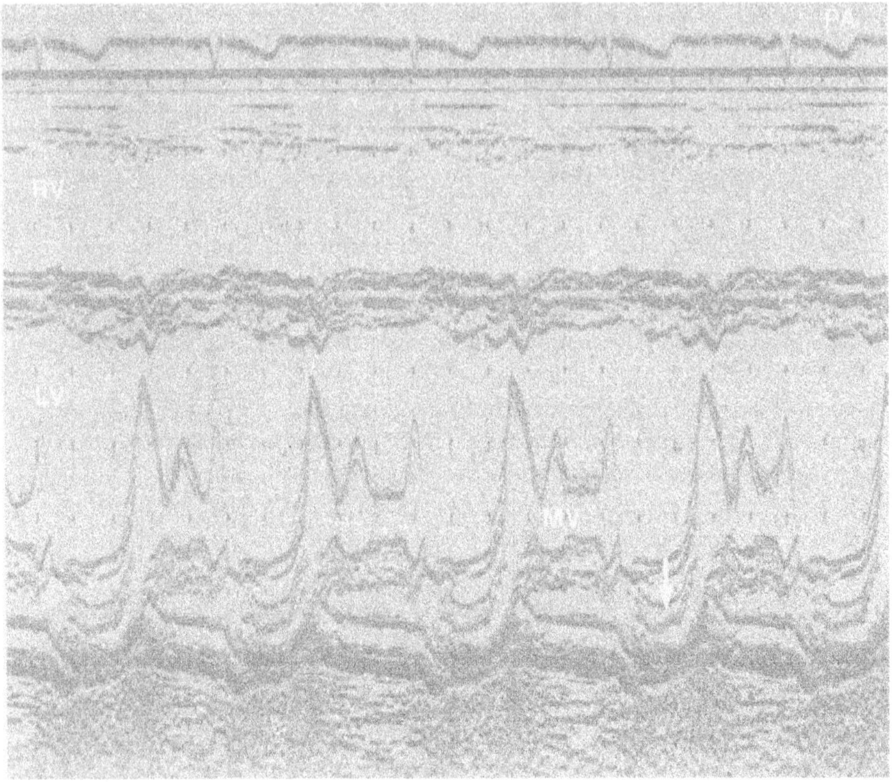

Fig. 13.8. PA: M-mode scan from a 14-year-old patient with MV prolapse. The *arrow* points to the late systolic posterior motion of the PMVL

A flat systolic motion of the MV, such as can be seen in dilated cardiomyopathies, should not be confused with a definite posterior valvular motion.

Suggestive features of MV prolapse include:
1) Multiple parallel MV echoes, resulting from beam spread and poor lateral resolution of redundant valvular tissue [77, 289],
2) Exaggerated leaflet mobility, producing diastolic contact with the IVS [77], and
3) The associated finding of a biconvex enlargement of the sinus of Valsalva with a significant increase in aortic root diameter. This was found by Sahn et al. [331] in 22 out of 26 patients with MV prolapse. A Marfan syndrome could not account for this abnormal enlargement as it occurred in only five of these patients.

Though only one cusp may be involved in MV prolapse, many authors have stressed the frequency of involvement of both leaflets [62, 212, 331].

If prolapse of the MV is documented, the TV should be carefully scanned, as TV prolapse is known to occur in association with MV prolapse [416]. According to some [50], the presence in a patient of a systolic click and a late systolic murmur may indicate either MV or TV prolapse, or a combination of the two.

Bidimensional echocardiographic features significantly enhance the noninvasive evaluation of MV prolapse and provide an explanation for many of the single cristal observations [331].

Conditions Associated with MV Prolapse

In the General Population

The MV prolapse syndrome is probably the most commonly encountered cardiac abnormality. Indeed, in an echocardiographic study of 136 volunteers, prolapse was documented in six cases, or 4.4% [29]. A still higher incidence of 6% was found by Procacci et al. [297] in an echocardiographic survey of presumably normal young females.

The anomaly is hereditary in some cases and a familial prevalence of 50% has been reported [20, 331, 413]. MV prolapse can occur in twins [112].

Asymmetric Septal Hypertrophy

Schmaltz et al. [341] angiocardiographically examined 45 patients (age 3–15.5 years) with the MV prolapse syndrome. Thirteen patients (30%) showed a thickened IVS.

Connective Tissue Disorders

MV prolapse is often related to connective tissue diseases, of which the most important is Marfan's syndrome [20, 36, 331, 364]. Classic Marfan's syndrome has been documented in approximately 4% of patients with mitral prolapse [77]. Conversely, up to 90% of patients with a Marfan's syndrome exhibit, in addition to aortic root dilatation, typical mitral leaflet prolapse [29, 36]. Furthermore, MV prolapse has been reported in up to 33% of first degree relatives of patients with Marfan's syndrome [281].

In addition to Marfan's syndrome, MV prolapse may complicate less serious skeletal abnormalities, such as pectus excavatum, high arched palate, arachnodactyly, hyperextensible joints [331], flat feet, kyphoscoliosis [310], and the straight back syndrome [293 a]. An increased frequency of thoracic skeletal anomalies with mitral prolapse has also been emphasized [337]. Finally, prolapse occurs more frequently in patients with muscular dystrophy, either the myotonic or Duchenne's type [305].

It is, therefore, tempting to speculate, as others have done, that a developmental abnormality of connective tissue underlies the various manifestations of MV prolapse.

In Association with Other Cardiac Anomalies

MV prolapse has been found in association with the following:

1. Atrial septal defect (ASD) (see 21.1.1), which has frequently been found to be associated with MV prolapse, although the reported incidence has varied with different authors from 5% [300] to 37% [77]. In 24 consecutive adult patients with ASD, the prevalence of MV prolapse was found to be as high as 95%, as determined by two-dimensional echocardiography [206].

2. Regarding truncus arteriosus (see 4.1.3) Assad-Morell et al. [14] echocardiographically recorded a pansystolic prolapse of the MV in three patients out of 20 with this anomaly.

3. Regarding tricuspid atresia (*see 7.1.3*) MV prolapse may be seen in two-thirds of patients with this condition; it is probably related to an increase in the size of the MV apparatus [431].

The echocardiographic demonstration of prolapse has been reported in other anomalies such as coarctation of the aorta [343].

We recently documented prolapse, both angio- and echocardiographically, in a 10-year-old boy, 4 years after surgical repair of tetrad of Fallot. Figure 13.9 is suggestive of prolapse in a child with an Ebstein's anomaly of the TV.

Caution must be exercised in interpreting associations with prolapse, because of its relatively high incidence in the general population.

In Association with Myocardial Disease

MV prolapse has been found in association with several myocardial diseases.

1. Regarding *coronary artery disease*, recent evidence suggests that MV prolapse, often without auscultatory features, may result from papillary muscle-left ventricular contraction abnormalities, secondary to this disease [77]. Raizada et al. [301] have shown that coexisting prolapse of the posterior MV leaflet with coronary artery disease usually indicated triple vessel obstructive lesions.

2. Prolapse of the mitral apparatus into the left atrium may accompany mitral incompetence due to *chordal rupture* or papillary muscle necrosis in *acute myocardial infarction.* In this situation, prolapse will be holosystolic and an irregular diastolic "flail" motion of the untethered leaflet will be documented [293 a].

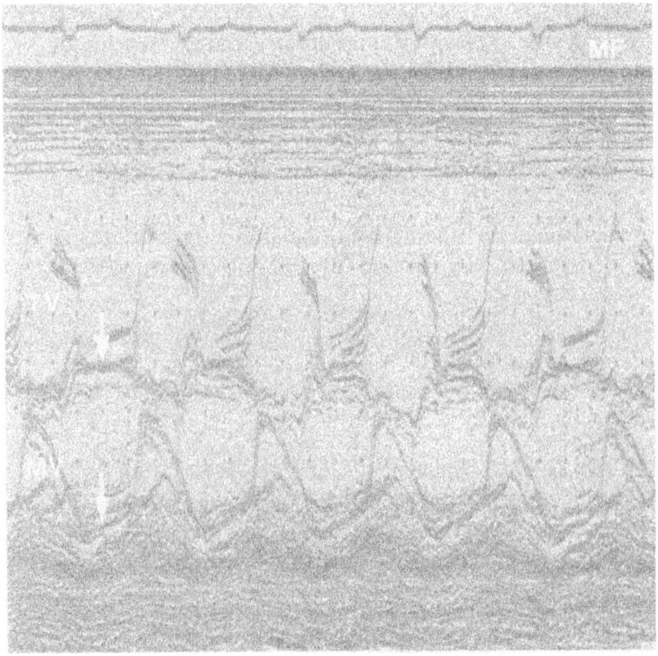

Fig. 13.9. MF: Same patient as in Fig. 8.1, but preoperatively. Mild TV and MV prolapse seem to be present (*arrows*). Note also the large amplitude of excursion of the ATVL

3. Regarding *Uhl's anomaly* (see 10.1.2), or congenital hypoplasia of the RV myocardium, an echocardiographic pattern of MV prolapse has been found at least once, in addition to ultrasonic signs of RV myocardial dysfunction [104].

4. Corya et al. [69] have described ultrasonic findings in five patients with carbon monoxide (CO) poisoning. Echocardiograms in three of the five patients showed MV prolapse, which was attributed to papillary muscle lesions known to occur in fatal cases of CO poisoning.

In Association with Infective Endocarditis

Patients with MV vegetations may have flail mitral leaflets, and a marked posterior motion into the left atrium, at the onset of systole, that may be recorded during echocardiography [405]. A coarse systolic flutter on the prolapsing segment seems to be an additional ultrasonic feature if prolapse is secondary to infective endocarditis [388].

In Primary Pulmonary Hypertension (see 10.5.2)

Goodman et al. [121] have found MV prolapse in four patients out of nine with primary pulmonary hypertension. The possibility of pulmonary hypertension should therefore be investigated in any patient with documented MV prolapse.

13.11.2 Pericardial Effusion (see 8.1.1)

Levisman and Abbasi [200] and Nanda et al. [266] found an abnormal posterior motion of the mitral leaflets typical for MV prolapse, in most patients with a chronic large pericardial effusion. A similar posterior motion of the anterior RV wall, the IVS, and the posterior LV wall occurred simultaneously [200]. It was thought that the congruous motion of the ventricular walls was more in line with a picture of pseudo-prolapse and did not reflect valvular dysfunction [266].

13.11.3 Cardiac Tamponade (see 16.2.3)

A similar echocardiographic picture of pseudo-prolapse affecting the MV has been encountered in cardiac tamponade following compression of the heart by a thymoma [43].

13.11.4 Premature Ventricular Contractions

MV prolapse can occur during premature ventricular contractions in apparently normal subjects [47].

13.12 Systolic Anterior Motion of the Mitral Valve

Systolic anterior motion (SAM) of the AMVL is an abrupt movement of the AMVL toward the septum at a rate greater than the endocardium of the left ventricular posterior wall (LVPW). The abnormal motion reaches its apex in mid systole and returns toward its origin in late systole [289]. In the most extreme forms of SAM, the AMVL may come into contact with the IVS for a variable period of time.

This abnormal motion is a characteristic feature of IHSS (see 20.1.1). In fact, if SAM cannot be demonstrated, even after provocative maneuvers such as amyl-

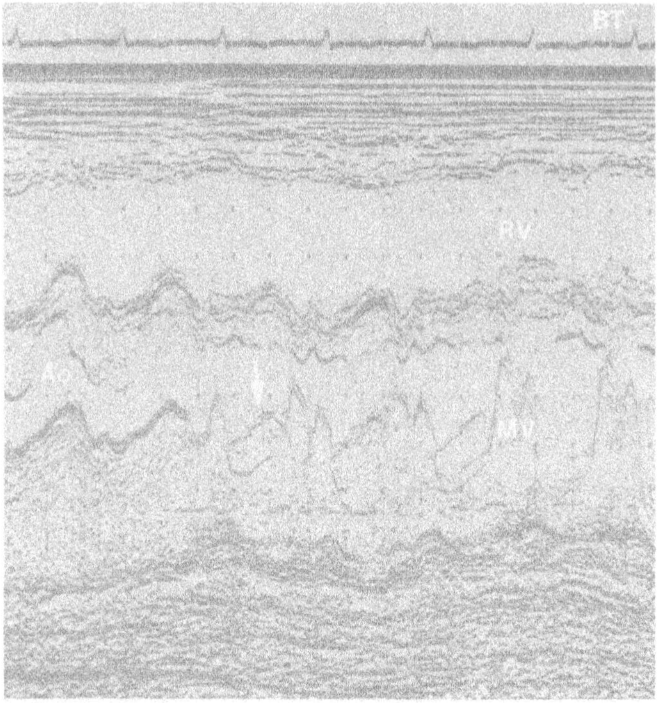

Fig. 13.10. BT: A SAM-like pattern of the AMVL (*arrow*) seems to be present on this echocardiogram obtained from a 22-year-old man with constrictive pericarditis (same patient as in Fig. 10.1). The SAM is, however, a phantom echo, and is caused by the projection in the MV area of posterior aortic wall echoes. Note also the abnormal septal motion diagnostic of constrictive pericarditis

nitrite, on a technically excellent echocardiogram, the LVOT is not obstructed and the diagnosis of IHSS is in doubt.

The exact mechanism of SAM in IHSS remains controversial, despite real-time cross sectional observations. We have documented, at least in some patients, a clear anterior motion of the AMVL during systole, a phenomenon we attributed to a Venturi-like effect in the narrowed, low-pressure LVOT. However, others have found, on dynamic imaging, that anterior-superior displacement of the posterior papillary muscle was a fundamental abnormality predisposing to the anterior motion of the leaflets and to LVOT obstruction [313].

Echocardiographic SAM with ASH are two of the most important diagnostic criteria for IHSS (see 20.1.1). However, SAM may occur in other conditions both with (13.12.2 to 13.12.6) and without (13.12.7 to 13.12.10) LVOT obstruction. In addition, SAM-like patterns of the AMVL may result from high output cardiac states or from spurious echoes (see Fig. 13.10).

13.12.1 Idiopathic Hypertrophic Subaortic Stenosis (see Fig. 13.11 and Sect. 20.1.1)

When a patient with IHSS has a pressure gradient, SAM of the AMVL is usually documented echocardiographically [118]. In addition, SAM causing dynamic LVOT obstruction, such as occurs in IHSS, has been described in the absence of

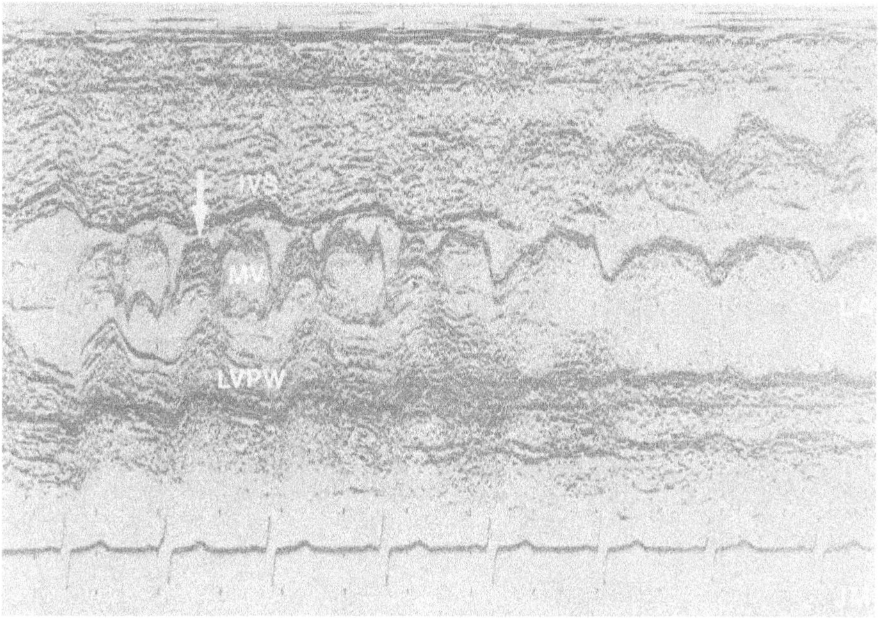

Fig. 13.11. JM: Echocardiogram obtained from a 8-year-old boy with classical IHSS. Note the thickened, immobile septum and the true SAM of the AMVL (*arrow*). The LV is reduced in size. This patient had a positive family history for IHSS

echocardiographic ASH, with normal septal thickness, thickening, and excursion [248]. Furthermore, echocardiographic evidence of stenosis may occur without hemodynamic obstruction or pressure gradient across the LVOT [178].

13.12.2 Tunnel Subaortic Stenosis

In this entity the most characteristic anatomic feature is a long fibromuscular narrowing of the LVOT, which remains relatively unchanged throughout the cardiac cycle [219].

Though ventricular hypertrophy is usually symmetric, ASH and SAM of the AMVL are sometimes documented.

13.12.3 Discrete Membranous Subaortic Stenosis (see 11.2.1)

This entity, in which LVOT obstruction is caused by a subvalvular membrane, may be associated with abnormalities of LV function, including SAM and delayed opening of the MV [245] (see Fig. 13.12).

Comment

IHSS, tunnel subaortic stenosis, and discrete membranous subaortic stenosis may thus share a common ultrasonic feature: SAM of the AMVL. Nevertheless, their echocardiographic differentiation remains possible (see Table 13.1). In both discrete and tunnel subaortic stenosis, concentric LVH with normal or hyperkinetic septal

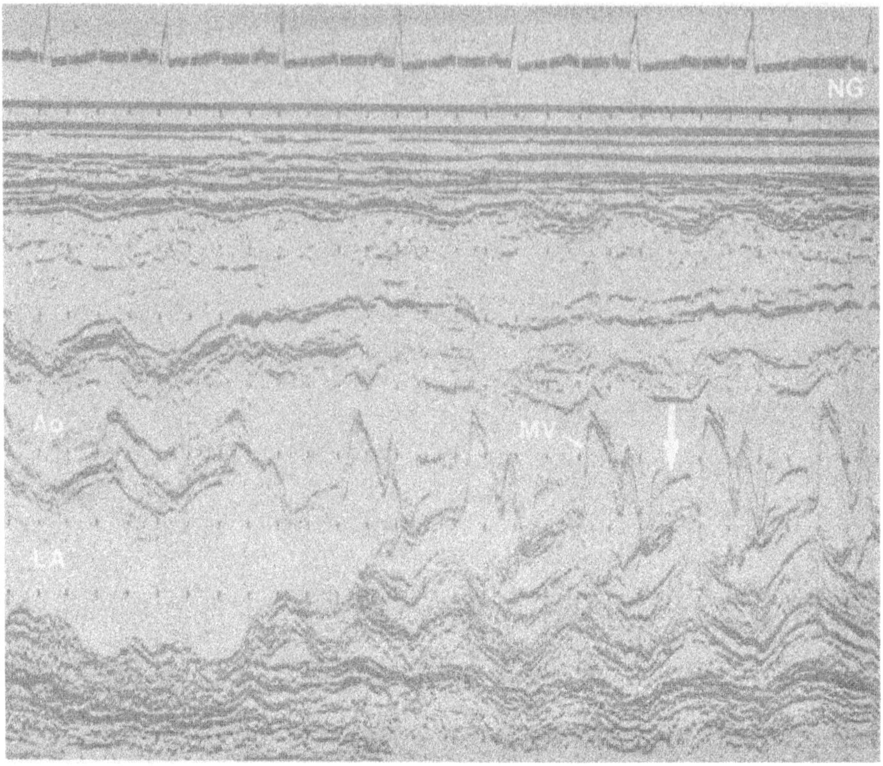

Fig. 13.12. NG: Echocardiogram obtained from a 8-year-old girl with subvalvular aortic stenosis (gradient 88 mm Hg) due to a fibromuscular diaphragm. IVS was, in addition, markedly hypertrophied. Note the SAM of the AMVL (*arrow*)

motion and systolic thickening is usually documented. In IHSS, symmetric LVH is occasionally encountered [321]; in these cases, however, septal contractions remain minimal. Discrete and tunnel subaortic stenosis may be further distinguished by other ultrasonic features (see Table 13.1).

Table 13.1. Differentiating echocardiographic features of IHSS, discrete subaortic stenosis (DSAS), and tunnel subaortic stenosis (TSAS)

Feature	IHSS	DSAS	TSAS
SAM	+(−)[a]	−(+)[b]	−(+)
ASH	+(−)	−(+)	−(+)
Septal systolic thickening and amplitude of excursion	Decreased	Increased	Increased
Narrow LVOT	Dynamic (systolic)	Fixed	Fixed
Abnormal aortic valve echogram	+	+	−
Anterior position of the mitral valve	+	−	+
Poststenotic dilatation of aorta	−	+	−
Unusual echoes in LVOT	−	+(?)	−

[a] (−) sometimes absent
[b] (+) sometimes present

13.12.4 Dynamic Obstruction in Concentric LVH

Dynamic LVOT obstruction with ultrasonic documentation of SAM of the AMVL can be documented occasionally in patients with concentric LVH [222].

13.12.5 Infiltrative Cardiomyopathy

LVOT obstruction in infiltrative cardiomyopathies such as glycogen storage disease of the heart, is a well-known occurrence. This may be documented echocardiographically by finding pronounced SAM of the AMVL [303].

13.12.6 d-TGA and Subpulmonary Obstruction (see 17.4.2)

Dynamic LVOT obstruction in patients with d-TGA is suggested if ASH and SAM of the MV is demonstrated [265]. However, these abnormalities have been observed in the absence of demonstrable hemodynamic obstruction [17, 278], probably as a consequence of the abnormally shaped left ventricle in d-TGA. In fact, SAM of the AMVL is more frequently found in patients with low LV pressure and without significant LVOT obstruction [278]. After a Mustard's operation, SAM may become even more prevalent [278]. In Fig. 13.13 SAM of the AMVL is well documented. This echo-trace was obtained in a 5-year-old boy with d-TGA and subpulmonary obstruction, 3 years after a Mustard's operation. LVOT obstruction persisted postoperatively, with a 50 mm Hg gradient.

SAM in these cases should not be confused with an abnormal cluster of echoes in the LVOT, corresponding to an aneurysm of the membranous ventricular septum in patients with d-TGA [347] (see 9.3.6).

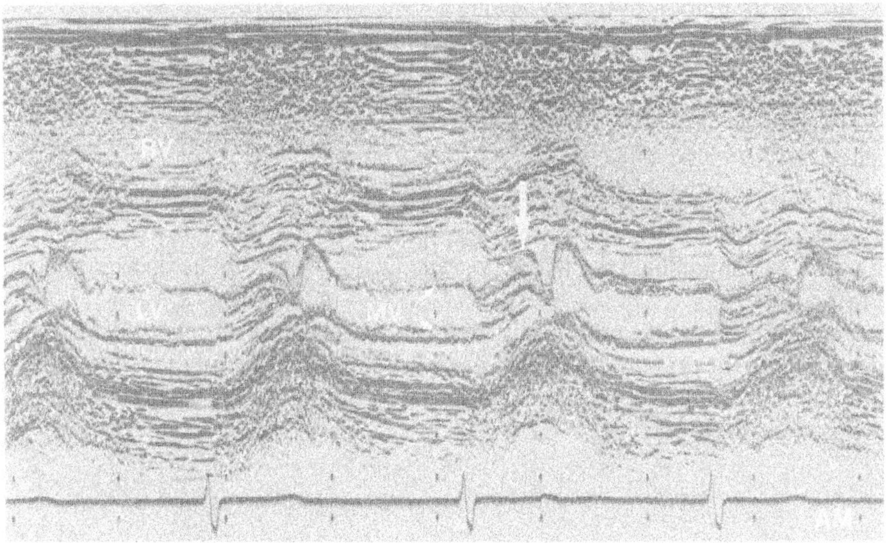

Fig. 13.13. AM: SAM in a patient with d-TGA after a Mustard's operation (see text) (*arrow*)

13.12.7 Coarctation of the Aorta (see 19.2.4)

Scovil et al. [343] studying 36 patients with coarctation of the aorta, found simultaneous IHSS and SAM in three patients, while a fourth patient exhibited SAM only.

13.12.8 Atrial Septal Defect (see 21.1.1)

Abnormal SAM of the AMVL, similar to that seen in patients with IHSS is occasionally reported in patients with ASD. Tajik et al. [381] reported such finding, along with RV dilatation and paradoxic septal motion, in a 30-year-old man.

13.12.9 Essential Pulmonary Hypertension

As in MV prolapse, SAM of the AMVL can sometimes be documented in essential pulmonary hypertension [387].

13.12.10 After Mitral Annuloplasty

SAM of the AMVL has been described at least once after this surgical procedure [387].
In addition, SAM-like patterns of the AMVL may result from high output cardiac states or spurious echoes.

High Output Cardiac States

SAM of the AMVL may result from an heterogeneous group of disorders in which hypercontractile cardiac action is the common denominator [64]. In these cases, rapid ventricular ejection may create a Venturi-like effect resulting in forward systolic motion of the MV [64].

However, this motion does not represent true SAM of the AMVL as (1) its amplitude is generally small and (2) its rate of motion in early systole does not exceed the rate of motion of the LVPW.

These pseudo-SAM patterns may be documented in entities such as (1) ventricular aneurysms [129]; (2) pericardial effusions [266]; (3) aortic regurgitation [289]; and (4) normal athletic hearts [289].

Spurious Echoes

Finally, because of limited lateral resolution of presently available echo systems, spurious echoes from the papillary muscles, chordae tendineae, or the posterior aortic wall may contaminate the MV echogram, giving it a SAM-like appearance (see Fig. 13.10).

These spurious echoes are more easily documented in cases of a prolapsing MV: in order to record the prolapse, the sound beam is usually directed more superiorly, close to the MV annulus, resulting in a superimposition of echoes from both the annulus and the valve leaflets [331].

Abnormal Dimensions and Wall Motion or Thickness

14 Abnormal Right Atrial Size

Index

Introduction

M-mode echocardiographic detection of the right atrial cavity remains difficult, for two reasons: (1) there are no clear-cut ultrasonic landmarks within the right atrium, and (2) its location behind the sternum renders it relatively unaccessible to ultrasound.

However, direct dynamic visualization of venous structures may be achieved using two-dimensional echocardiographic systems. With the transducer over the epigastrium, in the subxyphoid area, high quality images of the inferior vena cava, the right atrium, the interatrial septum, and the TV leaflets may be obtained [181]. The transducer can also be oriented through the long axis of the TV, revealing portions of the right atrium, tricuspid leaflets, and the right ventricle in long axis [181]. Peripheral vein injections with the appearance of contrast echoes further enhance visualization of these structures [207]. Sagittal views can also be obtained with the transducer at the cardiac apex and directed toward the right shoulder. Weinnert et al. [411], in so doing, were able to record several internal dimensions such as the long and short axes of the RV, the right atrial short axis (from the atrial septum to the right atrial free wall midway of long axis), and the right atrial long axis (from the base of the TV to the top of the right atrium).

14.1 Dilatation of the Right Atrium

14.1.1 Right Ventricular Diastolic Volume Overload (RVDVO)

Sagittal views using two-dimensional echocardiographic techniques have shown statistically significant increases in right atrial dimensions in patients with RVDVO [411].

14.1.2 Ebstein's Anomaly of the Tricuspid Valve (see 12.7.1)

Using two-dimensional echocardiography, detection in Ebstein's disease of a large RA cavity should not be difficult. However, it should be acknowledged that this cavity represents in part the "atrialized" portion of the RV. As identification of the displaced septal and enlarged anterior tricuspid leaflet is possible using two-dimensional echocardiography, the size of this atrialized right ventricle can be appreciated [294 a].

14.1.3 Atrial Tumors

The same two-dimensional echocardiographic technique should allow a clear visualization of any lesion within a dilated RA cavity. On the other hand, a right atrial tumor may be responsible for a mass of diastolic echoes within the RV, posterior to the ATVL [119, 285].

14.1.4 Tricuspid Stenosis or Atresia (see 12.4.1)

An enlarged RA cavity is an expected echocardiographic feature.

14.1.5 Tricuspid Regurgitation (see 22.1.3)

Depending on the degree of the regurgitation, RA dilatation may be documented.

15 Abnormal Left Atrial Size and Wall Motion

Index

Introduction

The left atrium can be measured along different axes: (1) an anterior-posterior axis (or Z axis) at the level of the aortic valve; (2) a superior-inferior axis (or Y axis) from the suprasternal notch; and (3) an oblique axis behind the interatrial septum [197].

When recorded from a parasternal position, or the Z axis, the LA appears echocardiographically as an echo-free space behind the AMVL, mitral ring, or aortic root. If a suprasternal transducer technique is used, the left atrium is seen posterior to the right pulmonary artery. These two transducer positions allow an evaluation of LA size according to two coordinates that are almost perpendicular to each other, the Z and Y axis respectively [118].

Assessment of LA size is routinely performed along the Z axis, or in an anterior-posterior direction. Most of the time this proves to be accurate and reproducible. However, a careful evaluation of LA dimensions should include assessment along two or three axes, as the LA may sometimes expand asymmetrically [197]. Two-dimensional echocardiography using a LV long axis cross section is then quite helpful, as it allows the entire LA cavity to be visualized.

Along the Z axis, or in an anterior-posterior direction, LA dimension is the maximal vertical distance, in mm, between the posterior surface of the posterior border of the aortic root and the anterior surface of the LA posterior wall. Measurement should be made at end-systole, when LA dimension is maximal. At least two aortic cusps within the aortic root should be visualized to ensure that the measured distance is a nearly transverse LA dimension.

Quantitative evaluation of the LA includes a determination of LA size (usually along the Z axis), and of the left atrial-aortic root ratio (LA/Ao). In addition, abnormalities in LA wall motion, including the posterior aortic wall, may be detected [372].

In this chapter anomalies characterized by abnormal LA dimensions and/or wall motion will be reviewed.

15.1 Increased Left Atrial Dimensions

The echocardiographic diagnosis of left atrial dilatation usually rests upon an abnormally elevated ratio of transverse atrial to transverse aortic root diameter [402]. Normally, this ratio is around one except in premature infants and in the immediate postnatal period, when a smaller ratio is found.

However, in anomalies involving the aortic arch or root, such as in tetrad of Fallot or in valvular aortic stenosis – conditions associated with a dilated and decreased aortic root, respectively – left atrial enlargement can only be diagnosed if left atrial dimensions exceed the normal age-related values.

15.1.1 Patent Ductus Arteriosus (PDA)

Ultrasonic diagnosis of PDA is usually based on indirect features such as LA enlargement. Contrast echocardiography may further substantiate the existence of a ductus (see 22.2.1).

Recently it has been shown that cross sectional imaging utilizing a mechanical sector scanner oriented so as to image the distal pulmonary artery and its bifurcation, can enable visualization of the PDA as a distal continuation of the pulmonary artery connected to the descending aorta [325].

An ultrasonic examination allows noninvasive follow-up of the fate of a ductal shunt [30] in either premature babies receiving indomethacin to close the ductus, or in cyanotic infants perfused with prostaglandins to maintain or improve lung perfusion through a patent ductus arteriosus (see Fig. 15.1).

15.1.2 Ventricular Septal Defect (VSD)

Left atrial dilatation is a secondary finding in children with uncomplicated VSD (or PDA), if pulmonary blood flow returning to the left side of the heart is markedly increased [83] (see Fig. 15.2).

Though an enlarged LA does not rule out an ASD, this occurrence is certainly not common [300]. In addition, the documentation of paradoxic septal motion in ASD

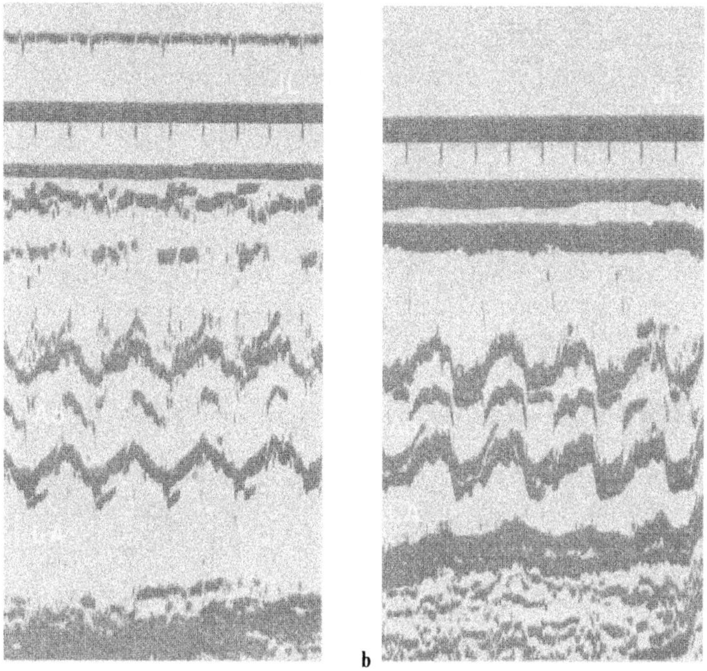

a b

Fig. 15.1 a, b. JL: Echocardiogram obtained from an infant with PDA. **a** Shows the echocardiogram before administration of indomethacine: the LA is enlarged, indicating a left-to-right shunt. **b** Shows the echocardiogram after administration of indomethacine: LA dimension has become normal

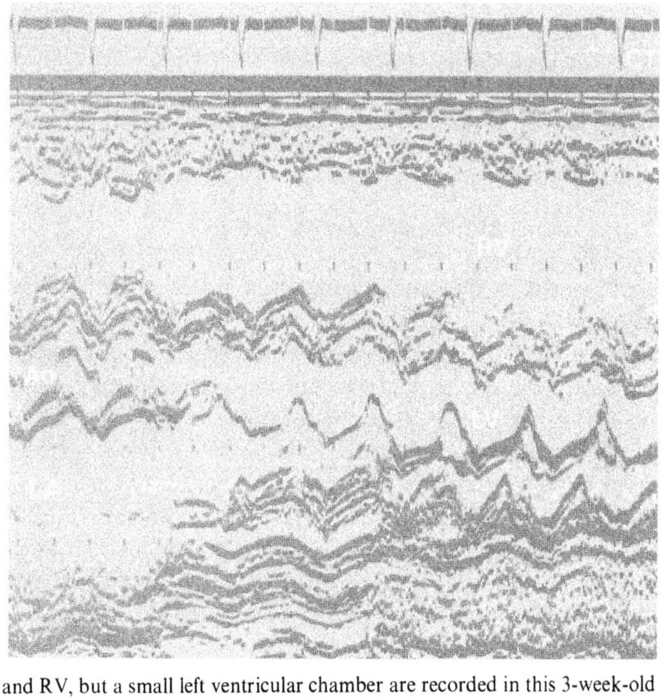

Fig. 15.2. CT: A large LA and RV, but a small left ventricular chamber are recorded in this 3-week-old infant with large left-to-right shunts at atrial, ventricular and ductal levels

should allow echocardiographic differentiation, since patients with uncomplicated VSD or PDA usually have normal septal motion.

The magnitude of a left-to-right shunt, at the ventricular or ductal levels, can be estimated echocardiographically, since there are good correlations between cineangiographically determined left atrial volumes and left atrial echo dimensions [30, 203, 436]. It is mostly to separate large from small shunts that echocardiography is useful [30, 304]. LA dimensions of 5 cm/M^2, or a LA/Ao ratio of up to 1.6 form an effective dividing line between small and large shunts [30]. Finally, large septal defects may be recognized directly by "drop-outs" in septal echoes (see Fig. 24.1)

15.1.3 Mitral Valve Regurgitation (see 13.1.2)

The importance of a mitral regurgitant jet can likewise be assessed noninvasively through the ultrasonic determination of left atrial size, as good correlations exist between this dimension and LA volumes determined cineangiocardiographically [436].

15.1.4 Increased Cardiac Output from Other Causes

LA dilatation may be a reflection of increased cardiac output, whatever its etiology, This is well illustrated by Fig. 15.3, which was obtained from a child with a markedly increased cardiac output secondary to a peripheral arteriovenous aneurysm.

15.1.5 Mitral Valve Stenosis (see 13.7.1)

15.1.6 Supravalvar Mitral Ring (see 9.8.1)

Increased left atrial size is a nonspecific finding in patients with LV inflow obstructive lesions and reflects to some extent the severity of the obstruction.

15.1.7 Diminished Left Ventricular Performance

LA enlargement is also documented in the presence of LV failure or poor LV compliance.

Therefore, it would seem impossible to echocardiographically separate infants with congestive heart failure from one another according to whether they had a large left-to-right shunt or impaired LV myocardial function secondary to hypoglycemia, sepsis, myocarditis, or hypoxemia. The LA/Ao ratio is abnormally increased in both situations. However, calculation of Vcf, or the mean velocity of circumferential fiber shortening, will allow such a separation [329]. In infants with a large left-to-right shunt, Vcf is significantly higher than in normal infants (Vcf = 2.12 $\pm$ 0.08 c/s vs. 1.51 $\pm$ 0.04 c/s) or in infants without structural heart disease but impaired LV function (VcF = 1.18 $\pm$ 0.06 c/s) [329]. Furthermore, as can be seen from Table 15.1, which is taken from Sahn et al. [329], if a distressed infant has a normal LA cavity and a normal Vcf, intrinsic pulmonary disease is more likely than myocardial failure.

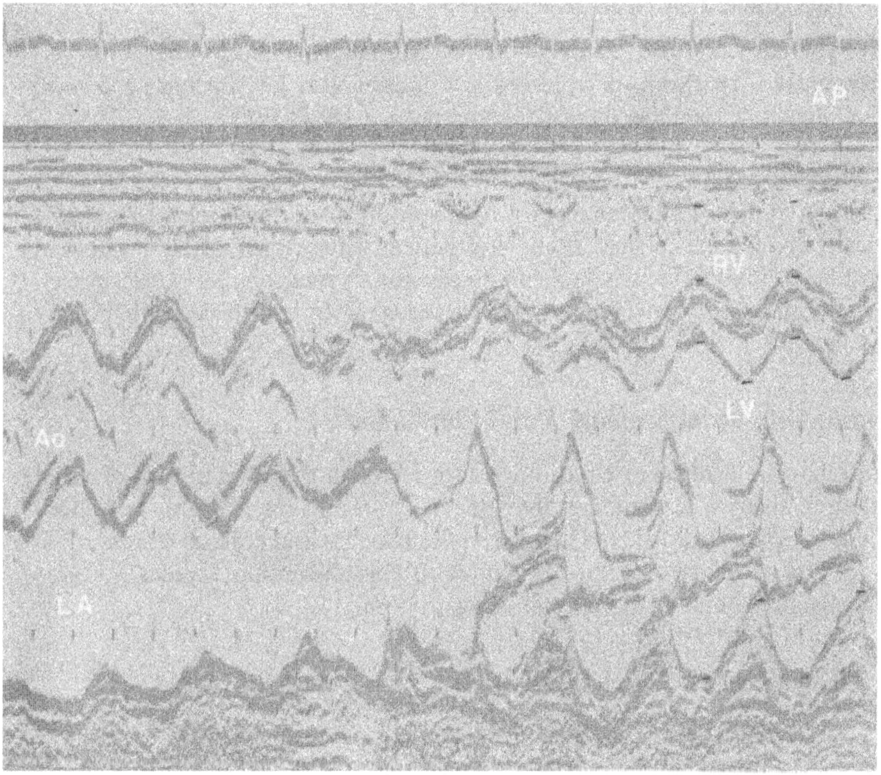

Fig. 15.3. AP: 2-year-old child with left atrial dilatation secondary to increased cardiac output (8.8 l/min), due to a peripheral AV fistula

Table 15.1. Diagnostic separation of infants in cardiorespiratory distress [329]

	LA/Ao ratio	Vcf
Normals	0.86 ± 0.10 [358]	1.51 ± 0.04 [329]
Intrinsic pulmonary disease	0.77 ± 0.01 [329]	1.51 ± 0.04 [329]
Left-to-right	1.28 ± 0.23 [358]	2.12 ± 0.08 [329]
shunt	1.14 ± 0.1 [329]	
Nonstructural heart disease	1.26 ± 0.2 [329]	1.18 ± 0.06 [329]

Comment

The difference in the reported LA/Ao ratio [329, 358] probably results from a different population. Silverman et al. [358] studied premature babies with birthweights from 700 to 2160 g., who where 1 to 35 days old at the time of the initial study, whereas Sahn et al. [329] included as normals 25 healthy prematures, 70 normal full-term infants, and 15 premature babies with respiratory distress syndrome. In addition, Sahn et al. [329] studied infants with a large left-to-right shunt whose weight ranged from 1.4 to 6.5 kg.

15.1.8 Hypoplastic Left Heart Syndrome (see 17.2.1)

In the hypoplastic left heart syndrome, left atrial enlargement may occur; however, this should not be taken to represent a well-developed LV. Recording of wall motion will show that it is the left LA and not the LV [83].

15.1.9 Systemic-to-Pulmonary Artery Anastomosis

Reitman et al. [307] have used the LA/Ao ratio to determine the patency of a surgically created left-to-right shunt in a patient with tetrad of Fallot who had undergone a Blalock-Taussig systemic-to-pulmonary anastomosis. After surgery, an increase in LA size could be documented, representing an increase in pulmonary blood flow.

Remark: Left Atrial Size and Atrial Fibrillation

LA size has been found to be an important factor in the development of atrial fibrillation and in determining the long term results of cardioversion once fibrillation has started. Patients (adults) whose LA dimension exceed 40 mm run a high risk of developing atrial fibrillation. If this dimension exceeds 45 mm, cardioversion is unlikely to maintain sinus rhythm [149].

15.2 Decreased Left Atrial Dimensions

15.2.1 Hypoplastic Left Heart Syndrome (see 17.2.1)

Although the left atrium is enlarged, in most infants with hypoplastic left heart syndrome, the LA cavity is small (15.1.8).

15.2.2 Total Anomalous Pulmonary Venous Return (see 8.3.3)

In this condition the LA is usually small because of a diminished inflow of blood into it [114, 140].

15.2.3 Extrinsic Compression of the Left Atrium

An extracardiac tumor, for instance in the mediastinum, may occasionally compress the left atrium and reduce its size.

15.2.4 After a Valsalva's Maneuver

In a recent echocardiographic study it was found that normal subjects submitted to Valsalva's maneuver decreased their LA dimension by an average of 30%. This normal response was found to be diminished or absent in severe congestive heart failure [311].

15.3 Increased Left Atrial Wall Motion

15.3.1 Mitral Valve Regurgitation (see 13.1.2) (see Fig. 15.4)

15.3.2 Increased Mitral Valve Flow Due to Left-to-Right Shunt

Exaggerated atrial wall motion, posteriorly during systole and in the opposite direction during ventricular filling, along with left atrial dilatation, is usually documented in the presence of increased flow through the MV (see Fig. 15.5).

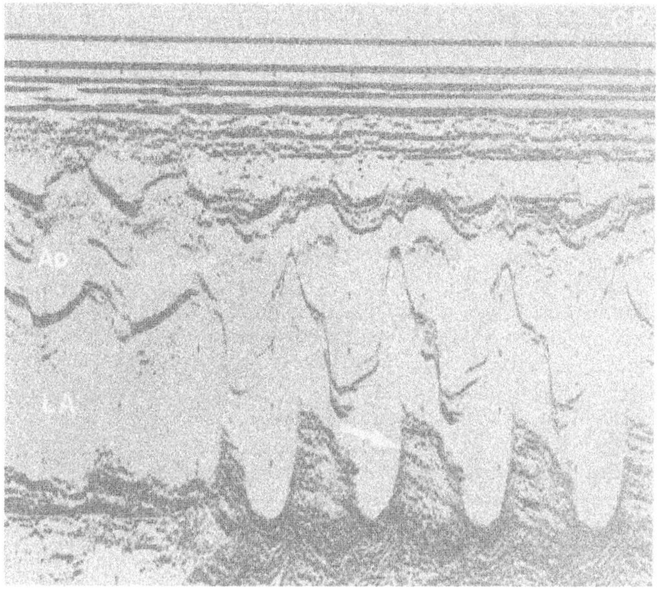

Fig. 15.4. CP: Vigorous LA contractions (*arrow*), and LA dilatation are documented in this 8-year-old girl with MV regurgitation

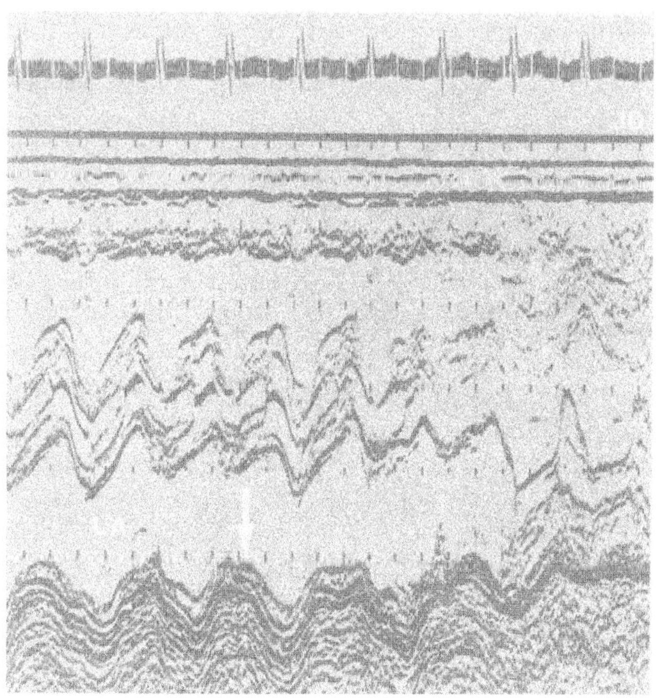

Fig. 15.5. JD: A slightly enlarged LA with vigorous contractions of its posterior wall (*arrow*); is recorded in this 6-week-old baby with left-to-right shunts at atrial, ventricular and ductal levels

16 Abnormal Right Ventricular Size and Wall Thickness

Index

Introduction

The RV is the first cardiac structure encountered by the ultrasonic beam in a standard echocardiographic examination. Both the inflow and outflow portions of the RV can be visualized, located anterior to the LV and to the aortic root, respectively [431].

Quantitative evaluation of the RV proves less satisfactory echocardiographically than that of the LV because of the flattened shape of the RV in the anterior-posterior dimension. However, information which can be derived to assess the RV is both anatomic and functional. Anatomic information includes the determination of RV dimensions; functional assessment is through the study of systolic time intervals including the right ventricular isovolumic contraction time (ICT).

Right Ventricular Dimensions

This represents the anterior-posterior distance, in mm, at end-diastole, between the RV anterior wall endocardial surface and the right septal surface. In general, this dimension is appreciated at the same transducer location as the LV internal dimension. As can be judged from reported values (see Appendix, p. 207), great variations exist within the same age groups. This variability is inherent to the RV shape and position as it is seen in an anterior-posterior direction. It is, therefore, more meaningful to follow serial measurements of RV dimension in the same patient rather than comparing RV dimensions among infants or children of the same age groups [431].

For the same reason, estimates of RV output, stroke volume, or ejection fraction are subject to error.

Right Ventricular Anterior Wall Thickness

This represents the shortest observed vertical distance, in mm, between the endo- and epicardial surface of the RV anterior wall at end-diastole. This is a difficult measure to make reliably because of problems involved in properly identifying these surfaces (see Appendix, p. 207).

Systolic Time Intervals

Noninvasive assessment of RV function using echocardiographically determined systolic time intervals (STI) has become a well-accepted procedure (see Chap. 23).

In this chapter, the most frequent causes of abnormal RV dimensions and anterior wall thickness will be reviewed.

16.1 Increased Right Ventricular Dimensions

16.1.1 Right Ventricular Dilatation Secondary to Diastolic Volume Overload (see Fig. 16.1 and Sects. 21.1.1 to 21.1.8)

16.1.2 Absence of Pericardium (see 21.1.11)

16.1.3 Right Ventricular Tumor (see 9.5.1)

16.1.4 Hypoplastic Left Heart Syndrome (see 17.2.1)

16.1.5 Ebstein's Anomaly of the Tricuspid Valve (see 12.7.1)

In this anomaly the RV proper is not dilated but there is a large anterior chamber which represents the "atrialized" portion of the RV (see Fig. 12.2).

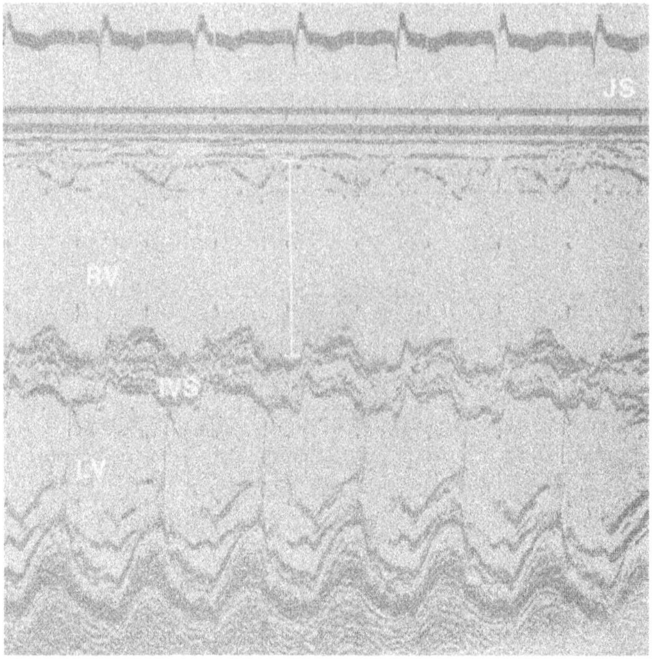

Fig. 16.1. JS: Echocardiogram obtained from a 6-year-old boy with secundum ASD. Note the dilatation of the RV, and an abnormal septal movement not completely paradoxial

16.1.6 Transposition of the Great Arteries (see 3.1.1)

RV end-diastolic dimensions are strikingly larger than normal in patients with TGA; a further increase follows a Mustard's operation [278]. To the contrary, LV dimensions are usually reduced.

16.1.7 Miscellaneous

RV dilatation may be a nonspecific finding in a variety of lesions, either acquired or congenital such as pulmonary hypertension, RV failure, myocarditis, persistent truncus arteriosus, etc. Most of these entities have specific and/or suggestive ultrasonic features.

In infants suffering from coarctation of the aorta, RV dimension is significantly greater than normal, becoming normal with increasing age [433].

16.2 Decreased Right Ventricular Dimensions

16.2.1 Pulmonary Atresia with Intact IVS

Although no definite ultrasonic features exist, pulmonary atresia with intact IVS should be suspected in a cyanotic child in whom an echocardiographic examination fails to detect pulmonary valve echoes in association with a diminutive RV, usually not exceeding in a neonate, 6 mm in its ultrasonic dimension [117]. The LV is usually dilated (see Fig. 16.2).

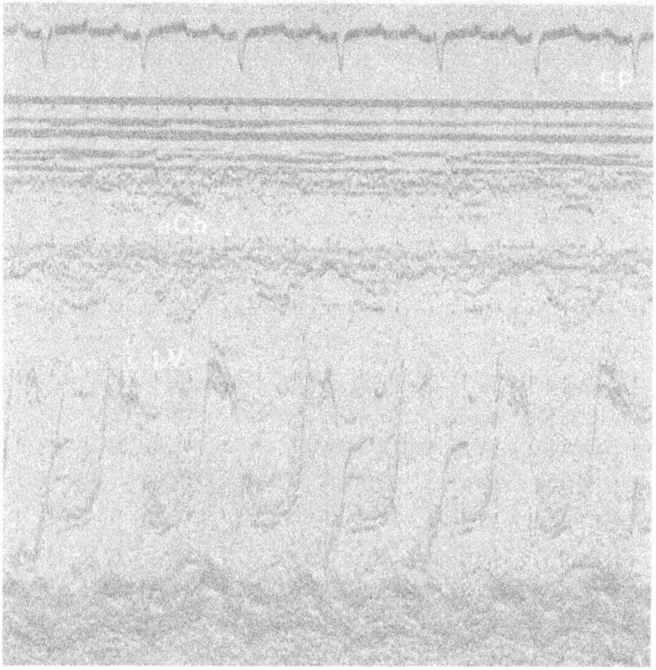

Fig. 16.2. EP: Echocardiogram obtained from a 9-year-old boy with pulmonary atresia and intact IVS. The anterior chamber is diminutive and the LV dilated

16.2.2 Tricuspid Atresia (see 7.1.3)

In a similar fashion, tricuspid atresia should be suspected in a cyanotic child in whom an echocardiographic examination fails to detect TV echoes in association with a diminutive RV, usually not exceeding in a neonate, 3 mm in its ultrasonic dimension [117]. The LV is usually dilated.

16.2.3 Cardiac Tamponade

Patients with pericardial effusion and tamponade demonstrate abnormally small right ventricles, as measured along the minor axis, at end-diastole, at end-expiration [340] (see Fig. 16.3).

Ventricular dimensional changes are specific for tamponade [340].

With Respiration

RV end-inspiratory dimensions in tamponade get larger, often becoming normal.

With the Direction of the Ultrasonic Beam

RV end-diastolic dimension is increased if the transducer is swept toward the outflow tract, but is still generally less at this level in patients with tamponade than in normal subjects. Other ultrasonic features have been described in cardiac tamponade, but are not specific for this condition [340, 346]. These are the following:

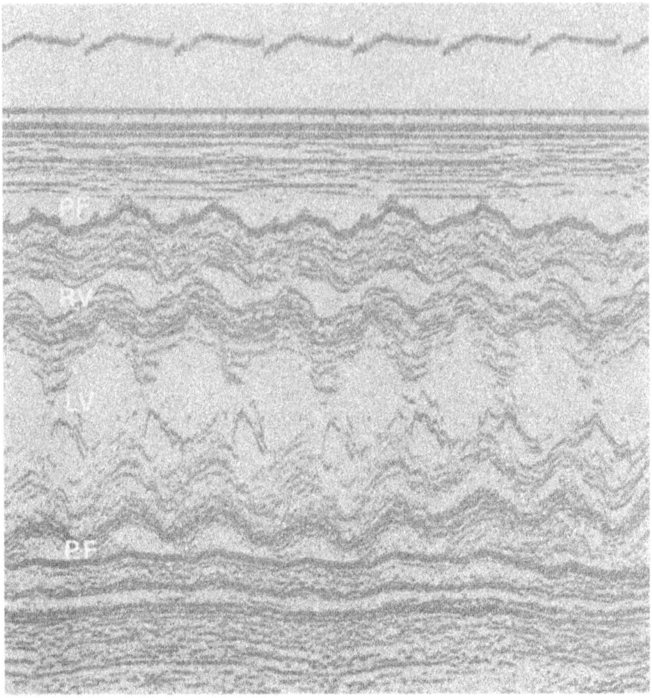

Fig. 16.3. Same patient as in Fig. 13.3. Pericardial tamponade is evidenced on this echo-trace by a marked reduction in size of a previously quite enlarged RV (see Fig. 13.9)

1) Changes in mitral valve motion, i.e., E–F_0 slope and D–E excursion,
2) Reciprocal respiratory variations in right and left ventricular end-diastolic dimensions. These variations should be pronounced knowing that a majority of normal children have augmentation of RV dimensions and diminution of LV diameter during inspiration [234].
3) A small cavity, with the LV end-diastolic diameter along the minor or anterior-posterior axis, at end-expiration, being at or just below normal limits [340].
4) A swinging or pendular motion of the whole heart within the pericardial sac. This is best visualized by real-time two-dimensional imaging.

16.2.4 Mediastinal Tumor

Compression of the heart and of the superior mediastinum by a tumor may mimic cardiac tamponade with a diminutive RV and prominent respiratory variations in the dimensions of the two ventricles [43].

A correct diagnosis should not be difficult, as an abnormal band of echoes originating from the tumor will be seen to occupy a space between the anterior chest wall and the RV wall.

16.2.5 Volume Depletion

RV narrowing may also appear with volume depletion, as in marked dehydration and blood loss [340]. Adequacy of fluid therapy can be monitored by the progressive increase in RV dimensions.

16.2.6 Marked Right Ventricular Hypertrophy

RV cavity narrowing can also be documented in the presence of marked hypertrophy of the RV anterior wall and/or of the IVS. However, RV narrowing in these cases occurs in systole only (see Fig. 16.4).

16.3 Increased Right Ventricular Anterior Wall Thickness

This is a nonspecific feature and may be documented in the following.

16.3.1 Obstructive Lesions to Normal Egression of Blood from the Right Ventricle (see Fig. 16.5)

16.3.2 Pulmonary Hypertension, Primary or Secondary (see 10.5.2)

16.3.3 Transposition Complexes with the Aorta Connected to the Anterior Ventricle

16.3.4 Infiltrative Cardiomyopathies (see Fig. 20.4)

16.3.5 Infants of Diabetic Mothers

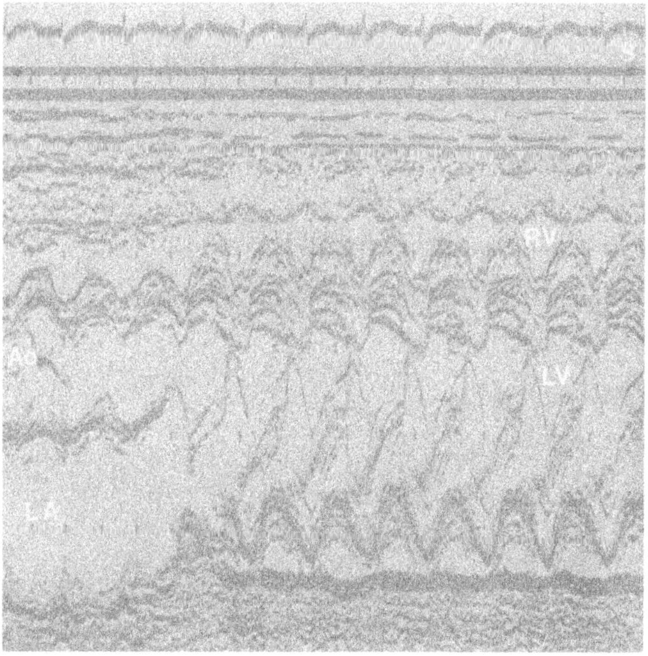

Fig. 16.4. S: A small right ventricular chamber is documented in this 8-month-old child, 2 weeks after pulmonary valvulectomy for severe stenosis. RV hypertrophy is still present. There is also some pericardial effusion. Note the abnormal septal motion following surgery

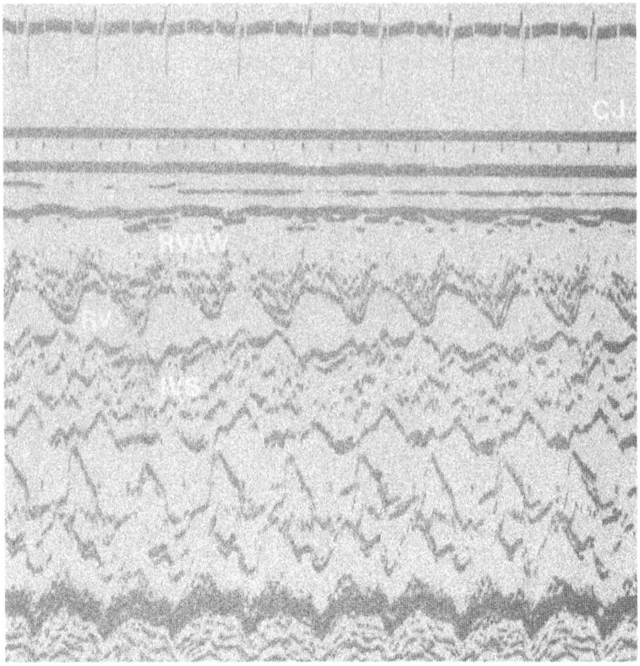

Fig. 16.5. CJ: This echo-trace showing RVH, and resulting in disproportionate septal thickening was obtained in a neonate with severe valvular pulmonic stenosis with a gradient of 80 mm Hg

16.4 Decreased Right Ventricular Wall Thickness

An abnormally thin right ventricular wall should suggest one of the following:

16.4.1 Uhl's Anomaly (see 10.1.2)

16.4.2 Ebstein's Anomaly (see 12.7.1)

In this anomaly measured anterior wall thickness represents the "atrialized" portion of the right ventricular wall.

16.4.3 Myocarditis

17 Abnormal Left Ventricular Size and Wall Motion

Index

Introduction

The Left Ventricle

The LV lends itself well to echocardiographic examination, using either conventional or two-dimensional ultrasonic systems.

Using conventional M-mode echocardiographic systems, the transducer is placed in the standard position on the chest wall and rotated slowly and uniformly from the aortic root to the LV apex. Several echo scans from different locations on the left precordium may be needed to correctly evaluate spatial relationships of LV structures.

There is no doubt that two-dimensional real-time systems can give this information more directly by displaying the motion of all echo signals of an entire cardiac cross section in their correct anatomic orientation.

However, M-mode echocardiography is generally preferred for the study of cavity size (diameter and volume) and wall thickness, essentially because of the availability of a strip chart recorder.

Left ventricular internal dimension (LVID) measured at the level of the chordae tendineae in adults and at the level of the posterior MV leaflet in children, is defined as the distance between the left septal surface and the posterior endocardial surface along the transverse plane. This distance is measured at end-diastole ($LVID_d$) and at end-systole ($LVID_s$). Normal age-related values for LVID, selected by Williams and Tucker [431] from a compilation of data, are listed in the Appendix (p. 207–208).

Gutgesell et al. [135] showed that the $LVID_d$ increases by about threefold during childhood and that this dimension correlates best with the logarithm of body weight ($r = 0.95$) and of body surface area ($r = 0.96$). The $LVID_d$ is thus proportionally greater in newborns than in adolescents or adults.

LV dimensions normally change with respiration: Meyer et al. [234] found an inspiratory diminution of LV dimensions, with inspiratory augmentation of RV dimensions, in the majority of normal children.

According to Feigenbaum [98], differences in LV internal dimension with respiration should not exceed 2 to 3 mm.

The Left Ventricular Outflow Tract

The LVOT is the area of the LV between the IVS and the AMVL; its width, measured between the C point of the MV echogram and the posterior aspect of the septum, ranges in the adult from 20 to 34 mm [315]. Normal values in children have not been published. However, it seems justified to relate the LVOT to the aorta and consider it to be narrowed or dilated if its dimension is smaller than or exceeds normal aortic width.

In this chapter, conditions or anomalies known to affect LV dimensions (cavity and/or LVOT) and/or amplitude of wall motion will be reviewed.

17.1 Increased Left Ventricular Dimensions

17.1.1 Left Ventricular Volume Overload

This can be documented in left to right cardiovascular shunts such as (a) ventricular septal defect (see 15.1.2) and (b) patent ductus arteriosus (see 15.1.1) as well as in valvular regurgitation such as (a) aortic regurgitation (see 11.8.2) and (b) mitral regurgitation (see 13.1.2). Regurgitation may be congenital or acquired (rheumatic heart disease, endocarditis, MV prolapse, etc.).

17.1.2 Dilated Cardiomyopathy

This can be documented in primary cardiomyopathy (see 13.2.3) and in cardiomyopathy secondary to (a) coronary artery disease, (b) aortic valve disease (see 23.3.1), (c) hypertensive heart disease, and (d) congestive heart failure from other causes (see 13.3.1).

17.1.3 Right Heart Hypoplasia

A dilated LV cavity is usually documented in patients with tricuspid atresia [135, 235, 350] (see 7.1.3) and pulmonary atresia with intact septum (see 16.2.1).

17.1.4 Resulting from Training

Enhanced training in athletes is accompanied by increases in both LV dimensions and mass as well as in LV shortening fraction and contraction velocity [8, 215].

17.2 Decreased Left Ventricular Dimensions

17.2.1 Hypoplastic Left Heart Syndrome

This syndrome includes varying degrees of underdevelopment of the left side of the heart. The anomalies include poorly developed left heart chambers, stenosis or atresia of the aortic and/or mitral orifices, and hypoplasia of the ascending aorta. If both valves are atretic, a LV cavity may not be found.

In the more severe form of the syndrome, the following echocardiographic features will be documented [83] (see Fig. 17.1):

1) Small LV cavity, with an end-diastolic dimension not exceeding 9 [95] to 11 mm [33, 117] in diameter,
2) Small to absent aortic root, not exceeding 5 [33] to 6 mm [95] in diameter,
3) Essentially one recordable AV valve, the tricuspid; the MV echo is grossly distorted (sometimes with multiple echoes) or absent [33],
4) LA usually small but sometimes dilated,
5) Enlarged RV chamber [235, 236], or a ratio of left ventricular to right ventricular end-diastolic dimension of under 0.6 [33, 95],
6) Increased pulmonary root diameter [431].

Two-dimensional echocardiography lends itself well to the diagnosis of hypoplastic left heart syndrome: a longitudinal echocardiographic cross section through the long axis of the heart will reveal a rudimentary LV chamber, without definite mitral or aortic valve motion (see Fig. 17.2).

17.2.2 Heart Tumors

Left heart tumors (see 9.2.1) can rarely fill the LV cavity, and give the impression of an hypoplastic left ventricle [118].

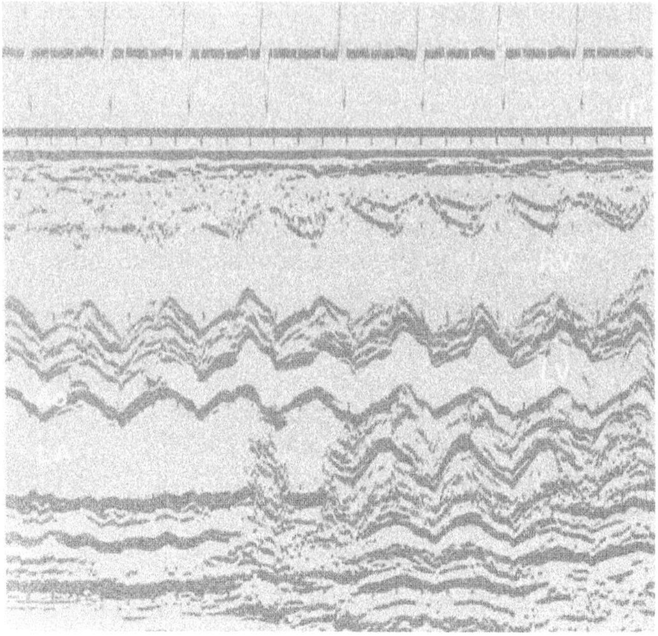

Fig. 17.1. JP: M-mode scan obtained from a 10-day-old infant with left heart hypoplasia. Note the absence of a well-identifiable MV. The exact diameter of the aorta is difficult to assess but the AoV shows a very small excursion. The child died some days later

Right heart tumors (see 9.5.1) such as a right ventricular tumor may displace the IVS posteriorly, compressing the LV to half its normal size [6].

In addition, it should be noted that in patients with severe aortic stenosis or coarctation of the aorta, concentric LV hypertrophy may give the impression of a small LV cavity. Sometimes, the LV may be difficult to find, especially if the right heart is severely dilated such as in an Ebstein's anomaly.

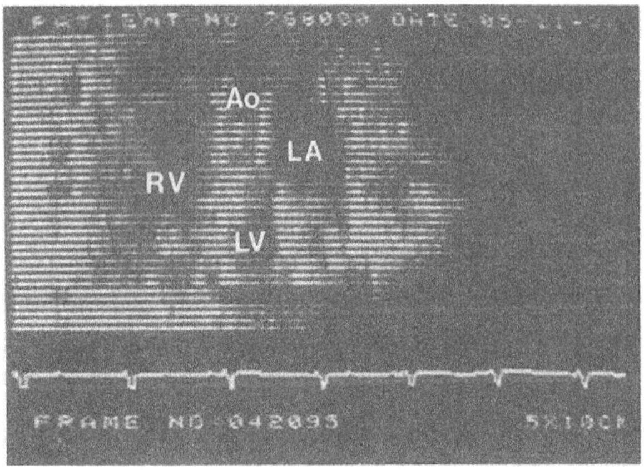

Fig. 17.2. Two-dimensional frame obtained from a neonate with a hypoplastic left heart syndrome. No MV motion could be visualized and the LV is diminutive. The left atrium, to the contrary, is enlarged

17.2.3 Valsalva's Maneuver

In a recent echocardiographic study it was found that normal subjects, submitted to Valsalva's maneuver, show a decrease in LV end-diastolic and end-systolic dimensions of 11.2% and 9.5%, respectively [311].

In this same study, LA dimensions decreased by 30%.

17.2.4 Transposition of the Great Arteries (see 3.1.1)

Most patients with d-TGA have LV end-diastolic dimensions below normal preoperatively, with a further reduction in this diameter after a Mustard's operation [278] (see Fig. 17.3).

In contrast, as seen in 16.1.6, RV end-diastolic dimensions are increased [278]. A linear relationship can be demonstrated between the ratio of $LVID_d/RVID_d$ and the ratio of peak systolic pressures in the left and right ventricles both before and after a Mustard's operation [278].

17.2.5 Total Anomalous Pulmonary Venous Return (see 8.3.3)

In this condition, the left heart chambers are usually small because of diminished blood flow to the left heart [140] (see Fig. 17.4).

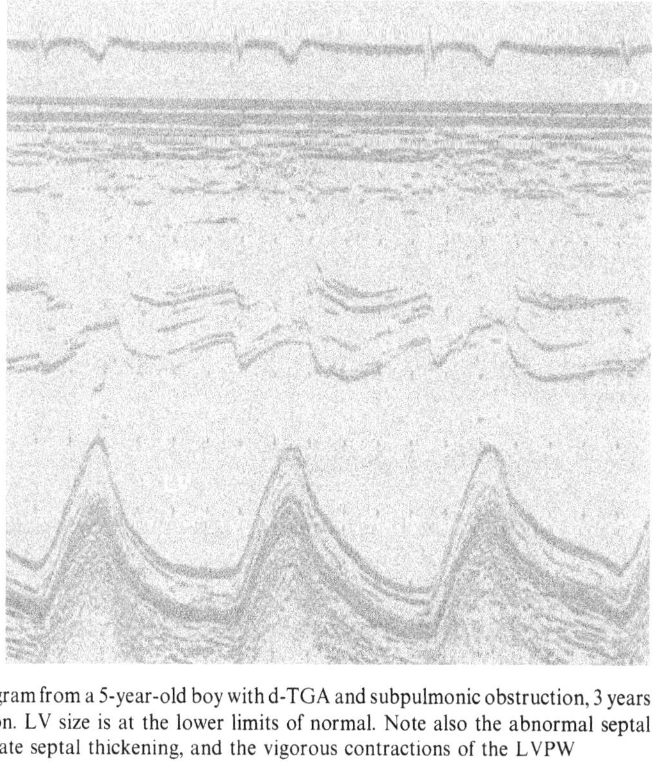

Fig. 17.3. VD: Echocardiogram from a 5-year-old boy with d-TGA and subpulmonic obstruction, 3 years after a Mustard's operation. LV size is at the lower limits of normal. Note also the abnormal septal motion, the disproportionate septal thickening, and the vigorous contractions of the LVPW

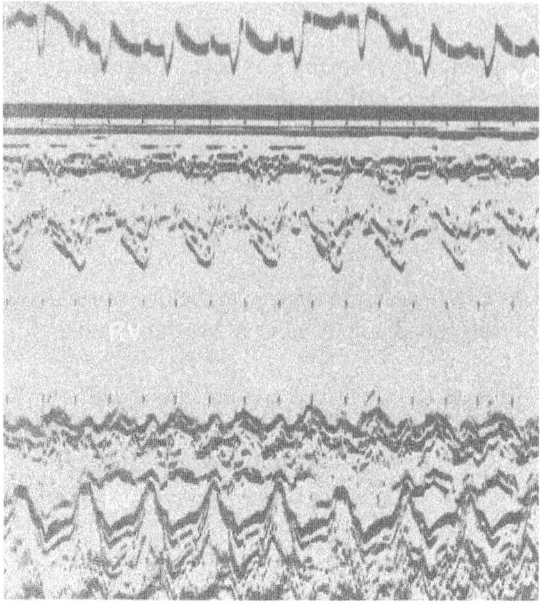

Fig. 17.4. PC: This echocardiogram obtained from a cyanotic neonate shows a dilated RV, paradoxical septal motion and a diminutive LV chamber. These findings suggest total anomalous pulmonary venous drainage. The diagnosis was confirmed at autopsy

17.2.6 Coarctation of the Aorta (see 19.2.4)

In infants suffering from coarctation of the aorta, LV diastolic dimension is significantly decreased. Gradually, however, this dimension will become normal with age [433].

17.3 Increased LVOT Dimensions

17.3.1 Aortic Valve Stenosis (see 11.5.1)

17.3.2 Aortic Valve Regurgitation (see 11.8.2)

17.3.3 Dilated Cardiomyopathy [314] (see 13.2.3)

17.3.4 Coronary Artery Disease [315]

17.4 Decreased LVOT Dimensions

A narrow LVOT may result from an obstruction to the egression of blood to the aorta (17.4.1, 17.4.3 to 17.4.5) or to the pulmonary artery (if TGA is present) (17.4.2).

17.4.1 Left Ventricular Obstructive Lesions to the Aorta

A narrow LVOT can be documented in the following:
1) Long segment subvalvar aortic stenosis, in which the obstruction is present throughout the cardiac cycle [219] (see 13.12.2, Table 13.1).

2) IHSS [289, 314] (see 20.1.1). Here the obstruction is dynamic and present during systole only.
3) Some forms of congenital aortic stenosis [362] (see 19.2.3).
4) Some VSDs [256]: subaortic stenosis may rarely accompany a VSD's, either below or above the level of the defect. Diagnosis of the subaortic obstruction is difficult and requires left heart catheterization. Echocardiography should enable noninvasive diagnosis by the demonstration of a narrowed LVOT and/or the demonstration of an abnormal aortic valve echogram.
5) Some heart tumors when they arise from the IVS [275].

17.4.2 Left Ventricular Obstructive Lesions to the Pulmonary Artery

Subpulmonary obstruction in d-TGA can result from a variety of causes and is most often located at the subvalvular level. Diagnosis of obstruction at this level can be made echocardiographically through the documentation of the following suggestive features [141, 265] (see Fig. 17.5):
1) The finding of an anterior root medially situated and a posterior root with a diameter of less than 75% of the anterior root [265].
2) Prolonged apposition of the MV with the IVS,
3) SAM of the AMVL,
4) Early closure and systolic fluttering of the pulmonary valve leaflets, and

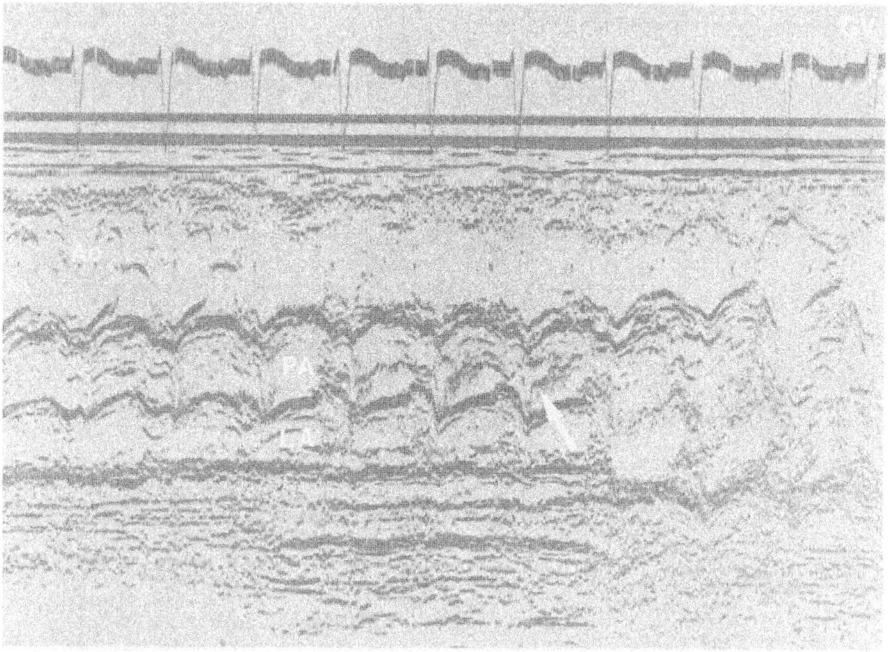

Fig. 17.5. GV: Echocardiogram obtained from a 3-month-old baby with d-TGA and subvalvular pulmonic stenosis. Both great arteries are visualized simultaneously. Note that the PA is smaller than the Ao. In addition, there is a premature PV closure and coarse fluttering of the leaflets *(arrow)*; all these features are diagnostic of subvalvular stenosis

5) Presence of multiple, fragmentary, posteriorly convex echoes in the LVOTof patients in whom the obstruction is caused by an aneurysm of the membranous ventricular septum [399].

To differentiate systolic, dynamic obstruction from a more severe anatomically fixed outflow tract stenosis, LVOT diameter and the LVOT/PA ratio must be studied. LVOT diameter corresponds to the anteroposterior dimension between the closure point on the MV below the pulmonary arterial root and the left endocardial surface of the IVS. In dynamic obstruction, the LVOT will be seen to be narrowed during systole only, whereas in fixed stenosis, narrowing of the LVOT persists throughout the cardiac cycle [18].

A small LVOT has also been described in d-TGA after a Rastelli's operation [312].

17.4.3 Ostium Primum Septal Defect (see 21.1.2)

The narrowed LVOT [257, 287] is here the echocardiographic equivalent of the angiographic appearance of a "gooseneck" deformity (see Fig. 17.6).

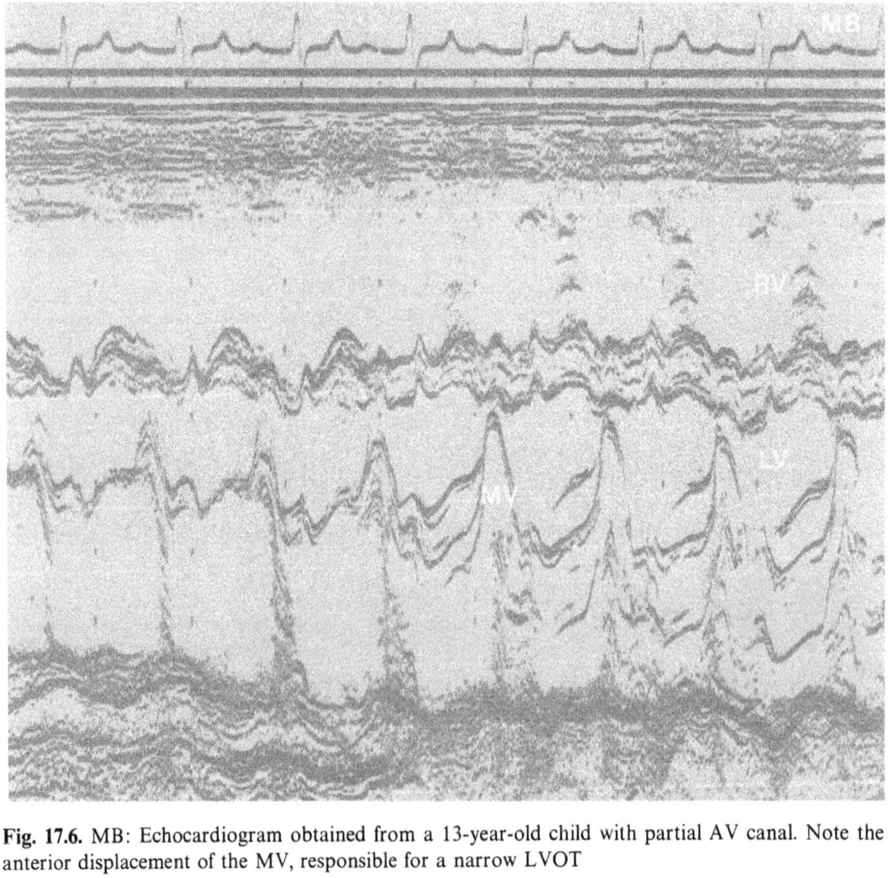

Fig. 17.6. MB: Echocardiogram obtained from a 13-year-old child with partial AV canal. Note the anterior displacement of the MV, responsible for a narrow LVOT

17.4.4 Pulmonary Artery Hypertension (see 10.5.2)

Prolonged apposition of the AMVL with the IVS has been described in patients with pulmonary artery hypertension. It then represents a nonspecific finding probably related to small LV dimensions.

17.4.5 In Some Acquired Cardiac Disorders

A narrow LVOT has been described in (1) some cardiomyopathies, including Pompe's disease, where anatomic ventricular outflow tract obstruction can develop secondary to myocardial hypertrophy [104], (2) in some patients with MV stenosis [315]; (3) in aortic valve vegetations [431] (see 9.3.4, (see Fig. 9.4 b) and (4) in aortic cusp prolapse [431] (see 9.3.3). In AoV vegetation and aortic cusp prolapse, narrowing of the LVOT occurs most often during diastole only.

17.5 Increased Wall Motion

LV posterior wall motion usually exceeds in amplitude the interventricular septal motion, which should have at least two-thirds of the excursion of the LVPW [315].

The interventricular septal motion is considered exaggerated when its excursion exceeds 10 mm [315].

Increased wall motion may result from the following:

17.5.1 Left Ventricular Volume Overload

LV volume overload can occur due to (a) forward flow, as in VSD and PDA; or (b) retrograde flow, as in aortic and mitral regurgitation.

17.5.2 Hyperkinetic Heart Syndrome

17.5.3 Overcompensation for Dyskinesia Elsewhere

The interventricular septal or LV posterior wall motion may be exaggerated as an overcompensation for dyskinetic segments elsewhere. This is well illustrated by Fig. 17.3, which was obtained from a 5-year-old child with d-TGA and subpulmonic obstruction. The child had undergone a Mustard's operation 3 years earlier, but a subpulmonic gradient of 50 mm Hg persisted. Septal motion is abnormal and practically nonexistent, whereas the LVPW contracts vigorously.

17.6 Decreased Wall Motion

Motion of the LVPW and the IVS is considered reduced when the excursion is less than 8 and 5 mm, respectively [315]. Decreased wall motion may be documented in the following:

17.6.1 Coronary Artery Disease

17.6.2 Congestive Heart Failure (see 13.3.1)

17.6.3 Myocardiopathies (see 13.2.3)

18 Abnormal Dimension of the Pulmonary Artery

Index

Introduction

The normally positioned PA is usually not well accessible to echocardiographic examination, except in infants and in older patients with PA dilatation, in whom both borders of the pulmonary root, at valvular level, may be seen [431] (see Fig. 18.1). Difficulties in defining PA dimensions are inherent to the normal posterior sweep of the main PA, which is oriented almost perpendicular to the chest wall. Only with the transducer in the suprasternal notch position [7] does it become easier to determine the normal width of the right PA. Normal age-related values for PA dimensions, determined at end-systole, can be found in the Appendix, p. 206. It should be noted that the pulmonary ostium is normally slightly larger than the aortic ostium, not only in infancy [136, 360], but in childhood as well [232].

The abnormally positioned pulmonary artery is often far easier to record. In d-TGA, for instance, the exact width of the PA can be determined (see Fig. 3.3). Abnormalities such as poststenotic dilatation or hypoplasia can also be recognized.

In this chapter, abnormalities characterized by an abnormal pulmonary root diameter and amenable to echocardiographic diagnosis, will be presented briefly.

18.1 Increased Pulmonary Artery Dimensions

18.1.1 Hypoplastic Left Heart Syndrome (see 17.2.1)

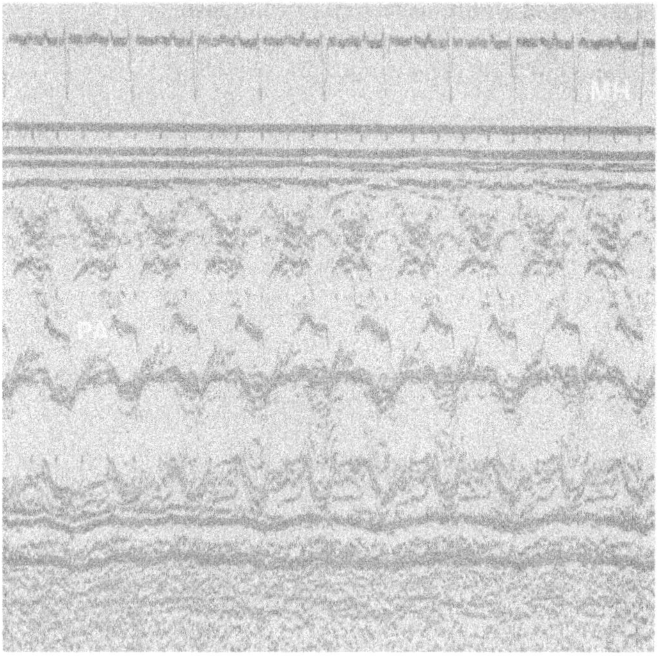

Fig. 18.1. MH: In some patients it is possible to record rather clearly both walls of the PA. This recording was made in a 2-month-old baby with coarctation of the aorta, PDA, and pulmonary artery hypertension. Pulmonary valve motion is abnormal and suggests pulmonary hypertension

18.1.2 Pulmonary Artery Hypertension (see 10.5.2)

18.1.3 Pulmonary Valve Stenosis (see 10.1.1)

18.1.4 Increased Pulmonary Blood Flow

If blood flow to the lungs is increased, such as in ASD or VSD, the pulmonary artery may dilate and its wall become accessible to ultrasound (see Fig. 18.1).

18.1.5 Idiopathic Dilatation of the Pulmonary Artery

The following ultrasonic features are expected in idiopathic dilatation of the pulmonary artery: (1) PA dilatation [421]; (2) normal echo pattern of pulmonary valve motion [421]; (3) right ventricular dilatation; (4) paradoxic septal motion; and (5) diastolic fluttering of the ATVL and/or of the IVS due to the regurgitant jet.

18.1.6 Congenital Absence of the Pulmonary Valve

The following ultrasonic features are expected in children with congenital absence of the pulmonary valve: (1) PA dilatation [421]; (2) absent PV echoes; (3) systolic expansion of the PA; (4) RV dilatation; and (5) paradoxic septal motion.

18.2 Decreased Pulmonary Artery Dimensions

18.2.1 Tetrad of Fallot (see 4.1.2)

18.2.2 Hypoplastic Right Heart Syndrome (see under Tricuspid Atresia) (7.1.3)

18.2.3 d-TGA with Subpulmonic Obstruction (see 17.4.2)

19 Abnormal Dimension of the Aorta

Index

Introduction

As seen in Chap. 11, the aorta is a stable intracardiac landmark represented by two dense parallel echoes separated by an echo-free space. These echoes are in continuity with the IVS anteriorly and the AMVL posteriorly.

The width of the echo-free space, at the level of the aortic cusps, with the transducer in the standard position, represents the aortic diameter at valvular level. This diameter does not change significantly throughout the cardiac cycle, so that reported values, which are not always obtained during the same portion of the cardiac cycle, may be compared to each other. Normal age-related values are given in the Appendix, p. 210.

This chapter will review conditions likely to be associated with an abnormal aortic width, either at the valvular level or distal to it.

19.1 Increased Aortic Dimensions

19.1.1 Marfan's Syndrome

Marfan's syndrome is a generalized connective tissue disorder affecting predominantly the eye, the skeletal and the cardiovascular systems. Important hemodynamic manifestations of the syndrome are (1) aortic regurgitation and/or dissection secondary to aortic root dilatation and (2) mitral regurgitation secondary to MV prolapse (see Fig. 19.1).

These complications may be responsible for the following echocardiographic features [36, 364]: (1) aortic root dilatation; (2) duplication of aortic wall echoes; (3) MV prolapse; and (4) flail posterior MV leaflet.

In addition, ultrasonic features commonly observed in patients with aortic and mitral regurgitation are also documented (see 11.8.2 and 13.1.2).

19.1.2 First Degree Relatives of Patients with Marfan's Syndrome

Aortic root dilatation can be documented in up to 18% of first degree relatives of patients with Marfan's syndrome [281].

19.1.3 Annulo-Aortic Ectasia (see 11.1.2)

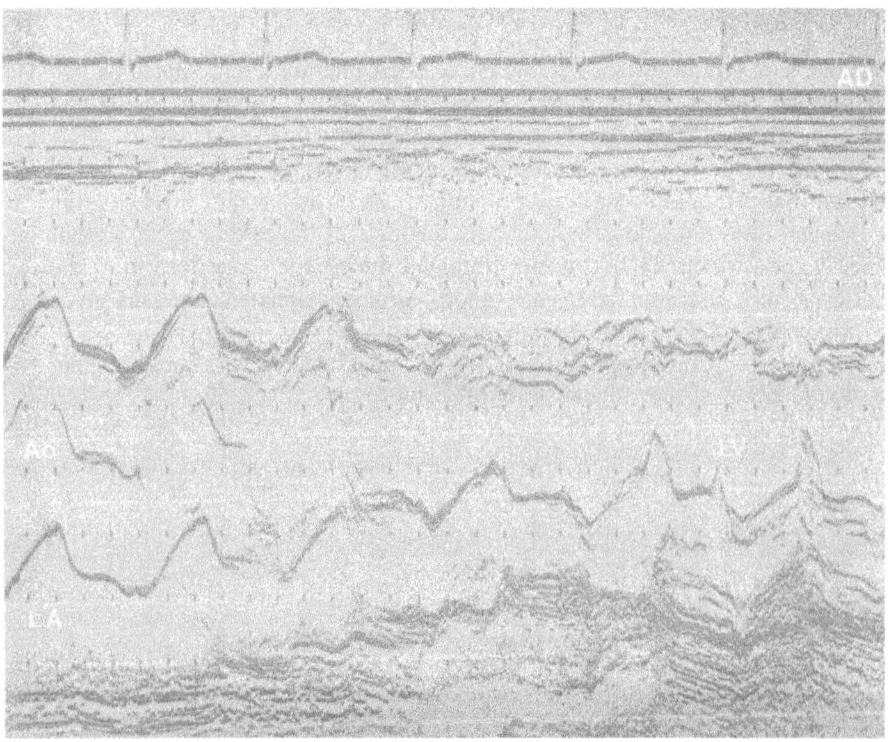

Fig. 19.1. AD: Echocardiogram obtained from a 14-year-old boy with a pseudo-Marfan's syndrome. Note the increased diameter of the aorta

19.1.4 Minor Musculoskeletal Anomalies

A majority of children with minor musculoskeletal abnormalities, such as pectus excavatum and arachnodactyly, have marked increases in aortic root dimension [331]; these children also have documented MV prolapse [331].

19.1.5 Mitral Valve Prolapse (see 13.11.1)

In an echocardiographic study of MV prolapse in children, 22 out of 26 were found to have a biconvex enlargement of the aortic sinuses of Valsalva and a significant increase in the diameter of the aortic root [331].

19.1.6 Aneurysm of the Ascending Aorta

Dissecting aneurysm of the ascending aorta may be observed in patients with Marfan's syndrome. Echocardiographically, this abnormality is characterized by a duplication of the echoes of one or both aortic walls and dilatation of the ascending aorta [251].

19.1.7 Aneurysm of the Right Aortic Sinus (see 9.3.5)

19.1.8 Valvular Aortic Stenosis (see 24.3.3)

The ascending aorta may be secondarily dilated in the presence of severe valvular aortic stenosis.

19.1.9 Discrete Subvalvar Aortic Stenosis (see 11.2.1)

19.1.10 Aortic Regurgitation (see 11.8.2)

19.1.11 Tetrad of Fallot (see 4.1.2)

In tetrad of Fallot, the aorta is usually large. Morris et al. [253] reported such a finding in 24 out of 25 patients. Aortic root dilatation becomes less striking, however, with advancing age.

19.2 Decreased Aortic Dimensions

A small hypoplastic aorta may be part of the hypoplastic left heart syndrome, or may represent an extreme form of supravalvar aortic stenosis.

19.2.1 Aortic Hypoplasia or Atresia (see Fig. 19.2)

A hypoplastic aorta may be part of the hypoplastic left heart syndrome (see 17.2.1). In this situation, the AoV is also hypoplastic, with diminished or absent aortic cusp motion

19.2.2 Supravalvar Aortic Stenosis

Supravalvar aortic stenosis may assume three forms [268, 395]: (1) the typical anatomic hourglass deformity, or localized narrowing of the ascending aorta; (2) the

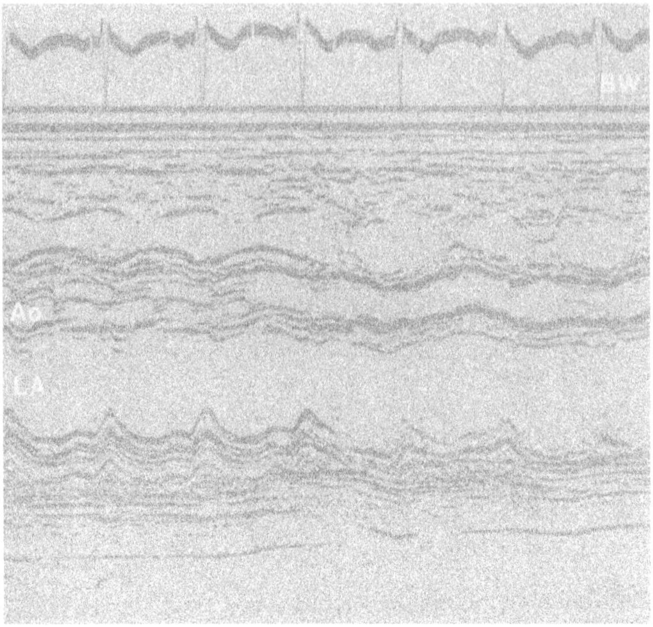

Fig. 19.2. BW: Echocardiogram obtained from a 3-week-old infant in congestive heart failure secondary to severe valvular aortic stenosis. Note the decreased aortic width (same patient as in Fig. 4.6)

membranous type, with a diaphragm-like structure in the ascending aorta; and (3) the hypoplastic type, with a diffuse narrowing of the entire ascending aorta.

Using M-mode echocardiography, the exact location and extent of the narrowing is difficult to define [425]. Cross sectional echocardiography provides this information more directly, although the degree of obstruction is often underestimated compared with data obtained during cardiac catheterization [427, 432]. The common form of supravalvar aortic stenosis (the hourglass deformity) is detected by delineation of echoes at the superior margin of the sinuses of Valsalva with clear impingement on the lumen of the aorta at that level [395, 432].

19.2.3 Some Forms of Congenital Aortic Stenosis

In some forms of congenital aortic stenosis [362] the AoV is thick and cartilaginous. The aortic root is small, often with a slight supravalvar narrowing and marked subvalvar hypertrophy. Biopsy of the ascending aorta usually shows intensive malalignment of the musculo-elastic media.

19.2.4 Coarctation of the Aorta

Coarctation of the aorta can be detected through a real-time cross sectional echocardiographic sector scan examination [333, 428]. The transducer is placed in the suprasternal notch and directed to the aortic arch which normally appears as an echo-free pulsating space. Coarctation in the descending aorta will appear as bright echoes within the aortic lumen with or without a change in the outer contour of the vessel. Both discrete and long-segment coarctation can be predicted [333].

20 Asymmetric Septal Hypertrophy

Index

Introduction

Echocardiography has become a standard procedure in the detection of disproportionate ventricular septal thickening, including genetically transmitted asymmetric septal hypertrophy (ASH). Disproportionate septal thickening is defined here as a ventricular septum to posterior wall thickness ratio of 1.3 or more. Septal thickness is measured at about one-third the distance from the AoV to the LV apex, while LVPW thickness is determined directly behind the posterior MV leaflet [221].

Not all cases of disproportionate septal thickening represent genetically transmitted ASH, or IHSS, as was thought initially [55]. To the contrary, a disproportionately thickened septum may be related to abnormalities of both the right and left heart [193]. Maron et al. [221], in echocardiographic and necropsy studies of 304 patients with various cardiac disorders, showed an overall prevalence of disproportionate ventricular septal thickening, with an abnormal thickness ratio, in 10%.

In order to avoid semantic confusion, we suggest the following abbreviations and definitions.

1. Disproportionate septal thickening refers to a septal to free wall thickness ratio at least equal to 1.3, regardless of its cause.

2. Asymmetric septal hypertrophy (*ASH*) refers to a genetically transmitted cardiomyopathy characterized by disproportionate thickening of the IVS, with numerous disorganized cardiac muscle cells on histologic examination. The specificity and significance of the disproportionate septal thickening and of the myocardial fiber disarray of ASH (and IHSS) remains, however, uncertain [38].

3. Idiopathic hypertrophic subaortic stenosis (IHSS) or *hypertrophic obstructive cardiomyopathy* (HOCM) refers to a more severe from of ASH, characterized by systolic anterior motion (SAM) of the AMVL responsible for LVOT obstruction.

Disproportionate septal thickening can occur in infants and young children without heart disease [193]. The resulting abnormal ratio usually resolves with time, through progressive thickening of the LVPW, to become normal by the age of 2 years. A diagnosis of ASH should, therefore, not be made in a small child whose echocardiogram shows disproportionate septal thickening but no other features suggestive of the cardiomyopathy.

Remarks

Only records with optimal resolution of the endocardial surfaces of both the IVS and the LVPW should be analyzed, and one should make certain that TV echoes are not included with the septal echoes.

Even with high quality recordings obtained using a correct transducer position, measurements are not always reproducible, which is especially troublesome in borderline cases [84].

20.1 Disproportionate Septal Thickness

20.1.1 Idiopathic Hypertrophic Subaortic Stenosis (IHSS) Including ASH

Definite Features

Asymmetric Septal Hypertrophy

A disproportionately thickened IVS is the constant and characteristic abnormality seen in a cardiomyopathic disease spectrum ranging from asymptomatic individuals to patients severely handicapped with the full-blown clinical picture of IHSS [84, 146, 218]. The introduction of echocardiography has greatly facilitated the documentation of this important anatomical feature, and hence the diagnosis of this cardiomyopathy.

Decreased Systolic Thickening and Amplitude of Excursion of the IVS

The IVS fails to contract or contracts very little in IHSS [375], not exceeding 22% of its diastolic thickness [321] (Fig. 20.1). This is in contrast to the normal systolic

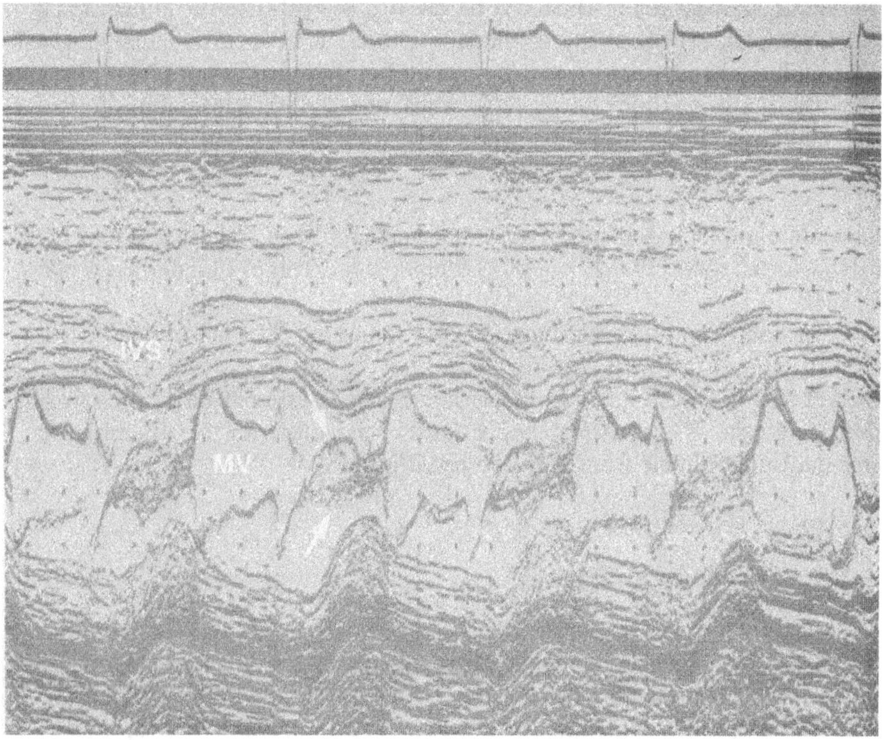

Fig. 20.1. Echocardiogram from a 18-year-old male with IHSS. Note the almost motionless IVS. SAM of the AMVL is also documented *(between arrows)*

increase in septal thickening, which ranges from 30 to 65% of the diastolic width [289, 321]. This poor contractility of the septum is of diagnostic importance in exceptional cases of IHSS with symmetric LVH [289]. Reduced or absent systolic septal thickening and motion is explained by the fact that IHSS is primarily a muscular disease characterized by a disorganized myocardial cellular arrangement.

Systolic Anterior Motion of the AMVL

There is apposition in systole of the asymmetrically hypertrophied septum and the AMVL [147] (see Fig. 20.1). Systolic apposition or obstruction may not necessarily be apparent, unless some provocative maneuvers such as amyl nitrite are used.

However, dynamic LVOT obstruction is possible in the absence of SAM [248] (see 13.12.1). In addition, the LVOT may be narrowed, during diastole, by displacement of the MV toward the IVS [147].

Secondary Features

Secondary features of IHSS include (1) increased contractions of the LVPW to compensate for the poor contractility of the septum [386] (see Fig. 20.1); (2) reduction in the E–F_0 slope of the AMVL: this reflects a diminished LV compliance and a reduced rate of filling of the LV [125, 214, 351]; (3) abnormal, partial mid-systolic closure, followed by late reopening, of the AoV leaflets [98]; (4) delayed opening of the MV [391]; and (5) normal ejection fraction [145].

The functional anatomy in IHSS can be assessed by real-time two-dimensional echocardiography: (1) the shape of the left ventricle is abnormal, resembling a "banana"; (2) the hypertrophied septum can be seen to bulge in the LVOT, for a variable distance beneath the aortic valve cusps; and (3) the abnormal position of the AMVL can be detected in cases with outflow obstruction [385].

Remarks

An echocardiographic examination should be made routine in relatives of patients with IHSS, for we found that 27 out of 73 examined relatives of 14 index cases had ASH [84].

Infants of diabetic mothers may have IHSS, or some kind of LVOT obstruction of a transient nature [134, 216] (see Fig. 20.2).

Smith et al. [359] recommend echocardiographic assessment of patients with Friedreich's ataxia, as approximately one-third of patients with this disease have features undistinguishable from those observed in IHSS.

20.1.2 Systemic Hypertension

20.1.3 Left-Sited Obstructive Lesions

Approximately 10% of patients with LV hypertrophy secondary to valvular aortic stenosis or systemic hypertension have a disproportionately hypertrophied septum [289] (see Fig. 20.3). Some rare forms of congenital aortic stenosis exist which are characterized by a thick cartilaginous valve, marked subvalvular hypertrophy, and a disproportionately thick ventricular septum [245].

As systemic hypertension and left-sited obstructive lesions may not give more specific echocardiographic features, differential diagnosis of ASH, as part of the IHSS syndrome, would seem impossible. However, it should be remembered that the IVS contracts poorly in ASH, whereas normal to strong contractions occur in the above-mentioned conditions.

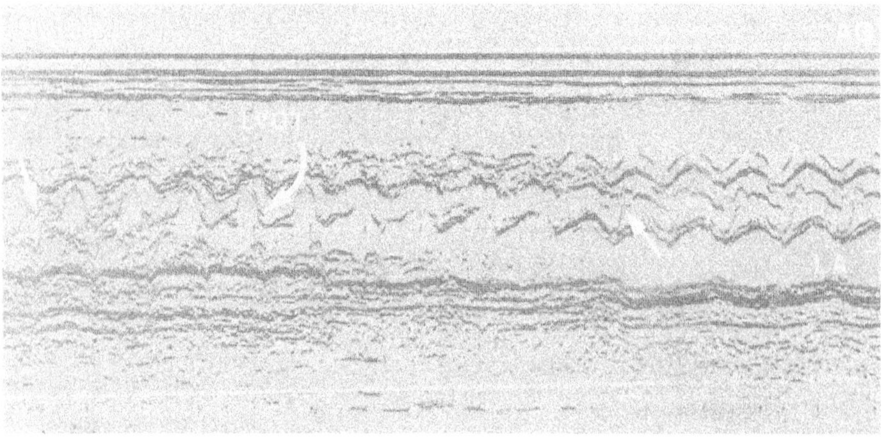

Fig. 20.2. AG: Echo-trace obtained from a 10-day-old infant born from a diabetic mother, with hemodynamically documented LVOT obstruction. Note the narrowed LVOT, a SAM-like pattern of the MV (*right arrow*) and the premature systolic closure of the AoV (*left arrow*)

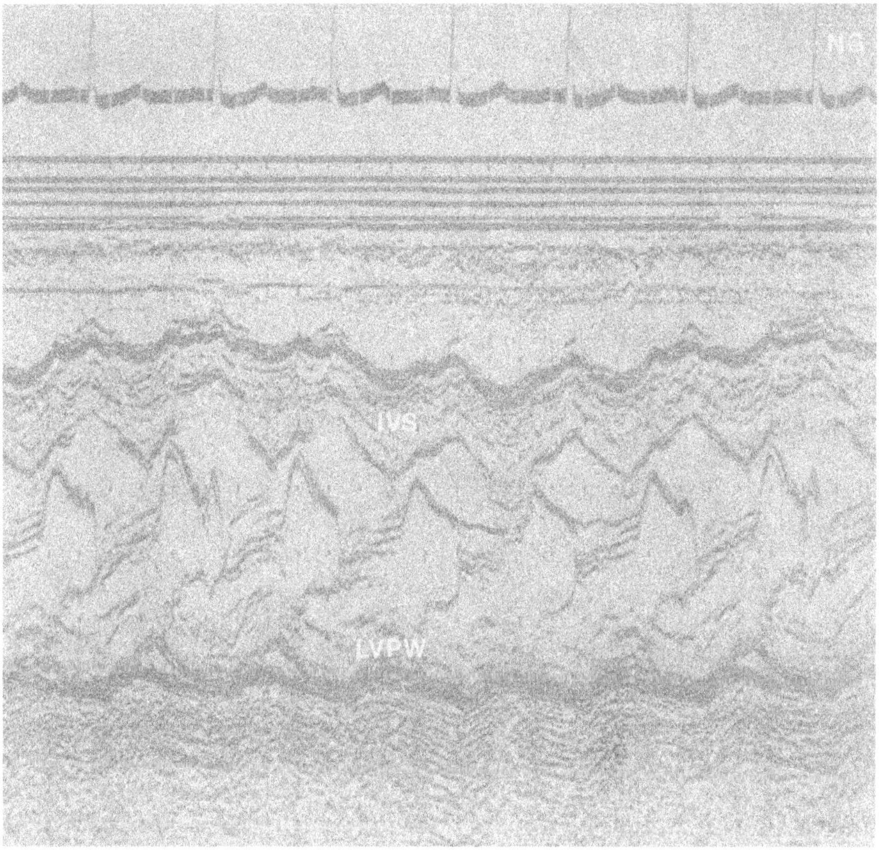

Fig. 20.3. NG: Disproportionate septal thickening in a 8-year-old patient with subvalvular aortic stenosis (gradient 88 mm Hg) (same patient as in Fig. 13.12)

Patients with AV canal defects often have a narrow LVOT because of MV displacement (see Fig. 17.6). Even in the absence of a pressure gradient, or before its appearance, LV hypertrophy may develop.

A similar finding can be documented in children with d-TGA and LVOT obstruction [265] (see Fig. 3.3).

Disproportionate septal thickening may also occur in infiltrative diseases [88], such as Pompe's disease [303]. This has been described in a 7-month-old black infant who, in addition, exhibited SAM of the AMVL. IHSS could be dismissed in this child, as septal motion remained normal.

20.1.4 Myocardial Infarction

Inferior myocardial infarction may lead to disproportionate septal thickening through either septal thickening or thinning of the LVPW [144]. In addition, patients with coronary artery disease may show disproportionate septal thickening of unknown etiology [223].

20.1.5 Mitral Valve Prolapse (see 13.11.1)

ASH is sometimes a concomitant feature of MV prolapse syndrome. However, in this situation, SAM of the AMVL cannot be documented, even after provocative maneuvers such as amyl nitrite [54].

20.1.6 Trained or Athlete's Heart

Athletes often have a septal-LVPW thickness ratio of over 1.3, along with increased ventricular internal dimensions [318]. Thus heart disease should not be erroneously diagnosed, as LV performance in the basal state remains normal.

ASH in athletes is thus to be considered as a normal variant, resulting from training.

20.1.7 Right Ventricular Hypertrophy

In the presence of RV hypertrophy, both the anterior free wall and the right side of the IVS may become thickened. As LV hypertrophy is not necessarily concomitant, a ventricular septum disproportionately thickened with respect to the LVPW may result (see Fig. 16.5).

This may be documented when (1) the RV works against increased vascular resistances; and (2) an obstructive lesion impedes egression of blood from the RV.

Indeed, to overcome increased vascular resistances, whether they are pulmonary, such as in primary [35] or secondary [220] pulmonary hypertension, or systemic, as in cases of d-TGA surgically corrected by a Mustard's operation [357], the RV will have to hypertrophy. An obstructive lesion will have the same effect on the RV musculature [193].

All these abnormalities responsible for disproportionate septal thickening are easily differentiated from IHSS (or ASH): other features of the cardiomyothy are not documented, while most of the other conditions have distinct echocardiographic and clinical findings:

1) Pulmonary hypertension (see 10.5.2),
2) d-TGA after a Mustard's operation. This is a postoperative condition without major diagnostic problems.
3) Pulmonic stenosis (see 10.1.1)
4) Tetrad of Fallot (see 4.1.2 and 4.1.3)

Generally, disproportionate septal thickening in RV hypertrophy correlates well with increasing ventricular systolic pressure [221].

20.2 Proportionate Septal Thickness

20.2.1 Left Ventricular Hypertrophy

Proportionate septal thickness or concentric LV hypertrophy will usually be documented if egression of blood from the LV is impeded. Examples abound, such as valvular aortic stenosis, systemic hypertension, etc.

In addition, the LV has been found to be symmetrically thickened in patients with a systemic disease associated with infiltrative cardiomyopathy even before clinically evident heart disease develops [31].

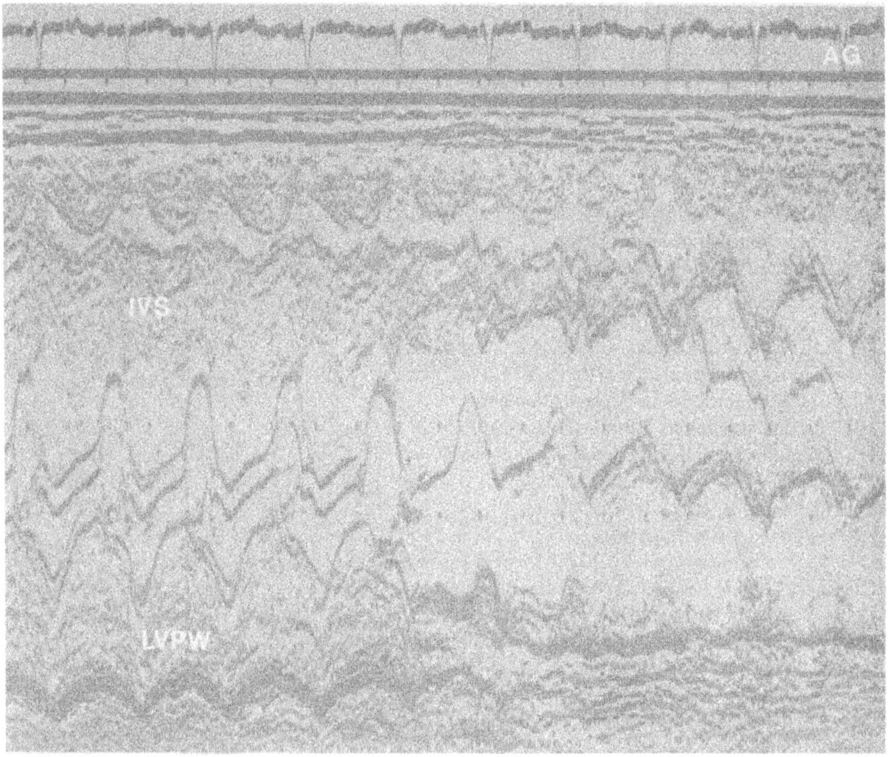

Fig. 20.4. AG: Echo-trace obtained from a 7-year-old child suffering from a cardiomyopathy of unknown etiology. Note the concentric ventricular hypertrophy of both the right and left heart

Echocardiography proves to be a powerful diagnostic test in determining the significance of an abnormal ECG suggestive of LVH, through its ability to directly measure wall thickness [252].

20.2.2 Combined Right and Left Ventricular Hypertrophy

In some cardiomyopathies both the right and left ventricle may be hypertrophied. Echocardiographically, the IVS, the RV anterior wall, and the LVPW may be grossly thickened (see Fig. 20.4).

21 Abnormal Septal Motion

Index

Introduction

The introduction of echocardiography as a noninvasive tool has proved to be of great interest in the study of septal motion, as this has been shown to be abnormal in various cardiac disorders.

Normal septal motion was first described in detail by Assad-Morell et al. [13]. In essence, the ventricular septum moves away from the sternum and toward the posterior LV wall during systole. The septum, and the LVPM moving anteriorly, thus move in opposite directions during ventricular ejection.

In the normal adult, the average amplitude of excursion of the LV septum is 0.5 cm (range 0.3 to 0.8 cm) [13]. No values seem to have been reported in normal children.

As stated by Hagan et al. [137] septal motion should be studied at the level of the chordae tendineae or below. Indeed, at mitral valve level, up to 54% of normal people do not demonstrate a normal posterior septal motion, but rather a motion which tends to be parallel to the LVPW. Thus no valid conclusions can be drawn from septal motion at that level.

Motion of the IVS can be abnormal in different ways: (1) the septum may move in an opposite direction, through most of the cardiac cycle; (2) initial septal motion may be affected because of abnormal septal activation; and (3) total excursion of the septum may be increased or decreased.

In this chapter, conditions with abnormal septal motion which are likely to be encountered in pediatric practice are presented. However, it should be realized that finding an abnormal septal motion is not specific, since so many disorders (see Index) can be associated with it. Abnormal septal motion should thus be interpreted in light of other echocardiographic features and the clinical setting [184].

21.1 Paradoxic Septal Motion with Right Ventricular Dilatation

Since the first description of paradoxic septal motion by Popp et al. [292], different types of abnormal septal motion have been recognized: (1) type A, where both the septum and LVPW move anteriorly during systole and posteriorly during diastole; (2) type B, where septal echoes become flattened during ventricular ejection; and (3) type AB, where minimal or no motion of the left side of the septum is documented during systole, whereas on its right side an anterior motion is noted [300].

The documentation of paradoxic septal motion, along with RV dilatation, is important clinically: upon this association is based an echocardiographic diagnosis of atrial septal defect [78, 175, 228, 237, 292, 378, 379], or more generally, of any right ventricular diastolic volume overload (RVDVO) state (see Index: 21.1.1 to 21.1.10).

However, paradoxic septal motion can also be documented in anomalies without increased diastolic blood flow to the RV, either with (21.1.11 to 21.1.13) or without (21.2) RV dilatation. Examples of the former include hypoplastic left heart syndrome, RV tumors, and congenital absence of the pericardium. All these entities are characterized by RV dilatation and paradoxic septal motion. In the absence of RV dilatation (21.2), paradoxic septal motion can still be encoutered.

An "echocardiographic" RVDVO state, or the association of RV dilatation with paradoxic septal motion, is thus not confined to "hemodynamic" RVDVO but includes any condition characterized by an enlargement, mostly and predominantly of the right ventricle.

Several mechanisms have been proposed to explain paradoxic septal motion [423]. In the absence of conduction disturbances or abnormal ventricular contraction patterns, it seems to be related, in most cases, to marked dilatation of the RV – irrespective of etiology – with displacement of the ventricular septum to a relatively posterior position within the ventricular mass, at end-diastole. This hypothesis assumes that geometric factors influence the direction of septal motion, so that during systole the septum moves back toward the center of ventricular mass [283]. Paradoxic septal motion depends thus upon two conditions: (1) RV dilatation must be significant, and (2) coexistent LV dilatation is either mild or nonexistent; this means that pressure or volume overload of either ventricle will influence the nature of septal motion only in so far as it causes RV dilatation [282].

This hypothesis has the advantage of explaining seemingly discordant observations e.g., (1) absence of paradoxic septal motion in some patients with "hemodynamic" RVDVO and associated LV dilatation; and (2) presence of paradoxic septal motion in unusual cases, such as in patients with tetrad of Fallot complicated by severe tricuspid or pulmonary insufficiency [14].

In patients with absent pericardium, paradoxic septal motion is probably due to altered cardiac position and motion within the thorax resulting from loss of normal pericardial restraint [83].

In the following paragraphs, conditions characterized by "echocardiographic" RVDVO are presented.

21.1.1 Secundum Atrial Septal Defect (ASD)

Paradoxic septal motion, along with RV dilatation, in patients with ASD and large left-to-right shunts (QP/QS over 2/1) was first reported by Popp et al. [292]. Diamond et al. [78] subsequently noted a direct linear relationship between the RV dimension index and the pulmonic-systemic flow ratio, in patients with ASD and normal pulmonary vascular resistance. In addition, 37 of their 39 patients showed an abnormal septal motion.

In some patients with ASD, however, a normal septal motion is preserved. As a rule, it concerns patients with additional cardiovascular anomalies such as VSD, PDA, pulmonary hypertension [377], aortic stenosis, or mitral regurgitation [378], which prevent a significant posterior displacement of the septum within the center of the ventricular mass [282]. The echocardiographic finding of "RVDVO" (i.e., the association of RV dilatation and paradoxic septal motion) (see Fig. 16.1), therefore suggests a shunt at the right atrial level or proximal to it, in a child with a pulmonary ejection murmur. Furthermore, the shunt should be considered important, as the magnitude of the left-to-right shunt is undoubtedly the factor causing the septum to move pardoxically in uncomplicated cases of ASD. However, a normal echocardiogram does not always rule out increased diastolic blood flow to the right heart and should not therefore be used to alter the indication for right heart catheterization in patients suspected of having an ASD [19, 61].

Though there is at present no general agreement concerning the reversal to normal septal motion after surgical correction of the defect causing RVDVO, it would seem reasonable to speculate that abnormal motion would persist as long as there is some RV dilatation in the absence of LV enlargement.

Persistence of RV dilatation and paradoxic septal motion postoperatively can be correlated with age at operation and length of postoperative follow-up; however, it cannot be correlated with the degree of preoperative RV enlargement, or with shunt size or RV pressures before or after operation [283]. There is no reason why, postoperatively, the motion of the septum would not, as before, be determined by its end-diastolic position, barring some particular circumstances such as abnormal ventricular activation. A recent echocardiographic study lends support to this hypothesis [400].

Other ultrasonic features of ASD are presented in relation to ostium primum septal defects (see 21.1.2).

21.1.2 Ostium Primum Septal Defect

Ostium primum septal defects are associated with RVDVO (right ventricular dilatation and paradoxic septal motion) in somewhat less than 50% of cases [139] (see Fig. 21.1).

Ostium primum defects can be differentiated from ostium secundum septal defects by the following ultrasonic features (see also Table 21.1).

The LVOT

In ostium primum, the LVOT is typically narrowed [124] because of the anterior displacement of the mitral valve (see Fig. 17.6). In ostium secundum (or ASD), the MV is not displaced and the LVOT remains normal.

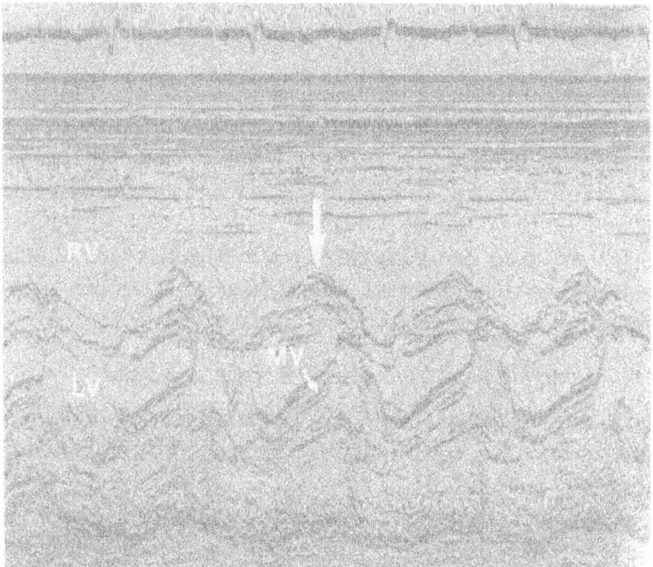

Fig. 21.1. IJ: Echocardiogram obtained from a 8-year-old girl with an ostium primum septal defect and a moderately large left-to-right shunt. Note the paradoxical septal motion: anterior motion of the septum occurs during systole (*arrow*)

Table 21.1. Ostium primum and ostium secundum septal defects: Differentiating features

	Ostium primum	Ostium secundum
Echocardiographic RVDVO	+	+
Narrow LVOT	+	–
Prolonged MSA[a]	+	–
Increased AV valve mobility	Mitral	Tricuspid
Reduced AV valve mobility	–	Mitral
Location AV valve	Abnormal	Normal
Atrial septal echoes	–	+
AV valve continuity	+	–
Associated anomalies		Mitral valve prolapse

[a] MSA = mitral septal apposition

Mitral-Septal Apposition in Diastole

Mitral-septal apposition is prolonged in ostium primum [124, 182] and absent or brief in ostium secundum [257]. This abnormal apposition is the echocardiographic equivalent of the angiographic gooseneck deformity.

The Atrioventricular Valve Leaflet Motion Pattern

In ostium secundum defects, diminished cardiac output [123, 288] is responsible for reduced velocity and excursion of the MV leaflets [172], whereas the TV shows increased mobility [257].

In ostium primum defects with mitral regurgitation, there is often, to the contrary, an increased MV mobility [257]. The AMVL may even appear to move through the ventricular septum [139] (see Fig. 6.4). This specific feature – originally ascribed to patients with the complete form of AV canal [430] – can be documented in over half of patients with partial AV canal.

Finally, abnormalities in MV motion, with multiple, sometimes fragmented and bizarre systolic and diastolic echoes, are also consistently observed in ostium primum septal defects [139, 182] (see Fig. 6.4). These abnormalities are probably related to the abnormal location of the MV and its unusual attachment to the IVS [430].

The TV may also seem to be displaced in partial AV canal: it lies posterior to the anterior aortic wall and, on an echocardiographic tracing, gives the impression of opening from within the ventricular septal echoes [139].

Echocardiographic Scan from Mitral to Tricuspid Valve

An ultrasonic sweep from one AV valve to the other is possible using both M-mode and cross sectional echocardiography along a horizontal section at the level of the membranous septum [26].

In ostium secundum defects, when scanning from mitral to tricuspid valves, echoes of the AMVL can be seen to continue with that of the interatrial septum (see Fig. 4.1). An echo interruption, indicating the defect itself, can sometimes be documented in the middle part of the interatrial septum [26].

In all cases of endocardial cushion defects, this ultrasonic sweep will not show atrial septal echoes in continuity with the AMVL, posterior to the TV [26] (see

Fig. 6.3) In addition, although more prevalent in complete AV canal [22], it may be possible to demonstrate in partial AV canal as well, an echocardiographic confluence between the two AV valves [139].

The Presence of Associated Anomalies

In ostium secundum septal defects, particular attention should be paid to the study of the MV, as up to 30% of patients with ASD may have MV prolapse [277]. A much higher prevalence figure of 95% was recently reported in patients with ASD, studied by two-dimensional echocardiography. Prolapse in these patients predominantly affected the AMVL [206].

Fine oscillations of the ATVL may suggests the association of pulmonary regurgitation [205].

21.1.3 Partial Anomalous Pulmonary Venous Return

There are at present no echocardiographic features allowing separation of atrial septal defects from partial anomalous pulmonary venous return to the right side of the heart.

21.1.4 Total Anomalous Pulmonary Venous Return (see 8.3.3)

Echocardiographic RVDVO in a cyanotic baby should suggest this diagnosis, certainly if, in addition, small left cavities are documented [277 a, 380] (see Fig. 17.4).

21.1.5 Ebstein's Anomaly (see 12.7.1)

Ebstein's anomaly will usually give an echocardiographic picture of "RVDVO" (see Fig. 12.2), although the RV per se is not dilated. Rather, its "atrialized" portion and the right atrium proper may be aneurysmally enlarged if (1) egression of blood is impeded through a diminutive RV, and (2) tricuspid regurgitation is associated.

Most patients with Ebstein's anomaly have type B septal motion. Type A is certainly much rarer and was documented in only one out of 16 patients studied by Farooki et al. [94]. Normal septal motion does not, however, exclude the diagnosis.

21.1.6 Tricuspid Regurgitation (see 22.1.3)

Severe tricuspid regurgitation is associated with RV dilatation and paradoxical septal motion.

After successful TV replacement, IVS motion promptly returns to normal [344].

21.1.7 Pulmonary Regurgitation

In addition to RV dilatation with paradoxic septal motion (RVDVO), fine oscillations of the ATVL may be documented in pulmonary regurgitation [98].

This finding should be looked for systematically in patients with ASD, as pulmonary regurgitation may occur in large atrial shunts even in the absence of pulmonary hypertension [205] (see 12.8.4).

21.1.8 Right Coronary Artery – Right Ventricular Fistula

Coronary arteriovenous fistula is a rare cause of congestive heart failure in the newborn. This was recently reported in a 2-day-old infant with a large fistula between the right coronary artery and the RV [398]. Volume overloading of the RV, responsible for fatal congestive heart failure was echocardiographically documented by an enlarged RV cavity and paradoxical motion of the IVS [398].

21.1.9 Idiopathic Dilatation of the Pulmonary Artery (see 18.1.5)

21.1.10 Congenital Absence of the Pulmonary Valve (see 18.1.6)

21.1.11 Congenital and Acquired Absence of the Pericardium

Echocardiographic findings in patients with congenital and acquired absence of the pericardium mimic RVDVO with increased right ventricular dimensions and abnormal septal motion. [280]. Congenital absence of the pericardium further resembles an atrial septal defect-like anomaly as physical, roentgenologic and electrocardiographic findings may be similar [280].

As in some cardiovascular centers, heart catheterization for atrial septal defects is no longer performed, it is not inconceivable that an occasional patient with congenital absence of the pericardium will be sent for surgical repair of an ASD. Any patient with echocardiographic features of RVDVO should, therefore, be catheterized.

21.1.12 Right Ventricular Tumors (see 9.5.1)

21.1.13 Hypoplastic Left Heart Syndrome (see 17.2.1)

21.2 Paradoxic Septal Motion not Necessarily Associated with Right Ventricular Dilatation

21.2.1 Idiopathic Hypertrophic Subaortic Stenosis (see 20.1.1)

Septal motion in IHSS could be called paradoxic, as no significant excursion may be documented throughout the cardiac cycle. In addition, the IVS fails to contract, or contracts very little in IHSS.

21.2.2 Dyskinetic Segments or Aneurysms Involving the IVS [137]

21.2.3 Pericardial Effusion (see 8.1.1)

21.2.4 Mitral or Aortic Valvular Prostheses [137]

In all these conditions (21.2.2 to 21.2.4) paradoxic septal motion can be documented in the absence of RV dilatation (see Fig. 21.2a, b).

21.2.5 Constrictive Pericarditis

Patients with constrictive pericarditis may have an abnormal septal motion not necessarily associated with RV dilatation [109, 289]. The abnormal pattern may consist in a flattening motion in systole followed by an unusual posterior motion in diastole [109]. An early IVS diastolic motion consisting of a sudden anterior displacement may often precede the posterior motion [42] (see Fig. 21.3). The

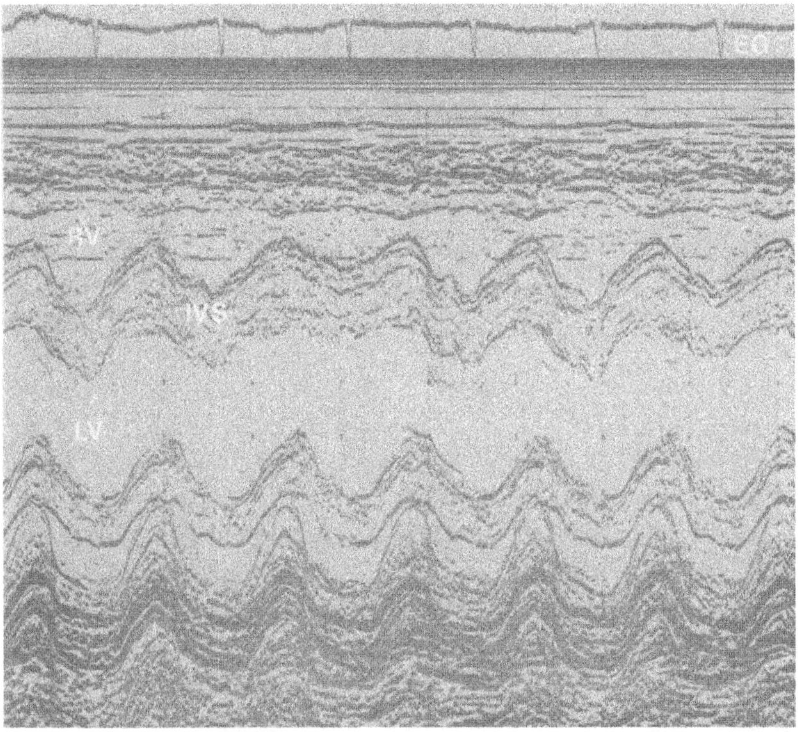

a

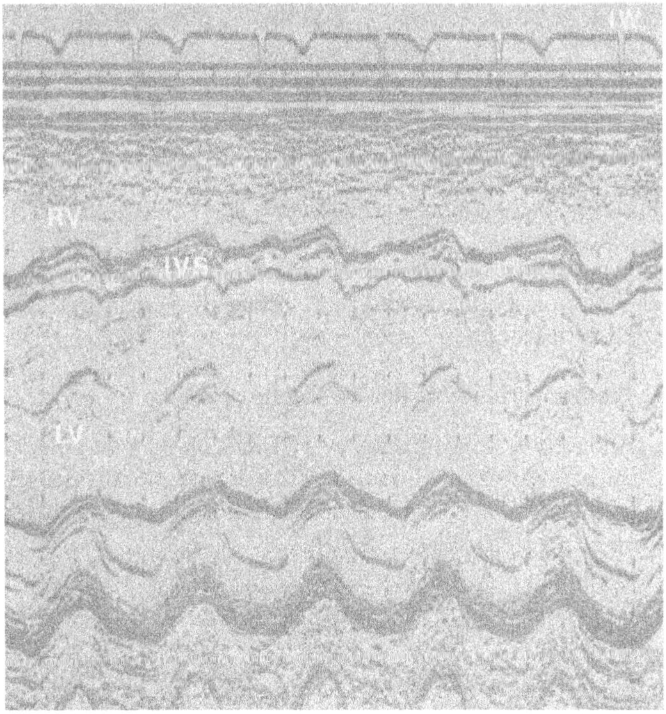

b

Fig. 21.2. a EG: Echocardiogram obtained from a 10-year-old boy 2 years following AoV replacement. Note the persistent paradoxic septal motion without right ventricular dilatation. **b** IW: Echocardiogram obtained from an 8-year-old girl 18 months following MV replacement. Paradoxic septal motion without right ventricular dilatation is well illustrated.

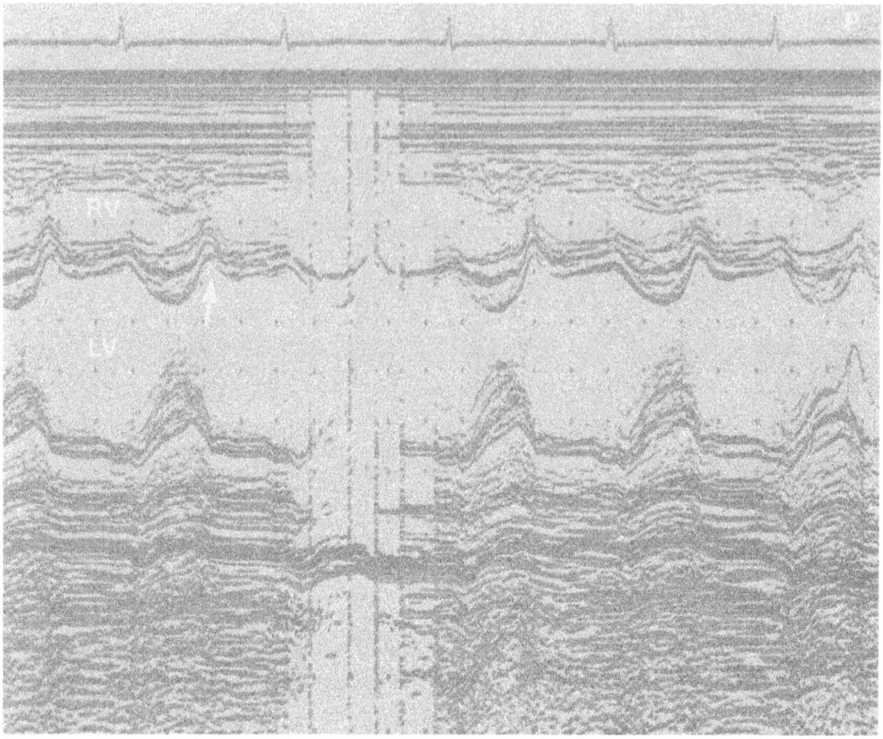

Fig. 21.3. P: Illustration of septal motion in constrictive pericarditis. Early in diastole, there is a sudden anterior displacement of the septum (*arrow*) followed by a brisk posterior rebound. Some pericardial fluid is also present

amplitude of excursion is variable, greater than normal in some [109], and hypokinetic in others [42]. The degree of systolic thickening is diminished.

Other ultrasonic features of constrictive pericarditis include [109] (1) flat diastolic motion of the LVPW; (2) posterior pericardial thickening; and (3) epicardial-pericardial separation.

21.2.6 Abnormal Motion Following Cardiac Surgery

Echocardiographic abnormalities of IVS motion may be noted following cardiac surgery, mostly during the first two postoperative months (see Fig. 21.4a, b) [40]. Septal ischemia, RV adhesions, and reduction of intrapericardial tension have been suggested as possible causes [280].

21.3 Abnormal Initial Septal Motion

21.3.1 Left Bundle Branch Block

In the presence of left bundle branch block (LBBB) there is a paradoxical septal motion very similar to that seen in patients with RVDVO [81]. There is, however, an important distinguishing feature, namely, an early rapid posterior motion of the septum following the onset of electrical depolarization. This motion lasts for about

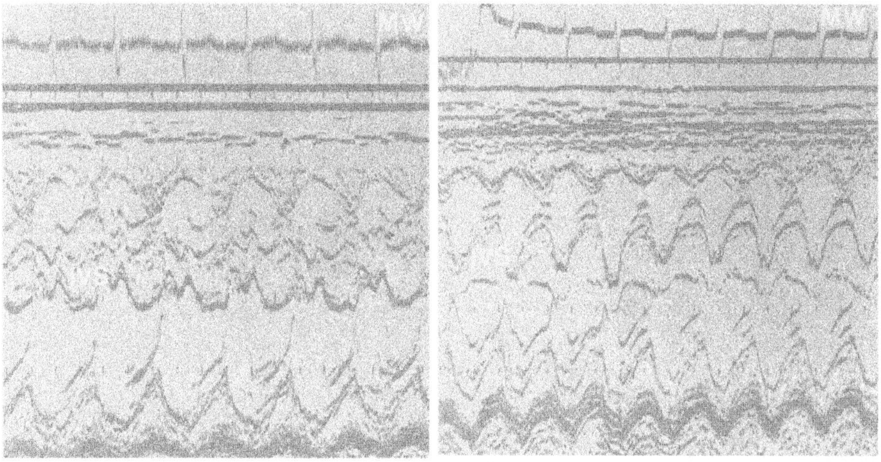

a b

Fig. 21.4. MW: Pre- (a) and postoperative echocardiograms (b) obtained from a 7-month-old baby with severe valvular pulmonic stenosis. Septal motion is normal preoperatively and paradoxical postoperatively

0.04 s, or until the onset of ventricular ejection, at which time it moves anteriorly [81].

21.3.2 d-TGA After Mustard's Operation

The abnormal motion pattern characteristic of LBBB (see 21.3.1) is frequently observed in children with TGA surgically corrected by a Mustard's operation (see Fig. 21.5).

A likely explanation is that septal depolarization is electrically reversed with LBBB, and functionally reversed with surgically corrected d-TGA.

21.3.3 Type B Ventricular Pre-Excitation

21.3.4 Right Ventricular Premature Beats

A similar abnormal septal motion may be documented in type B ventricular pre-excitation [102, 158, 289, 389] and with RV premature beats [412].

21.3.5 Right Ventricular Pacemaker

In most patients with a RV pacemaker, an initially very active posterior motion of the IVS occurring within 70 ms of the pacemaker artifact and followed by a posterior, or more rarely, a flat or anterior movement of the septum during the remainder of the ejection period, can be documented [438] (see Fig. 21.6).

21.3.6 Right Bundle Branch Block (RBBB)

Patients with a postoperative RBBB pattern may also exhibit an early systolic anterior septal notch similar in location, depth, and duration, but opposite in direction to the early systolic motion seen in patients with complete LBBB [352] (see Fig. 21.7)

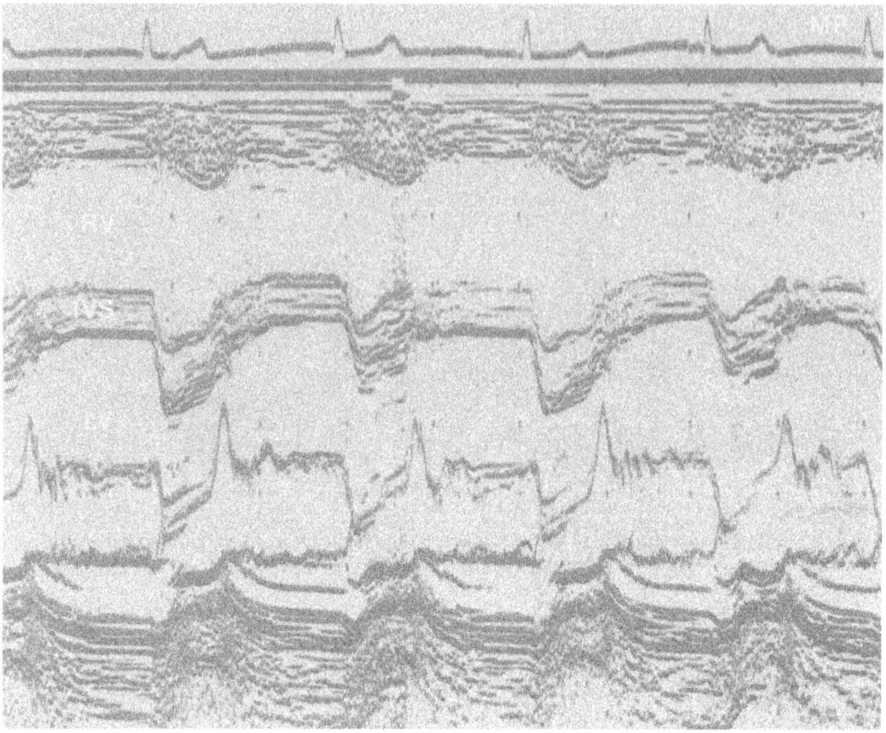

Fig. 21.5. MP: LV echogram in a 5-year-old patient with d-TGA after a Mustard's operation. Septal motion is abnormal, contributing mainly to the right (systemic) ventricle

21.4 Decreased Total Excursion of the IVS

21.4.1 Coronary Artery Disease

In patients suffering from coronary artery disease, septal motion is essentially flat during systole, with only slight motion away from the LVPW. This represents hypo- or akinesia of the septum; its differentiation from type B septal motion will rest upon the assessment of RV dimensions, usually normal in patients with coronary artery disease [13], and upon the observation of compensatory hyperkinetic contractions of the LVPW [164].

21.4.2 Congestive Cardiomyopathy

In congestive cardiomyopathy, generalized hypokinesis with poor interventricular septal and posterior wall motion is documented.

However, an apparently normal or increased septal motion will be documented, although septal systolic thickening will remain decreased if significant mitral regurgitation complicates the cardiomyopathy [199, 230].

Other ultrasonic features consistent with congestive cardiomyopathy include: (see Fig. 13.2) (1) dilated LV cavity with a wide LVOT [2, 68]; The left ventricle

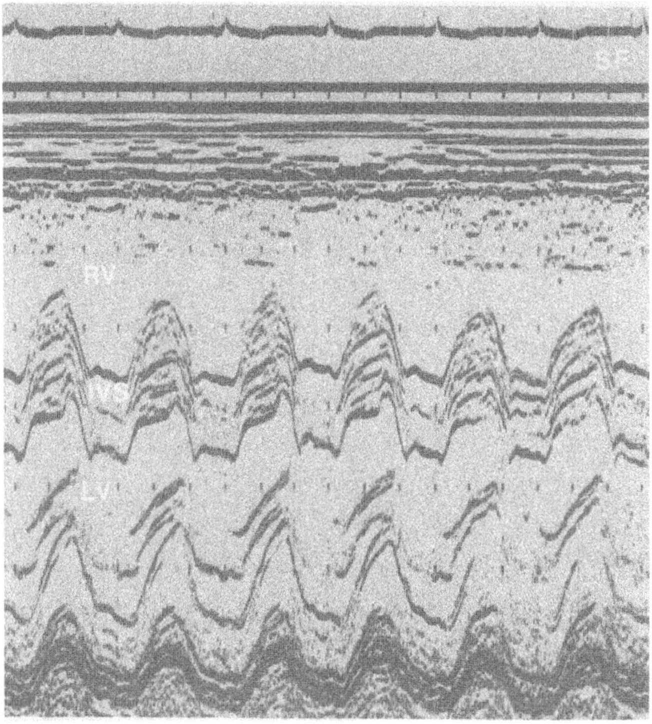

Fig. 21.6. SF: Echocardiogram obtained from a 4-year-old girl with a lithium-powered pacemaker inserted because of a complete heart block following intracardiac repair of a VSD 18 months earlier. Note the abnormal systolic septal motion

acquires a globular shape, well documented on cross sectional echocardiographic pictures; (2) low ejection fraction; (3) reduced MV excursion [68]; and (4) decreased A-C slope on the MV echogram [273].

21.5 Increased Total Excursion of the IVS

Septal motion may be abnormal if its total excursion is increased. This can be documented in the following conditions.

21.5.1 Left Ventricular Volume Overload States [314]

LV volume overload may occur in (1) patent ductus arteriosus; (2) VSD; (3) mitral regurgitation (see Fig. 21.8); and (4) ruptured chordae tendineae [184].

21.5.2 LV Posterior Wall Infarction

Increased septal motion compensates here for the reduced contractility of the LVPW.

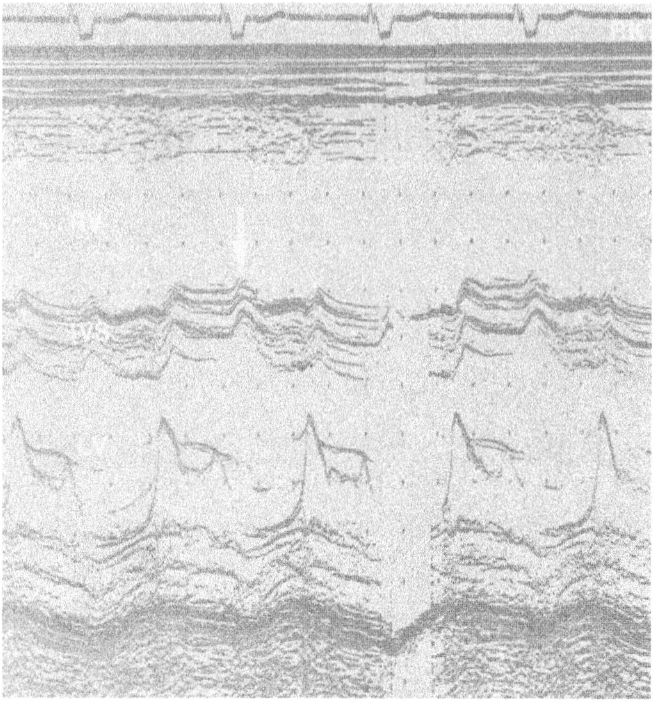

Fig. 21.7. RK: Recording from a 11-year-old boy with a postoperative complete RBBB. The child had undergone repair for tetrad of Fallot 5 years before. Note the early systolic anterior septal motion (*arrow*)

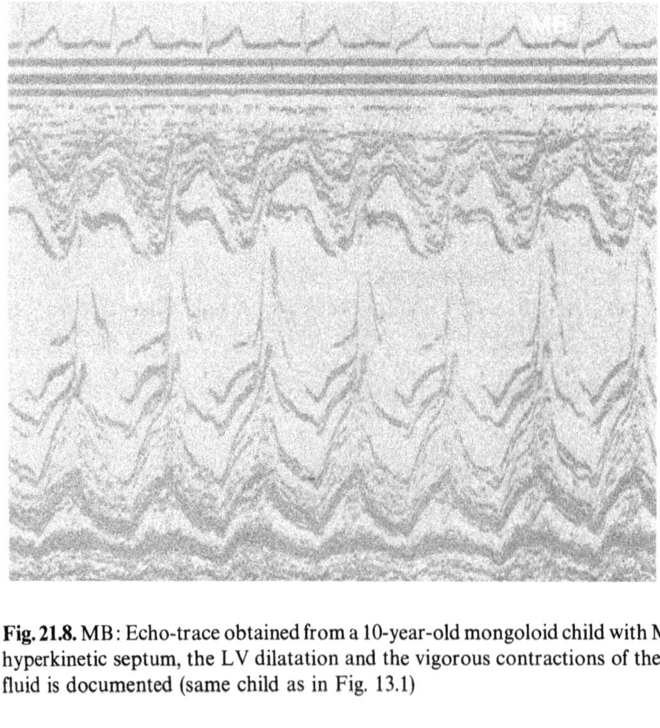

Fig. 21.8. MB: Echo-trace obtained from a 10-year-old mongoloid child with MV regurgitation. Note the hyperkinetic septum, the LV dilatation and the vigorous contractions of the LVPW. Some pericardial fluid is documented (same child as in Fig. 13.1)

Function

Contrast Echocardiography

22 Abnormal Contrast Pathways

Index

Introduction

Contrast echocardiography records the presence of intracardiac echoes generated by different types of fluid injected rapidly into normally echo-free vessels or heart chambers. Virtually any fluid, including the patient's own blood, can produce echoes through the formation of microbubbles.

Contrast echocardiography was first used clinically to identify and dilineate heart structures. Subsequently, the technique proved useful in the detection and localization of intracardiac shunts and in the study of blood flow patterns [126].

The possibilities of contrast echocardiography depend on the equipment available (M-mode vs 2D echocardiography), the site of the injection (intracardiac vs. a peripheral vessel), and to a lesser extent on the contrast agent used. In clinical practice, echoes generated by injection of saline in the right antecubital vein are quite sufficient as an acoustic contrast agent [138].

In this chapter, the most important clinical applications of contrast echocardiography will be discussed: abnormalities in contrast pathways both after peripheral vessel injection and after central injections through an indwelling catheter will be described.

To the best of our knowledge, only one other totally noninvasive method exists which allows detection and quantitation of a left-to-right intracardiac shunt, namely, the single breath inhalation of O_2-15 labeled carbon dioxide ($C^{15}O_2$) [384].

22.1 Contrast Echoes After Peripheral Venous Injections

22.1.1 Contrast Echoes Crossing the Atrial Septum in Atrial Septal Defects

In the presence of a right-to-left atrial shunt, snowflake-like echoes produced after a peripheral venous injection, will cross the interatrial septum to arrive in the LA [138]. This passage occurs during the rapid filling phase of ventricular diastole, as well as at the onset of LV contraction [396]. Shunted blood then enters the LV via the mitral orifice. This flow pattern can be detected by single-element echocardiographic systems when beam axis is directed either through the Ao and the LA or the MV funnel. Cross sectional echocardiographic techniques provide additional information, as they allow the left atrium and part of the right atrium to be visualized simultaneously.

Even in the absence of cyanosis and the presence of left-to-right atrial shunting the passage of acoustic contrast from right to left can sometimes be observed after a peripheral vein injection [138]. It is likely that during a very short part of the cardiac cycle the direction of the shunt is reversed, permitting contrast echoes to reach the LA cavity. (see Fig. 22.1).

Furthermore, it is possible using contrast cross sectional echocardiography, to visualize a left-to-right atrial shunt after a rapid peripheral venous injection through the documentation of a negative contrast echo pattern in the RA: contrast echoes which appear in the RA are seen to be pushed away by unmarked blood streaming through the atrial septal defect into the RA.

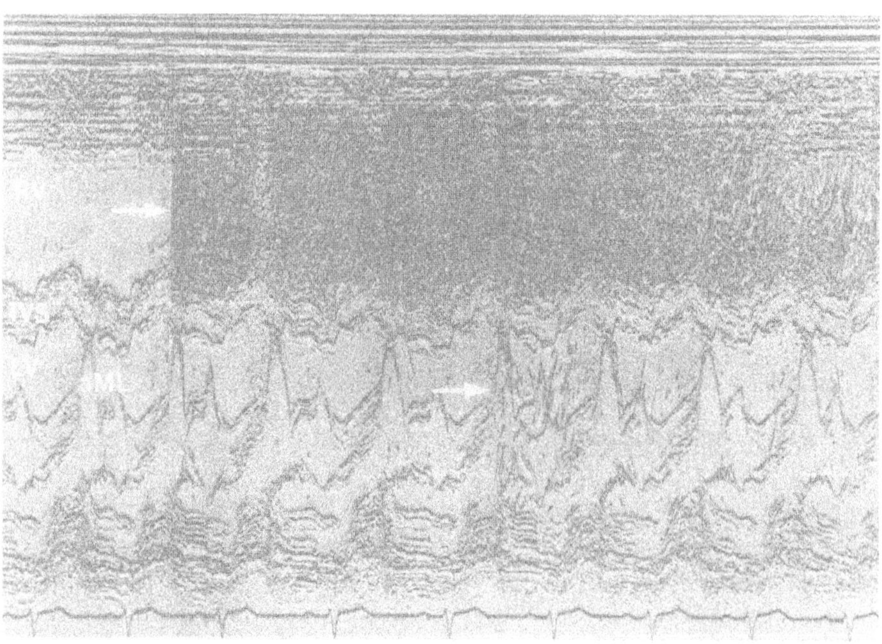

Fig. 22.1. *Upper arrow* indicates the arrival of contrast echoes within the RV cavity after an IV injection of contrast material, in an 18-year-old male with ASD. Some right-to-left atrial shunting is evidenced by the appearance of contrast echoes, some beats later, in the MV funnel and LV cavity (*lower arrow*)

22.1.2 Contrast Echoes Crossing the Ventricular Septum in Ventricular Septal Defects (see Fig. 22.1)

Right-to-left shunting may occur through a VSD when the peak RV systolic pressure reaches or exceeds 70 mm Hg [396]. A right-to-left ventricular shunt is amenable to ultrasonic diagnosis by contrast echocardiography after a peripheral vein injection: echoes are observed to pass from the right into the left ventricular cavity at a time when the MV is still closed. Contrast echoes are thus not observed within the LA cavity and the MV orifice is spared from echoes.

In patients with VSD, Serwer et al. [345] found that with peripheral injection contrast echocardiography, RV pressures could be estimated and resistance to pulmonary blood flow evaluated: with RV pressures not exceeding 60–80% of systemic, dye may appear in the RV and in the LV anterior to the MV, but not in the aorta. However, with large left-to-right shunts and RV pressures at systemic levels, dye will enter the aorta. If outflow resistance to pulmonary blood flow is increased, such as in tetrad of Fallot or with increased pulmonary vascular resistances, diastolic appearance of dye within the LV, anterior to the MV, will occur earlier than it would if pulmonary resistance was low.

Dynamic cross sectional images through the long axis of the LV allow a rapid ultrasonic diagnosis of a right-to-left ventricular shunt, as both ventricles and the LA are visualized simultaneously.

Contrast echocardiographic techniques with peripheral venous injections have proved valuable in the detection of residual right-to-left intracardiac shunts in the early postoperative period [87] (see Fig. 22.2).

Left-to-right ventricular shunting can be visualized either by a negative contrast echo pattern in the RV after a peripheral venous injection, or more reliably, by a

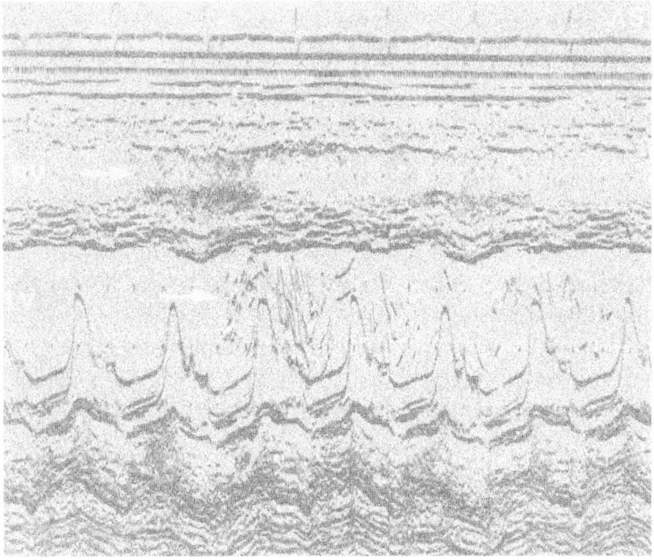

Fig. 22.2. AS: Echo trace obtained from a 2-year-old child 24 h after surgical closure of a VSD. *Upper arrow* indicates the arrival of contrast echoes within the RV after an IV injection. *Lower arrow* indicates the appearance of contrast echoes within the LV cavity. The MV funnel remains contrast-free

positive contrast echo pattern in the RV after an intracardiac injection through an indwelling catheter in the LA or LV.

22.1.3 Back and Forth Movements of Contrast Echoes Across the Tricuspid Valve in Tricuspid Valve Regurgitation

Appearance of contrast echoes in the inferior vena cava, with a back and forth movement of these echoes across the TV, has been described as diagnostic of tricuspid regurgitation [207]. To visualize the inferior vena cava, TV and RA, a two-dimensional phased array imaging system was used, with the transducer in the subxyphoid area. Contrast material was injected in an antecubital vein. In patients without tricuspid regurgitation, no contrast echoes appeared in the inferior vena cava. This method was considered to be more reliable in detecting tricuspid regurgitation than other more conventional noninvasive techniques.

22.1.4 As a Diagnostic Aid in d-TGA (see 3.1.1)

The combination of a suprasternal notch approach and contrast echocardiography after a peripheral vein injection has been shown to contribute to the identification of most patients with discordant ventriculo-arterial connections through the documentation of an early, more intense opacification of the aorta [255]. Naturally, the method is valid only when the two great arteries and the semilunar valves have been identified unequivocally.

22.2 Contrast Echoes After Arterial Injections

22.2.1 Detection of Patent Ductus Arteriosus (see 15.1.1)

In the presence of a PDA, echo contrast agents injected into the descending aorta will pass into the PA. This passage can be detected by suprasternal notch echocardiography, which allows a simultaneous visualization of both the aorta and the right PA [9, 332].

22.3 Contrast Echoes After Intracardiac Injections

22.3.1 Detection of Intracardiac Shunts

Injections of contrast agents directly into cardiac cavities through an indwelling catheter allow an accurate assessment of both the site and the direction of an intracardiac shunt. Kerber et al. [176] and Sahn et al. [332] describe this technique in the detection of shunts in patients with ASD, VSD, and tetrad of Fallot. The technique is often useful in the immediate postoperative period, when an indwelling catheter in the left atrium, placed at the time of surgery, allows injection of contrast agents for the detection of a residual postoperative shunt [397].

22.3.2 Detection of Specific Pathways in Common Ventricle with One or Two AV Valves

In patients with single ventricle and two AV valves, a central or peripheral venous injection of contrast material will result in the appearance of a cloud of echoes in the ventricle, anterior to the MV, during the rapid inflow phase of ventricular diastole [349].

To the contrary, if there is only one AV valve, all dye will arrive posterior to the only demonstrable AV valve [349].

Tricuspid atresia, however, should be excluded in this last situation, as it is characterized by an identical echocardiographic flow pattern [349] (see also 7.1.3).

Functional Parameters

23 Systolic Time Intervals

Index

Introduction

Simply stated, the systolic time intervals (STI) consist of the two major components of the systolic cycle of the heart: the pre-ejection phase and the ejection period. Together they make up the total electromechanical systole or "QP_2."

The duration of the STI depends on four basic factors [153], the same that are responsible for the extent of cardiac fiber shortening [34]: (1) the preload; (2) the afterload; (3) the contractile or inotropic state of the myocardium; and (4) the rate and sequence of intraventricular electrical conduction.

STI therefore allow an evaluation of ventricular performance. Clinically, left ventricular STI are derived from the simultaneous high speed recording of the ECG, the phonocardiogram, and the indirect carotid pulse tracing. It is not possible to measure the right ventricular STI in a similar fashion because of the inability to accurately define the onset of RV ejection. Clinical applications of left ventricular STI have not achieved widespread popularity in the pediatric age group, as high quality recordings are usually hard to get in small children.

The introduction of ultrasound as a noninvasive tool for the assessment of cardiac function will undoubtedly extend the diagnostic possibilities of the STI to this difficult age group. Indeed, both right and left ventricular STI can be accurately determined from echocardiographic tracings [152, 153, 368], more specifically, from the pulmonary and aortic valve echogram with a concomitant ECG. Right (R) and left (L) ventricular ejection time (VET) are defined from pulmonary and aortic valve opening to closure (see 23.1). Ideally, two cusps of either valve should be recorded at the time of leaflet separation and coaptation. However, if only one cusp can be registered, as often occurs for the PV, onset and termination of ejection can still be determined. Pulmonary ejection is then considered to start at the point on the tracing of rapid outward leaflet motion at which point the closed valve echo changes from a thick to a very fine echo trace; likewise, the junction of the fine leaflet echo trace with the thick, closed valve echo line, following rapid inward leaflet motion, indicates the termination of ejection [153, 242].

Right and left PEPs are measured from the initial ventricular depolarization of the ECG, usually the Q-wave, to the onset of valve opening (see Fig. 11.1). In order to minimize the influence of respiratory variations on right STI, measurements should be made during the expiratory phase whenever possible, or the shortest STI should be selected and averaged.

Spitaels et al. [365] have shown that the PEP/LVET ratio represents a simplified expression of alteration in the STI, as it requires no correction for heart rate or age. The PEP/LVET ratio is thus a useful single expression of LV performance [415].

The mean PEP/LVET ratio for 76 normal children studied by Spitaels et al. [365] was 0.313 (SD ± 0.05). An identical ratio was recently obtained by Gutgesell et al. [135]. To the contrary, regression equations for LPEP and LVET were respectively [365]:

$$\text{LPEP} = 65 + 0.169\ \text{M (M: months), and}$$
$$\text{LVET} = 373 - 1.291\ \text{R (R: heart rate per minute).}$$

The same insensitivity to age or heart rate for the PEP/RVET ratio has been found by Hirschfeld et al. [153] and Riggs et al. [309] and their respective collaborators. The mean PEP/RVET ratio in their normal patients, from 2 months to 21 years of age, was 0.24, with a range of 0.17 to 0.33.

Given the constant PEP/VET values for both ventricles in normal children, it is not surprising that determination of these intervals have found numerous applications in addition to the study of LV performance (see Index).

Classical M-mode recordings are quite adequate to determine STI and related parameters. Recently, however, a dual M-mode registration system has allowed the echocardiographic recording of different valves simultaneously on a beat-to-beat basis [334]. This is possible through the independent selection of two crystals from known locations within the array of a multiscan echocardiographic system, and their registration in a rapid alternating fashion, along with the ECG, by a strip chart recorder. This greatly facilitates calculation of STI and related parameters from one cardiac cycle. The quality of this type of registration should be higher, as both single element transducers can be directed optimally to specific cardiac structures. Parameters on both sides of the circulation derived, for instance, from the simultaneous recording of the AoV and PV echogram, can be compared with each other without having to correct each separately for variation in respiration and heart rate [334].

This dual M-mode technique also allows a more sophisticated analysis of hemodynamic parameters which, until now, have been difficult to delineate, such as the isovolumic relaxation period for either ventricle.

A major limitation to the clinical application of STI derived from M-mode echocardiography is that a one-dimensional view is used to evaluate motion and volume changes in a three-dimensional cavity. More accurate data might be expected using long axis cross sectional images of the left ventricle, which are theoretically amenable to long axis and surface area measurements using formulas tested in quantitative single plane angiography [315]. However, due to poor visualization of the cardiac apex and some distortions present in two-dimensional cardiac images, results using this techniques are at present not reproducible.

23.1 Assessment of Pulmonary Artery Pressure and Pulmonary Vascular Resistance

The PEP/RVET ratio allows echocardiographic assessment of PA pressure and pulmonary vascular resistance in patients of all ages and heart rates including neonates [308] Hirschfeld et al. [153], studying a series of patients with a variety of congenital heart lesions, showed that the PEP/RVET ratio correlated well with the pulmonary artery diastolic pressure (PADP): patients with ratios less than or equal to the normal mean (i. e., 0.25) have a greater than 97.5% chance of having a PADP of less than 25 mm Hg; a ratio less than 0.30 virtually assures a normal PADP; if a ratio greater than 0.35 is obtained, PADP usually exceeds 30 mm Hg.

An elevated PEP/RVET ratio may thus be indicative of more severe lung disease. This is well illustrated in newborns suffering from respiratory distress syndrome: the more severe the disease, the higher the PEP/RVET ratio [143].

More recently, quite good correlations have been found between right ventricular isovolumic contraction time (RVICT) and pulmonary artery end-diastolic pressure (PAEDP). With a RVICT of less than 25 ms, PAEDP is predictably below 18 mm Hg. The RVICT is defined echocardiographically as the time from TV closure to PV opening [243].

The PEP/RVET ratio, or the RVICT, also allows a sequential examination of the pulmonary vascular bed in selected patients (see 23.1.1), the differentiation of fixed from reversible pulmonary hypertension (see 23.1.2), and the follow-up of patients after PA banding (see 23.1.3).

23.1.1 Sequential Assessment of Individual Patients

This will permit detection of early development and/or progression of pulmonary vascular disease, for instance, in patients with a large left-to-right cardiovascular shunt, or in patients with d-TGA, who are at particular risk.

A significant increase in pulmonary vascular resistance should be strongly suspected if the RPEP/RVET ratio increases: heart catheterization should then be repeated [309].

In patients with d-TGA, assessment of PA pressure will rest upon the PEP/LVET ratio. Gutgesell et al. [133] has recently shown that a PEP/LVET ratio of less than 0.26 is consistently associated with PA diastolic pressures of less than 20 mm Hg, and in most patients with a pulmonary artery pressure less than one-third of the mean systemic arterial pressure [132]. To the contrary, pulmonary hypertension was present in most patients with a PEP/LVET ratio of at least 0.30. Abnormalities of cardiac rhythm, conduction, and/or myocardial dysfunction should have been ruled out previously.

23.1.2 Fixed Versus Reversible Pulmonary Hypertension

Regarding the differentiation of fixed (organic) from reversible (vasoconstrictive) pulmonary hypertension with oxygen inhalation, if the RPEP/RVET fails to decrease during oxygen administration, fixed pulmonary hypertension is probable [155].

23.1.3 After Pulmonary Artery Banding

Although resistance to ejection remains high, by the very presence of the pulmonary artery band, several authors have found the RPEP/RVET ratio to be reduced in the postoperative period of patients in whom banding had been effective in lowering pulmonary vascular resistances [155, 309].

23.2 Diagnostic Use in Congenital Heart Disease

23.2.1 Semilunar Valve Identification

Hirschfeld et al. [152] have shown that the LVET is shorter than the RVET in normal children, with a mean LVET/RVET ratio of 0.80, while the LPEP generally exceeds the RPEP. As long as pulmonary resistance does not exceed systemic, this is documented clinically by PV closure after aortic closure [361].

In uncomplicated d-TGA the situation is reversed [152]: RVET is shortened and RPEP prolonged, as the RV now contracts against systemic resistance [34]. The LVET/RVET ratio is also reversed, having an average value of 1.22, regardless of a previous Mustard's operation [152].

Thus the shortest ejection time generally points to the systemic ventricle. This feature helps in the identification of the semilunar valves in complex heart lesions, such as in double outlet RV, in which the semilunar valves classically lie along approximately the same transverse plane [366]. It further allows identification of the semilunar valve that is in continuity with an atrioventricular valve [361].

However, STI become unreliable in semilunar valve identification in the presence of increased afterload affecting the pulmonary circuit. Under these circumstances RVET may eventually become shorter than LVET, or vice-versa in cases of transposition. This can be documented in at least two different clinical situations:

1) In obstructive pulmonary hypertension, and

2) During the neonatal period, if complicated by factors known to affect pulmonary vascular resistance, such as hypoxia and acidemia [323]. The expected dramatic fall in pulmonary vascular resistance following expansion and ventilation of the lungs might then be delayed and a shortened RVET, or prolonged PEP, documented. This has recently been corroborated by Gutgesell et al. [133], who found RVSTI to be similar in neonates suffering from a respiratory distress syndrome (RDS) with normally related great arteries, and those afflicted with d-TGA, conditions whereby the right ventricle is subjected to an increased afterload. The same authors [133] found, however, that even in the first 48 h of life, LVSTI were similar in normals and infants with RDS, while infants with d-TGA had shorter LPEP and longer LVET.

23.2.2 Alteration of STI in Volume Overloading of the Right Ventricle

In patients with ASD, Curtiss et al. [71] have shown a significant prolongation of the QP_2 interval due to a significant increase in RVET. Unfortunately, in contrast to normal right ventricles, a linear correlation of RVET and stroke index could not be documented [277 b].

23.3 Functional Assessment in Acquired Heart Disease

STI are useful parameters in the functional assessment of a variety of acquired heart diseases.

23.3.1 Aortic Valve Disease

Patients with compensated aortic valve disease (stenosis and/or insufficiency) are characterized by shortened PEP (in aortic regurgitation) and by lengthened LVET (in aortic stenosis). The PEP/LVET ratio is thus decreased [414].

This has allowed a noninvasive estimation of the severity of the obstruction in adults with aortic stenosis [4, 105]. Paradoxically, normal STI are found in these patients with the development of LV failure, as PEP will then get longer and LVET shorter [414].

23.3.2 Mitral Valve Regurgitation (see 13.1.2)

In this situation the PEP/LVET ratio will be characteristically increased up to 0.50, even if ventricular performance is not diminished [403, 414]. A ratio of over 0.50, however, usually points to a reduction in LV performance [403]. The elevated ratio in mitral regurgitation is probably due to the systolic leak into the left atrium during the PEP of systole, which results in a diminished rate of LV pressure development during that period [403]. This causes the PEP of systole to be prolonged with a commensurate abbreviation of the ejection phase through the aortic valve. A diminished contractile performance of the LV may be an additional factor [403].

23.4 Study of Left Ventricular Performance (see Chap. 24)

24 Left Ventricular Performance

Index

Introduction

One of the most promising clinical applications of echocardiography consists in the noninvasive assessment of LV performance.

This can be achieved in several ways:
1) Through determining left ventricular volumes, stroke volume and ejection fraction (24.1).
2) Through determining different kinds of parameters, such as (a) STI's (24.2); (b) ejection phase indices of contractility (24.3), which include fractional shortening (FS) and mean velocity of circumferential fiber shortening (VcF); and (c) endocardial velocity parameters (24.4), which include maximal systolic endocardial velocity (SEVM) and maximal diastolic endocardial velocity (DEVM),
3) By studying left ventricular dimensional changes in relation to MV motion (24.5), and
4) By assessing left ventricular function by computer analysis of the echocardiogram (24.6).

In children, particularly useful indices of LV function that remain relatively constant throughout chilhood [135], are (1) the STI, more specifically the PEP/LVET ratio; as seen in chapter 23, the PEP/VET ratio normally averages 0.31 for the left ventricle [135, 365]; and (2) the index of fractional shortening.

In this chapter it will be shown how in a variety of conditions, LV performance can be assessed noninvasively.

24.1 Left Ventricular Volumes, Ejection Fraction, and Stroke Volume

The minor axis of the LV cavity, defined as the distance between the left septal surface and the posterior endocardial surface, in mm, at the level of the PMVL, or of the chordae tendineae in the older child, can easily be determined at end-diastole ($LVID_d$) and end-systole ($LVID_s$). These measurements are quite important clinically. Indeed, from these dimensions, LV volumes, stroke volume, ejection fraction, and cardiac output can be estimated reliably [173, 240]. This is based on the assumption that the LV cavity is a prolate ellipsoid with a major axis twice the length of the two minor axes.

Commonly used formulas, derived and simplified from the above assumptions, are:
1) LV end-diastolic volume: $LVEDV = LVID_d^3$,
2) LV end-systolic volume: $LVESV = LVID_s^3$,
3) Stroke volume: $SV = LVEDV - LVESV$ (in cc),
4) Cardiac output (l/min): $CO = SV\ (cc/beat) \times HR\ (beats/minute) \times 10^{-3}$, and
5) Ejection fraction: $EF = \dfrac{LVEDV - LVESV}{LVEDV}$

These unsophisticated formulas are simple, reliable, and easy to use in serial evaluation of patients.

24.2 Systolic Time Intervals (STI)

The STI have been applied in the functional assessment of a variety of cardiovascular conditions.

24.2.1 Differentiation of Constrictive Pericarditis from True Myocardial Failure

Constrictive pericarditis, whose differentiation from cardiomyopathy is difficult on clinical grounds, even after sophisticated procedures such as cardiac catheterization and angiography, can be clearly differentiated from myocardial disease by the determination of STI [106, 277 b].

In the absence of a structural abnormality of the heart, the finding of a long PEP followed by a short LVET, or a PEP/LVET ratio over 0.44, which is typically associated with a low ejection fraction and heart failure [277 b], will favor a cardiomyopathy. In constrictive pericarditis, where filling rather than emptying is impaired, these intervals usually remain normal. Ghose et al. [106] showed a clear discrimination between these two entities, with 0.5 as the dividing line both for the PEP/LVET ratio and for the ejection fraction. In general, the level of abnormality in ventricular performance will parallel an increasing PEP/LVET ratio, as can be judged from Table 24.1, taken from Ghose et al. [106].

Table 24.1. Ventricular performance and PEP/LVET ratio

Ventricular performance	PEP/LVET ratio
Mildly abnormal	0.44–0.52
Moderately abnormal	0.53–0.60
Severely abnormal	Over 0.60

24.2.2 Appreciation of Sequential Changes in Left Ventricular Performance Following Drug Administration

Sequential changes in LV performance, for instance after the administration of vasoactive drugs, can be readily appreciated by determination of the STI.

Digitalis

After digitalis administration, improved LV performance is reflected in a reduction of a previously elevated PEP/LVET ratio, although rarely to normal [414]. The reduction in this ratio is brought about by a reduction in the PEP, as ejection time alone does not change [44, 120].

Beta-Receptor Stimulators

These agents, more than digitalis, prove effective in lowering an abnormally elevated PEP/LVET ratio. A hallmark of the effects of positive inotropic agents, such as isoproterenol and to a lesser extent digitalis, is an abbreviation of the total electromechanical systole [414]. Although the PEP/LVET ratio has the advantage of being self-corrected for sex and heart rate [365], some authors advocate heart rate correction when the inotropic action of various interventions is studied serially in single patients [63].

24.2.3 Appreciation of Sequential Changes Pre- and Postoperatively

Patients with atrial septal defects have a shorter LVET index (i.e., ejection time corrected for heart rate), a longer mean PEP index, and a higher ratio of PEP/LVET as compared to normals [404]. There is a direct linear relation between both the PEP index and the PEP/LVET ratio and the size of the shunt.

This mildly diminished overall LV performance, as shown by the STI, appears to be related to the volume overload of the RV and the concomitantly diminished volume of the LV, as LV performance returns to normal after closure of the defect [404].

24.2.4 Left Ventricular Failure in Valvular Heart Disease

The effect of failure on LV function in AoV and MV disease can be assessed by the determination of STI (see Chap. 23).

In summary, the PEP/LVET ratio tends to become normal when aortic valvular disease decompensates, whereas a ratio of over 0.50 is usually documented in the presence of decompensated mitral regurgitation.

24.2.5 Left Ventricular Performance After Acute Myocardial Infarction

As myocardial infarction is rare in children, the interested reader is referred to the appropriate literature.

Before concluding the chapter on STI, STI and ventricular conduction disturbances, and clinical applications of isovolumic contraction time (ICT), one of the component intervals of the PEP, should be considered.

STI and Ventricular Conduction Disturbances

STI cannot be relied upon for a functional assessment if ventricular conduction is altered, as in complete left and right bundle branch block.

Left Bundle Branch Block (LBBB)

A LBBB will characteristically prolong the left PEP selectively [414]. As LBBB is a very rare occurrence in a pediatric population, this may not prove bothersome in clinical practice.

Right Bundle Branch Block (RBBB)

A complete RBBB, if not affecting left ventricular STI, does prolong the RPEP [153], which would seem to preclude the use of right ventricular STI in the assessment of postoperative patients with complete RBBB [153]. However, this difficulty can be circumvented by the separate determination of the two component intervals of the PEP: the electromechanical delay and the isovolumic contraction time (ICT). Indeed, the ICT is less influenced by conduction abnormalities than are other measures of ventricular performance [167, 415].

Clinical Applications of ICT

Clinical applications of ICT have so far been limited due to technical difficulties in delineating this subinterval [414]. Echocardiography has made it possible to reliably determine the length of the ICT, from mitral leaflet coaptation to aortic cusp opening, using different cardiac cycles at similar R-R intervals [154] or more easily using a dual M-mode registration system [334].

Hirschfeld et al. [154] have recently determined the ICT and have found vast differences between normal children (mean ICT = 29 ms ($\pm$9 ms)) at a mean heart rate of 107 (± 27), and those with patent ductus arteriosus (marked shortening) and left ventricular myocardial disease (marked lengthening), when analyzed as groups. Indeed, in 20 children suffering from myocardial disease, Hirschfeld et al., [154] found a mean ICT of 57 ms (± 17), far above the normal regression for normal children, despite the fact that 13 of these children had been treated with digitalis prior to echocardiographic evaluation.

Johnson et al. [167] showed that serial echocardiographic evaluation of RV ICT can give an accurate reproducible assessment of RV afterload in many children with congenital heart disease and complete RBBB. In normal children, mean RV ICT ranged from 1 to 20 ms (mean ± SD = 10.2 ± 5.2 ms).

24.3 Ejection Phase Indices of Contractility

The echocardiographic recording of septal and LV posterior wall motion has been shown to be a reproducible method of evaluating LV function [135].

Essentially, two indices of contractility may be derived from this recording: (1) fractional shortening, and (2) mean velocity of circumferential fiber shortening.

Fractional Shortening (Fs)

Fractional shortening is determining by the formula:

$$Fs = \frac{LVID_d - LVID_s}{LVID_d} \times 100\ (\%)$$

where LVID = left ventricular internal dimension during diastole (d), or systole (s).

Reported normal values have varied from 30 to 40%, e.g., 32 ± 6% [334]; 34 ± 3% [431]; and 36 + 4% [135].

This index represents the percentage of shortening of the LV internal dimension, or minor axis, during systolic contraction. Provided that the LV is approximately circular on cross section, fractional shortening is the same as shortening of the internal circumference of the chamber, i.e., circumferential shortening [101]. The calculation of Fs, on a M-mode recording, is simple and involves no assumptions about the axis ratio of the LV [230]. Fs can be assessed, even more precisely, from two-dimensional transverse cross sections of the left ventricle even if this cavity lacks a circular shape on cross section. This is made possible by high resolution two-dimensional systems, which allow correct tracing of the LV endocardial circumference, in systole as in diastole, at different levels within the ventricular chamber.

As discussed before (Chap. 23), Fs is of particular value in the assessment of LV function in children because of its constancy throughout childhood [135], and its independence of heart rate [334].

Mean Velocity of Circumferential Fiber Shortening (Vcf, Vd)

The mean velocity of circumferential fiber shortening is determined from the formula

$$Vcf = \frac{LVID_d - LVID_s}{LVID_d \times ET}$$

where Vcf is expressed in circumferences per s, LVID is expressed in mm, and ET is expressed in s.

This index represents the rate or mean velocity of circumferential fiber shortening, normalized for LV end-diastolic dimensions. A significant correlation ($r = 0.91$) has been found between angiographic and echocardiographic estimates of this parameter [173].

The reported normal values are (1) for normal infants [326, 334], 1.51 ± 0.04 circumferences/s; (2) for children aged 2 to 10 years [431], 1.34 ± 0.03 circumferences/s; and (3) for children aged 5.4 ± 0.07 years [135], 1.01 ± 0.02 circumferences/s.

The mean Vcf is thus higher in younger children with a faster heart rate, as LVET is directly related to age and inversely to heart rate [135]: younger subjects with a faster heart rate have a shorter LVET and thus a higher value of Vcf [135].

It is now possible to determine Vcf more accurately by simultaneous dual M-mode echocardiograms, including a MV and AoV echo-trace; this makes possible the calculation of the LVET combined with the calculation of the simultaneously derived LV diastolic and systolic dimensions [334].

Fs and Vcf represent ejection phase indices of contractility and may be used to evaluate the basal contractile state even in patients with chronic changes in cardiac loading. However, because they are affected by acute changes in preload and afterload [320], these indices are of less value in the detection of acute changes in contractility. The isovolumetric phase indices (PEP) then prove to be more accurate [34].

Fs and Vcf prove valuable in the assessment of a number of clinical situations: (1) the study of LV function in mitral and aortic valve disease; (2) the study of left ventricular function in acute rheumatic fever; (3) the evaluation of digoxin therapy on LV performance; (4) the estimation of the severity of the obstruction in children with fixed valvular aortic stenosis; and (5) as an aid in the differential diagnosis in infants with congestive heart failure.

24.3.1 Study of Left Ventricular Function in Mitral and Aortic Valve Disease

McDonald recently used the Fs index to echocardiographically assess LV function in MV [230] and in AoV disease [229].

Mitral Valve Disease

In *mitral regurgitation* without LV failure, myocardial contraction is abnormally increased; if failure is documented, myocardial contractions are not so vigorous but remain within normal limits [230]. As McDonald states, these findings contrast strikingly with those in other forms of chronic heart disease with LV failure, which are characterized by a marked reduction in myocardial contractions. The value of echocardiography in MV disease is thus to allow a differentiation of primary mitral regurgitation from regurgitation secondary to other causes such as myocardiopathies. A LV angiocardiogram can thus be advantageously avoided. Wanderman et al. [403] have subsequently shown that there is an inverse relation between the PEP/LVET ratio and the percent change in minor axis diameter. An increase in the PEP/LVET ratio to greater than 0.50 is consistently associated with abnormal LV performance, whereas a normal ratio reflects normal or supernormal LV performance.

In *mitral stenosis*, to the contrary, myocardial contraction is reduced in about one-third of patients [230]. This reduction is perhaps of prognostic value in the postoperative course of patients undergoing MV surgery.

Aortic Valve Disease

In AoV disease, myocardial contraction generally remains normal in the absence of failure. If failure supervenes, reduced myocardial contraction is documented by a substantial reduction in Fs [229].

24.3.2 Study of Left Ventricular Function in Acute Rheumatic Fever (RF)

VcF is increased at the onset of acute RF in children suffering from mitral regurgitation without failure (Vcf = 1.90 ± 0.31 circumferences/s); in the presence of failure, however, Vcf is decreased (Vcf = 1.18 ± 0.25 c/s) [339]. Subsequently, Vcf decreases progressively in the first group, staying above normal levels, whereas in the second group, with failure, Vcf increases to exceed the expected normal values. This suggests that in this last group of children, the carditis is healing but that mitral regurgitation persists.

The echocardiogram thus facilitates the serial assessment of the severity of the carditis in acute RF; in addition, the documentation of an initial decrease in Vcf may be an important prognostic factor [339].

24.3.3 Estimation of the Severity of Obstruction in Children with Fixed Aortic Stenosis

In congenital aortic stenosis, the normal box-like configuration of the AoV echogram is usually preserved. In addition, the severity of the obstruction cannot be deduced from the AoV orifice, except in infants with critical aortic stenosis, as the echocardiographic orifice depends more on transducer position and the angle at which the ultrasonic beam intersects the doming valve orifice.

Nevertheless, estimation of the transvalvular gradient is possible and can be approached in different ways.

From the Index of Fractional Shortening (Fs)

Johnson et al. [165] showed that the Fs index permits excellent separation of patients with mild to moderate obstruction from those with moderate to severe obstruction: if Fs stayed under 40%, the authors could never document a LV-aortic peak systolic pressure gradient of over 45 mm Hg; if Fs was in excess of 40%, a 0.96 likelihood existed for the obstruction to be at least equal to 45 mm Hg; and if Fs was over 45%, the likelihood of a gradient of over 70 mm Hg was 0.90 However, Blackwood et al. were not able to confirm the above findings [128].

From the Relative Left Ventricular Wall Thickness

Glanz et al. [113], in patients with normal myocardial function, demonstrated a consistent relationship between LV peak systolic pressure and the echocardiographically measured relative LV wall thickness, which is one of the major determinants of the percent shortening fraction.
This relationship was expressed as follows:

$$\text{pressure (mm Hg)} = 225 \times \frac{\text{Ws}}{\text{LVES}}$$

where Ws = systolic wall thickness, and
LVES = systolic LV internal diameter.

Interestingly, Johnson et al. [166] found an identical relationship between end-systolic wall thickness and cavity transverse dimension to predict the severity of aortic obstruction in children.

For Blackwood et al. [28] this relationship was only slightly different:

$$\text{pressure (mm Hg)} = 245 \times \frac{\text{Ws}}{\text{LVES}}.$$

From Cross Sectional Echocardiographic Analysis

Cross sectional echocardiography, more than M-mode examination, helps in the detection of congenital valvular aortic stenosis, through its ability to visualize the entire AoV area. Curvature of the aortic cusps toward the center of the aortic lumen, reflecting systolic doming of the valve, and responsible for limited aortic cusp separation, can be visualized using either a sector scanner [429] or two-dimensional cross-sectional echocardiography.

The severity of the obstruction can be graded by looking at the ratio of maximum aortic cusp separation (MACS) to aortic root diameter (AOD) [429]. A MACS/AOD ratio of 0.42 to 0.62 indicates mild stenosis, while a ratio of under 0.35 is consistent with severe aortic obstruction.

Finally, in the presence of severe aortic obstruction, secondary supportive echocardiographic features will be documented, such as (see Figs. 11.4–11.6):

1) Decreased intercusp distance during systole,
2) Multiple diastolic echoes (usually with bicuspid valves),
3) An eccentric diastolic closure line (usually with bicuspid valves),
4) Concentric LVH,
5) Dilatation of the ascending aorta, except in neonates with critical stenosis who may have a decreased aortic root dimension (see 19.2),
6) Reduced MV diastolic closure slope.

Aortic valve disease may sometimes exist simultaneously with hypertrophic subaortic stenosis [262].

24.3.4 Evaluation of Digitalis Therapy on Left Ventricular Performance

Vcf proves quite useful in evaluating the effects of digitalis therapy on LV performance. An increase in the percent shortening of the LV minor dimension, and in Vcf, both in the basal state and after acute pressure loading, without changes in ejection time, is documented during digoxin therapy [70]. These results are in keeping with the reported reduction in the PEP/LVET ratio after digitalis therapy [76, 414].

24.3.5 Differential Diagnosis of Congestive Heart Failure in Full-Term and Preterm Infants

The determination of either Vcf [329] or Fs [23] in infants with signs of cardiac failure is of diagnostic interest. Indeed, if one of these parameters is increased, a large left-to-right shunt should be suspected; to the contrary, nonstructural heart disease such as myocarditis becomes more likely in the opposite situation. Finally, if cardiac failure is related to a respiratory distress syndrome, the above-mentioned parameters are usually not affected [23, 329]. As Table 24.2, taken from Sahn et al. [329], shows, the LA/Ao ratio further helps in this diagnostic separation.

Table 24.2. Diagnostic separation of infants with congestive heart failure due to left-right shunts or to nonstructural heart disease

	LA/Ao ratio	Vcf
Normal	0.77 ± 0.01	1.51 ± 0.04
Left-right shunt	1.14 ± 0.01	2.12 ± 0.08
Nonstructural heart disease	1.26 ± 0.1	1.18 ± 0.06

In older children suffering from cardiomyopathies, similar diminished values for ejection phase indices are reported [334].

24.4 Maximal Systolic and Diastolic Endocardial Velocity Parameters

Maximal systolic endocardial velocity (SEVM) and maximal endocardial diastolic velocity (DEVM) are determined by taking a tangent of the steepest portion of the systolic or diastolic endocardial excursion of the LV posterior wall and measuring the slope in cm/s.

New developments in echocardiography, such as the computer assisted processing of two-dimensional images, allow the reconstruction in M-mode of the echo information from any line through the two-dimensional image. This implies that M-mode recordings may be obtained from many well-delineated parts of the LVPW. SEVM and DEVM may be assessed from all these locations, making it possible to describe in quantitative terms areas of hypo- or hyperkinesia.

Normal values for these indices are [185]: SEVM $= 6.2 \pm 1.4$ cm/s, and DEVM $= 18 \pm 3$ cm/s.

Both indices are reduced in patients with muscular dystrophy, even when other criteria of myocardial performance are still unrevealing [185]. The DEVM, reflecting muscular relaxation, is the more reliable of the two indices.

24.5 Left Ventricular Dimensional Changes in Relation to Mitral Valve Motion

In normal subjects, maximum wall thickness, minimum dimension of the LV, and MV opening are synchronous [392]: the onset of MV opening thus coincides with the start of the increase in LV dimension [107].

However, when segmental abnormalities of contraction are present, a characteristic disturbance may be documented with the onset of outward wall movement preceding the start of MV opening [394] (see Fig. 24.1).

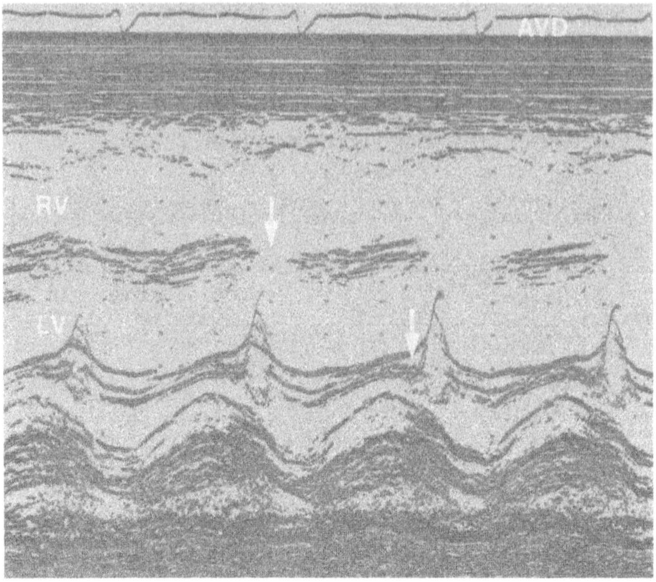

Fig. 24.1. AVD: Echocardiogram obtained from a 19-year-old male with d-TGA, VSD, subpulmonary obstruction, and partial pulmonary venous return to the superior vena cava. Note that the onset of outward wall movement preceeds the start of MV opening (*lower arrow*). (*Upper arrow* points to the presence of a VSD)

Such information can be gained from direct inspection of the original echo trace, or more precisely, from digitizing the various echoes using a simple computer technique [107].

24.6 Left Ventricular Function by Computer Analysis of the Echocardiogram

Left ventricular echoes can be digitized. Computer analysis allows a continuous measurement of cavity size, and a study of diastolic filling, wall motion, and variations in thickness. Using this technique abnormal LV function can be readily recognized. Such studies are possible even in newborns [373].

Appendix

Normal Echocardiographic Values

In this appendix, normal age-related values for most important echocardiographic measurements are listed. These include values for RV anterior wall thickness, RV end-diastolic dimension, septal and LVPW thicknesses, LV end-diastolic dimension, LA and aortic dimensions at valvular level, and pulmonary root diameter.

Some of these data are from Dr. P. J. Voogd, who studied 425 healthy school children (207 boys and 218 girls) between the ages of 3 and 17 years in Leiden, Holland. Echocardiograms were obtained by experienced technicians using an Echocardiovisor 03 (Organon Teknika), at the time of a regular yearly physical check-up by the school physician. Children afflicted with any disease process or congenital anomaly were excluded from the study. Measurements were made as follows: aortic and left atrial diameters were obtained at end-systole, the aortic dimension being determined between the anterior aspects of both aortic walls. LV end-diastolic dimensions were obtained at the tip of the PMVL at the point of the greatest vertical distance, at which place LVPW and septal thicknesses were also determined. Echocardiographic dimensions were measured semiautomatically and data were computerized. Formulas based on linear as well as on exponential regression equations were derived for most important echocardiographic measurements. Linear regression equations were possible for various body parameters such as body weight, length, and surface area, and for age. They offer the advantage of simple use. The exponential equations derived for body weight (see Table A1) are more sophisticated, as they provide fifth and 95th percentile values. Though less practical, their correlation coefficient is often better. The interested reader is referred to Dr. P. Voogd's complete study:

Voogd P, Rijsterborgh H, Zwieten G van, Lubsen J: Percentiles of echocardiographic dimensions in healthy children and young adolescents. In: Lancée C (ed). Echocardiology. Proceedings of the 3rd Symposium on Echocardiology. Nijhoff, The Hague 1979, p. 299-307.

Missing data are taken from the available literature. All these data are of interest as they allow to follow the growth pattern of a particular cardiac structure [319].

Table A1. Table of exponents (B) and coefficients (A) for boys and girls, allowing calculation of the fifth, 50th, and 95th percentiles (P) in mm, of various echocardiographic dimensions, in relation to body weight (in kg)[a]

Echo parameter	Exponents and coefficients for boys			
	B	A5	A50	A95
IVS (ED)	0.379	1.51	1.97	2.47
LVID (ED)	0.263	15.48	17.27	19.13
LVPW (ED)	0.362	1.42	1.80	2.29
IVS (ES)	0.297	3.09	3.87	4.81
LVID (ES)	0.303	7.87	9.41	10.96
LVPW (ES)	0.342	2.56	3.33	4.06
Ao	0.334	6.55	7.71	8.93
LA	0.247	10.49	12.35	14.61
Echo parameter	**Exponents and coefficients for girls**			
	B	A5	A50	A95
IVS (ED)	0.346	1.60	2.08	2.69
LVID (ED)	0.228	16.85	18.86	20.91
LVPW (ED)	0.382	1.27	1.57	2.03
IVS (ES)	0.235	3.40	4.37	5.46
LVID (ES)	0.247	9.79	11.32	13.00
LVPW (ES)	0.339	2.51	3.21	3.98
Ao	0.272	7.86	9.18	10.67
LA	0.150	13.94	16.72	20.08

[a] For instance: LVID (ED), P5 (boy, 30 kg) $= A5 \times (\text{weight})^B = 15.48 \times (30)^{0.263}$

Table A2. Normal values for pulmonary root diameter

Group	Weight (kg)[a]	No.	Measurement	Diameter (mm)[b]	References
Neonates	2.6–4.6	200	Outside diameter at end-systole	9.4–13.0	Hagan [136]
	2.27	21	At end-diastole	10.7–13.3 (12)	Solinger et al. [360]
	2.73	28		11.2–13.8 (12.5)	
	3.18	25		11.7–14.3 (13.0)	
	3.64	22		12.2–14.8 (13.5)	
	4.09	23		12.7–15.3 (14.0)	
	1.9.–4.3	38	At end-systole	9.2–12.8	Godman et al. [117]
Adults			At end-systole	20–40	Weyman, cited by Williams and Tucker [431]

[a] Mean values

[b] Mean values in brackets

Table A3. Right ventricular anterior wall thickness

Group	Weight (kg)[a]	No.	Measurement	Ant. wall thickness (mm)[b]	References
Neonates	2.6–4.6	200	Endocardium to epicardium at level of MV	2–4.7	Hagan [136]
	2.27	21	Endoc. to epic.	1.1–2.9 (2)	
	2.73	28	at level of TV	1.3–3.1 (2.2)	Solinger et al. [360]
	3.18	25		1.6–3.4 (2.5)	
	3.64	22		1.8–3.6 (2.7)	
	4.09	23		2.0–3.8 (2.9)	
Infants, children (0.5–18 years)		102	"Inner chest" or peric. to endocardial surf. at end-diastole	1.3–3.5	Epstein et al. [90]

[a] Mean values [b] Mean values in brackets

Table A4. Normal values for Right ventricular dimensions

Group	Weight (kg)[a]	No.	Measurement	RV dimension (mm)[b]	References
Neonates	2.6–4.6 (mean: 3.4)	200	Endocardium to RSS[c] at end-diastole, at level of MV	6.4–15.0 (11.4)	Hagan [136]
	1.9–4.3	50	Endocardium to RSS at end-diastole, with LV posterior	10–17.5	Godman et al. [117]
Infants, Children	8–11.5	26	Ant. RV wall to	3–15 (9)	
	11.6–22.9	26	RSS, at end-diastole	4–15 (10)	
	23–34.3	20		7–18 (11)	Feigenbaum [98]
	34.4–45.7	15		7–16 (12)	
	45.8–57	11		8–17 (13)	
Adults			At end-diastole	Under 30 7–23 (supine) 10–26 (left lateral position)	Roelandt [315] Feigenbaum [98]

[a] Mean values [c] RSS = right septal surface
[b] Mean values in brackets

Table A5. Normal values for LV end-diastolic dimensions

Group	Weight (kg)[a]	No.	Transducer position	$LVID_d$ (mm)[b]	References
Neonates	2.6–4.6 (mean: 3.4)	200	AMVL and PMVL level	12–23 (18.7)	Hagan [136]
	2.27	21	Mitral valve level	16.1–21.7 (18.9)	
	2.73	28	(top of the QRS)	16.5–22.1 (19.3)	
	3.18	25		17.0–22.6 (19.8)	Solinger et al. [360]
	3.64	22		17.5–23.1 (20.3)	
	4.09	23		18.0–23.6 (20.8)	

[a] Mean values
[b] Mean values in brackets

Continued next page

Table A5 (continued)

Group	Weight (kg)[a]	No.	Transducer position	$LVID_d$ (mm)[b]	References
Infants	0–11.5	26	Inferolateral to maximal AMVL excursion	13–32 (24)	Feigenbaum [98]
Older	11.6–22.9	26	AMVL or chordae	24–38 (34)	
children	23.0–34.4	20	still visible	33–45 (38)	
	34.4–45.7	15		35–47 (41)	Feigenbaum [98]
	45.8–57.0	11		37–49 (43)	
Boys	15–82	208	Just below MV	32.16–57.04	
Girls	14–77	218	at onset of QRS	30.08–54.59	
Adults			Just below MV on top of R wave	39–56	Roelandt [315]

Table A6. Linear regression equations to find $LVID_d$, for both boys and girls, 4 to 17 years old, weighing 14 to 82 kg, were derived by P. Voogd, from age, body length and weight, and body surface area

Boys:	LVIDd	=	1.17 (age in years) + 31.46 (R: 0.80)
		=	0.21 (length in cm) + 14.26 (R: 0.86)
		=	0.31 (weight in kg) + 32.66 (R: 0.85)
		=	13.55 (BSA in M^2) + 27.42 (R: 0.86)
Girls:	LVIDd	=	1.00 (age in years) + 31.90 (R: 0.76)
		=	0.18 (length in cm) + 16.94 (R: 0.79)
		=	0.27 (weight in kg) + 32.58 (R: 0.79)
		=	11.93 (BSA in M^2) + 28.01 (R: 0.81)

Similarly, P. Voogd found exponential regression equations derived from body weight, for both boys and girls (see Table A1).

Table A7. Normal values for septal thickness

Group	Weight (kg)[a]	No.	Measurement	Septal thickness (mm)[b]	References
Neonates	2.6–4.6 (mean: 3.4)	200	At MV or TV	1.8–4.0 (2.7)	Hagan [136]
	2.27	21	End-diastole, at MV	2.1–3.3 (2.7)	
	2.73	28		2.4–3.6 (3.0)	
	3.18	25		2.6–3.8 (3.2)	Solinger et al. [360]
	3.64	22		2.9–4.1 (3.5)	
	4.09	23		3.1–4.3 (3.7)	
Infants	0–11.5 (mean: 7.7)	26	End-diastole	4–6 (5)	Feigenbaum [98]
Older	11.6–22.9	26	End-diastole	5–7 (6)	
children	23.0–34.3	20		6–7 (7)	
	34.4–45.7	15		7–8 (7)	Feigenbaum [98]
	45.8–57.0	11		7–8 (7)	
	57.1–91.0	5		7–8 (8)	
Adults			On top of R wave	6–12	Roelandt [315]

[a] Mean values

[b] Mean values in brackets

Table A8. Linear regression equations to find septal thickness in boys and girls

	Septal thickness (mm)
Boys[a]	0.05 (length in cm) +0.32 (R: 0.72)
	0.08 (weight in kg) +4.84 (R: 0.72)
	3.36 (BSA in M^2) +3.55 (R: 0.73)
Girls[b]	0.26 (age in years) +4.41 (R: 0.63)
	0.07 (weight in kg) +4.76 (R: 0.62)
	2.91 (BSA in M^2) +3.67 (R: 0.62)

[a] In boys, 4 to 17 years old, weighing 15 to 82 kg, linear regression equations were derived by Dr. P. Voogd from body length and weight, and body surface area.
[b] In girls, aged 4 to 17 years, weighing 14 to 77 kg, linear regression equations prove less accurate. The best correlations are found with age, weight and body surface area (Dr. P. Voogd).
Exponential regression equations, derived by Dr. P. Voogd, from body weight are listed in Table A1.

Table A9. Normal values for LVPW thickness (at end-diastole)

Group	Weight (kg)[a]	No.	Wall thickness (mm)[b]	References
Neonates	2.6–4.6 (mean: 3.4)	200	1.6–3.7 (2.6)	Hagan [136]
	2.27	21	2.0–3.4 (2.7)	
	2.73	28	2.3–3.7 (3.0)	
	3.18	25	2.5–3.9 (3.2)	Solinger et al. [360]
	3.64	22	2.8–4.2 (3.5)	
	4.09	23	3.0–4.4 (3.7)	
Infants	0–11.5 (mean: 7.7)	26	4–6 (5)	Feigenbaum [98]
Older children	11.6–22.9 (mean: 17.7)	26	5–7 (6)	
	23.0–34.3 (mean: 28.1)	20	6–7 (7)	
	34.4–45.7 (mean: 40.5)	15	7–8 (7)	Feigenbaum [98]
	45.8–57.0 (mean: 51.3)	11	7–8 (7)	
	57.1–91.0 (mean: 75.0)	5	7–8 (8)	
Adults			6–12	Roelandt [315]

[a] Mean values
[b] Mean values in brackets

Table A10. Linear regression equations to find LVPW thickness, in both boys and girls, aged 4 to 17 years, weighing 14 to 82 kg, were derived by Dr. P. Voogd, from body weight and surface area

Boys	LVPW	= 0.07 (weight in kg) + 4.09 (R: 0.74)
		= 2.92 (BSA in M^2) + 3.05 (R: 0.73)
Girls	LVPW	= 0.06 (weight in kg) + 3.87 (R: 0.70)
		= 2.75 (BSA in M^2) + 2.86 (R: 0.70)

Exponential regression equations derived by Dr. P. Voogd from body weight are listed in Table A1.

Table A11. Normal values for aortic root diameter

Group	Weight (kg)[a]	No.	Measurement	Aortic root diameter (mm)[b]	References
Neonates	2.6–4.6 (mean: 3.4)	200	External diameter	8.1–12 (10)	Hagan [136]
	2.27	21	Outside diameter	9.3–11.3 (10.3)	
	2.73	28	at end-systole	9.7–11.7 (10.7)	
	3.18	25		10.2–12.2 (11.2)	Solinger et al.
	3.64	22		10.7–12.7 (11.7)	[360]
	4.09	23		11.1–13.1 (12.1)	
	1.9–4.3	50		8–11	Godman et al. [117]
Infants	0–11.5 (mean: 7.7)	26	At end-diastole	7–17 (13)	Feigenbaum [98]
Older children	11.6–22.9 (mean: 17.7)	26	At end-diastole	13–22 (17)	
	23.0–34.3 (mean: 28.1)	20		17–23 (20)	
	34.4–45.7 (mean: 40.4)	15		19–27 (22)	Feigenbaum [98]
	45.8–57.0 (mean: 51.3)	15		17–27 (23)	
	57.1–91 (mean: 75)	5		22–28 (24)	
Adults			At end-diastole (onset of QRS)	20–37	Feigenbaum [98] Roelandt [315]

[a] Mean values
[b] Mean values in brackets

Table A12. Linear regression equations to find the aortic root diameter, in boys and girls, 4 to 17 years old, weighing 14 to 82 kg, were derived by Dr. P. Voogd from age, body length and weight, and body surface area

In boys:	Aortic width	= 0.90 (age in years) + 15.72 (R: 0.81)
		= 0.15 (length in cm) + 3.64 (R: 0.83)
		= 0.22 (weight in kg) + 17.25 (R: 0.80)
		= 9.80 (BSA in M^2) + 13.39 (R: 0.82)
In girls:	Aortic width	= 0.69 (age in years) + 16.88 (R: 0.74)
		= 0.12 (length in cm) + 7.15 (R: 0.74)
		= 0.18 (weight in kg) + 17.55 (R: 0.75)
		= 7.95 (BSA in M^2) + 14.53 (R: 0.76)

Exponential regression equations derived by Dr. P. Voogd from body weight are listed in Table A1.

Table A13. Linear regression equations to find LA diameter in boys, 4 to 17 years old, weighing 15 to 82 kg, were derived by Dr. P. Voogd from body weight and body surface area

LA dimension: 0.20 (weight in kg) + 22.27 (R: 0.71)
8.81 (BSA in M^2) + 19.03 (R: 0.71)

In girls such formulas prove unsatisfactory.
Exponential regression equations derived by Dr. P. Voogd from body weight are listed in Table A1.

Table A14. Normal values for left atrial dimensions

Group	Weight (kg)[a]	No.	Measurement	LA dimension (mm)[b]	References
Neonates	2.6–4.6 (mean: 3.4)	200	Posterior surface of	5–10 (7)	Hagan [136]
	2.27	21	PAW to LA endocardium	6.8–10.5 (8.7)	
	2.73	28	at end-systole	7.4–11.1 (9.3)	
	3.18	25		8.0–11.7 (9.9)	Solinger et al. [360]
	3.64	22		8.6–12.3 (10.5)	
	4.09	23		9.2–12.9 (11.1)	
	1.9–4.3	50	Aortic root to LA wall at end-systole	4–10.5	Godman et al. [117]
Infants	0–11.5 (mean: 7.7)	26	Anterior surface of PAW or mitral ring to LA wall at end-systole	7–23 (17)	Feigenbaum [98]
Older children	11.6–22.9 (mean: 17.7)	26	Anterior surface of PAW or mitral	17–27 (22)	
	23.0–34.3 (mean: 28.1)	20	ring to LA wall at end-systole	19–28 (23)	
	34.4–45.7 (mean: 40.4)	15		20–30 (24)	Feigenbaum [98]
	45.8–57.0 (mean: 51.3)	11		21–30 (27)	
	57.1–91.0 (mean: 75.0)	5		21–37 (28)	
Adult			End systole, largest diameter	15–40	Roelandt [315]

[a] Mean values
[b] Mean values in brackets

References

1 Abbasi AS (1976) Echocardiography in the differential diagnosis of the large heart. Am J. Med 60: 677–686

2 Abbasi AS, Chahine RA, MacAlpin RN, Kattus AA (1973) Ultrasound in the diagnosis of primary congestive cardiomyopathy. Chest 63: 937–942

3 Acar J, Kulas A, Grimberg D, Brun P, Luxereau P (1976) L'échocardiographie chez les malades atteints de valvulopathie aortique. Nouv Presse Med 5: 93–94

4 Ahmed SS, Levinson GE, Schwartz CJ (1972) Systolic time intervals as measures of the contractile state of the left ventricular myocardium in man. Circulation 46: 559–571

5 Akgün G, Layton C (1977) Aortic root and left atrial wall motion. An echocardiographic study Br Heart J 39: 1082–1087

6 Allen HD, Blieden LC, Stone FM, Bessinger FB, Lucas RV (1974) Echocardiographic demonstration of a right ventricular tumor in a neonate. J Pediatr 84: 854–856

7 Allen HD, Goldberg SJ, Sahn DJ, Ovitt TW, Goldberg BB (1977) Suprasternal notch echocardiography. Assessment of its clinical utility in pediatric cardiology. Circulation 55: 605–612

8 Allen HD, Goldberg SJ, Sahn DJ, Schy N, Wojcik R (1977) A quantitative echocardiographic study of champion childhood swimmers. Circulation 55: 142–145

9 Allen HD, Sahn DJ, Goldberg SJ (1978) New serial contrast technique for assessment of left-to-right shunting in patent ductus arteriosus in the neonate. Am J Cardiol 41: 288–294

10 Allen JW, Harrison EC, Camp JC, Borsari A, Turnier E, Lau FYK (1977) The role of serial echocardiography in the evaluation and differential diagnosis of pericardial disease. Am Heart J 93: 560–567

11 Andriange M (1974) L'échocardiographie. Rev Med Liege 29: 193–201

12 Assad-Morell JL, Tajik AJ, Giuliani ER (1974) Aneurysm of membranous interventricular septum. Echocardiographic features. Mayo Clin Proc 49: 164–171

13 Assad-Morell JL, Tajik AJ, Giuliani ER (1974) Echocardiographic analysis of the ventricular septum. Prog Cardiovasc Dis 17: 219–237

14 Assad-Morell JL, Seward JB, Tajik AJ, Hagler DJ, Giuliani ER, Ritter DG (1976) Echo-phonocardiographic and contrast studies in conditions associated with systemic arterial trunk overriding of the ventricular septum. Truncus arteriosus, tetralogy of Fallot, and pulmonary atresia with ventricular septal defect. Circulation 53: 663–673

15 Atsuchi Y, Nagai Y, Komatsu Y, Nakamura K (1977) Echocardiographic demonstration of anomalous septum in cor triatriatum. Jpn Heart J 18: 266–271

16 Atsuchi Y, Nagai Y, Komatsu Y, Nakamura Y, Shibuya M, Hirosawa K (1977) Echocardiographic manifestations of annulo-aortic ectasia: its "paradoxical" motion of the aorta and premature systolic closure of the aortic valve. Am Heart J 93: 428–433

17 Aziz KU, Paul MH, Muster AJ (1976) Echocardiographic localization of interatrial baffle after Mustard operation for dextro-transposition of the great arteries. Am J. Cardiol 38: 67–72

18 Aziz KU, Paul MH, Muster AJ (1978) Echocardiographic assessment of left ventricular outflow tract in d-transposition of the great arteries. Am J. Cardiol 41: 543–551

19 Bahler AS, Meller J, Brik H, Herman MV, Teichholz LE (1976) Paradoxical motion of the interventricular septum with right ventricular dilatation in the absence of shunting. Report of two cases. Am J. Cardiol 38: 654–657

20 Barlow JB, Pocock WA (1975) The problem of non-ejection systolic clicks and associated mitral systolic murmurs: emphasis on the billowing mitral leaflet syndrome. Am Heart J 90: 636–655

21 Barlow JB, Pocock WA, Marchand P, Denny M (1963) The significance of late systolic murmurs. Am Heart J 66: 443–452

22 Bass JL, Bessinger FB, Lawrence C (1978) Echocardiographic differentiation of partial and complete atrioventricular canal. Circulation 57: 1144–1150

23 Baylen B, Meyer RA, Korfhagen J, Benzig GIII, Budd ME, Kaplan S (1977) Left ventricular performance in the critically ill premature infant with patent ductus arteriosus and pulmonary disease. Circulation 55: 182–188
24 Beardshaw JA, Gibson DG, Pearson MC, Upton MT, Anderson RH (1977) Echocardiographic diagnosis of primitive ventricle with 2 atrioventricular valves. Br Heart J 39: 266–275
25 Becker AE, Tynan MJ, Anderson RH (1977) Cardiac anatomy in congenital heart disease. In: Bom N (ed.) Echocardiology. Nijhoff, The Hague
26 Beppu S, Nimura Y, Nagata S, Ramai M, Matsuo H, Matsumoto M, Kawashima Y, Sakakibara H, Abe H (1976) Diagnosis of endocardial cushion defect with cross-sectional and M-mode echocardiography. Differentiation from secundum atrial septal defect. Br Heart J 38: 911–920
27 Bini RM, Bloom KR, Culham JAG, Freedom RM, Williams CM, Rowe RD (1978) The reliability and practicality of single crystal echocardiography in the evaluation of single ventricle. Angiographic and pathological correlates. Circulation 57: 269–277
28 Blackwood RA, Bloom KR, Williams CM (1978) Aortic stenosis in children. Experience with echocardiographic prediction of severity. Circulation 57: 263–268
29 Bloch A (1976) L'échocardiographie. Applications cliniques. Med Hyg (Geneve) 34: 777–784
30 Bloom KR, Rodrigues L, Swan EM (1977) Echocardiographic evaluation of left-to-right shunt in ventricular septal defect and patent ductus arteriosus. Br Heart J 39: 260–265
31 Borer JS, Henry WL, Epstein SE (1977) Echocardiographic observations in patients with systemic infiltrating disease involving the heart. Am J Cardiol 39: 184–188
32 Boucher CA, Fallon JT, Myers GS, Hutter AM, Buckley MJ (1977) The value and limitations of echocardiography in recording mitral valve vegetations. Am Heart J 94: 37–43
33 Bozio A, Payot M, Vela-Espelta F, Kratz C, Normand J, Davignon A (1977) Le syndrome d'hypoplasie du coeur gauche. Corrélations anatomo-échocardiographiques. Arch Mal Coeur 71: 1–8
34 Braunwald E (1977) Current concepts in cardiology. Determinants and assessment of cardiac function. N Engl J Med 296: 86–89
35 Brown OR (1973) Echocardiographic study of right ventricular hypertension producing asymmetric septal hypertrophy. Circulation 47/48: Suppl V: 47
36 Brown OR, Demots H, Kloster FE, Roberts A, Menashe VD, Beals RK (1975) Aortic root dilatation and mitral valve prolapse in Marfan's syndrome. An echocardiographic study. Circulation 52: 651–657
37 Brown OR, Popp RL, Kloster FE (1975) Echocardiographic criteria for aortic root dissection. Am J Cardiol 36: 17–20
38 Bulkley BH, Weisfeldt ML, Hutchins GM (1977) Asymmetric septal hypertrophy and myocardial fiber disarray. Features of normal developing, and malformed hearts. Circulation 56: 292–298
39 Burges J, Clark R, Kamagaki M, Cohn K (1973) Echocardiographic findings in different types of mitral regurgitation. Circulation 48: 97–106
40 Burggraf GW, Craige E (1975) Echocardiographic studies of left ventricular wall motion and dimensions after valvular heart surgery. Am J Cardiol 35: 473–480
41 Calder L, Praagh R van, Praagh S van, Sears WP, Corwin R, Levy A, Keith JD, Paul MH (1976) Truncus arteriosus communis. Clinical, angiocardiographic and pathologic findings in 100 patients. Am Heart J 92: 23–38
42 Candell-Riera J, Garcia del Castillo H, Permanyer-Miralda G, Soler-Soler J (1978) Echocardiographic features of the interventricular septum in chronic constrictive pericarditis. Circulation 57: 1154–1158
43 Canedo MI, Otken L, Stefadouros MA (1977) Echocardiographic features of cardiac compression by a thymoma simulating cardiac tamponade and obstruction of the superior vena cava Br Heart J 39: 1038–1042
44 Carliner NH, Gilbert CA, Pruitt AW (1974) Effects of maitenance digoxin therapy on systolic time intervals and serum digoxin concentrations. Circulation 50: 94–98
45 Casaneda AR, Anderson RC, Edwards JE (1969) Congenital mitral stenosis resulting from anomalous arcade and obstructing papillary muscles. Am J Cardiol 24: 237–240
46 Chandraratna PAN, Langevin E (1977) Limitations of the echocardiogram in diagnosing valvular vegetations in patients with mitral valve prolapse. Circulation 56: 436–438
47 Chandraratna PAN, Lopes JM, Litman BB, Gupta JD, Samet P (1974) Abnormal mitral valve motion during ventricular extrasystoles: an echocardiographic study. Am J Cardiol 34: 783–786

48 Chandraratna PAN, Bhaduri U, Littman BB, Hildner FJ (1974) Echocardiographic findings in persistent truncus arteriosus in a young adult. Br Heart J 36: 732–736
49 Chandraratna PAN, Balachandran PK, Shah PM, Hodges M (1975) Echocardiographic observations on ventricular septal rupture complicating acute myocardial infarction. Circulation 51: 506–510
50 Chandraratna PAN, Lopes JM, Fernandez JJ, Cohen LS (1975) Echocardiographic detection of tricuspid valve prolapse. Circulation 51: 823–826
51 Chandraratna PAN, Samet P, Robinson MJ, Byrd C (1975) Echocardiography of the "floppy" aortic valve. Report of a case. Circulation 52: 959–962
52 Chandraratna PAN, Robinson MJ, Byrd C, Pitha JV (1977) Significance of abnormal echoes in left ventricular outflow tract. Br Heart J 39: 381–389
53 Chandraratna PAN, SanPedro S, Elkins RC, Grantham N (1977) Echocardiographic, angiocardiographic and surgical correlations in right ventricular myxoma simulating valvar pulmonic stenosis. Circulation 55: 619–622
54 Chandraratna PAN, Tolentino AO, Mutucumarana W, Gomez AL (1977) Echocardiographic observation on the association between mitral valve prolapse and asymmetric septal hypertrophy. Circulation 55: 622–626
55 Chanine RA, Raizner AE, Ishimori T, Montero AC (1977) Echocardiographic, hemodynamic, and angiographic correlations in hypertrophic cardiomyopathy. Br Heart J 39: 945–953
56 Chesler E, Joffe HS, Vecht R, Beck W, Schrire V (1970) Ultrasound cardiography in single ventricle and the hypoplastic left and right heart syndromes. Circulation 42: 123–129
57 Chesler E, Joffe HS, Beck W, Schrire V (1971) Echocardiographic recognition of mitral-semilunar valve discontinuity. An aid to the diagnosis of origin of both great vessels from the right ventricle. Circulation 43: 725–732
58 Chesler E, Joffe HS, Beck W, Schrire V (1971) Echocardiography in the diagnosis of congenital heart disease. Pediatr Clin North Am 18: 1163–1190
59 Chung KJ, Alexon CG, Manning JA, Gramiak R (1973) Echocardiography in truncus arteriosus. The value of pulmonic valve detection. Circulation 48: 281–286
60 Clarkson PM, Brandt PWT, Barratt-Boyes BG, Neutze JM (1972) "Isolated atrial inversion". Visceral situs solitus, visceroatrial discordance, discordant ventricular d-loop without transposition, dextrocardia: diagnosis and surgical correction. Am J Cardiol 29: 877–881
61 Cody MC, Giuliani ER, Mair DD (1973) "Paradoxical" septal motion by echocardiography in a patient with normal right heart hemodynamics. Mayo Clin Proc 48: 31–34
62 Cohen MV (1976) Double mitral leaflet prolapse: echocardiographic-phonocardiographic correlation. Am Heart J 91: 168–177
63 Cokkinos DV, Heimonas ET, Demopoulos JN, Haralambakis A, Tsartsaus G, Gardikas CD (1976) Influence of heart rate increase on uncorrected pre-ejection period/left ventricular ejection time (PEP/LVET) ratio in normal individuals. Br Heart J 38: 683–688
64 Come PC, Bulkley BH, Goodman ZD, Hutchins GM, Pitt B, Fortuin NJ (1977) Hypercontractile cardiac state simulating hypertrophic cardiomyopathy. Circulation 55: 901–908
65 Cooperberg P, Hazell S, Ashmore PG (1976) Parachute accessory anterior mitral valve leaflet causing left ventricular outflow tract obstruction. Circulation 53: 908–911
66 Cope GD, Kisslo JA, Johnson ML, Behar VS (1975) A reassessment of the echocardiogram in mitral stenosis. Circulation 52: 664–670
67 Cope GD, Kisslo JA, Johnsosn ML, Myers S (1975) Diastolic vibration of the interventricular septum in aortic insufficiency. Circulation 51: 589–593
68 Corya BC, Feigenbaum H, Rasmussen S (1974) Echocardiographic features of congestive cardiomyopathy compared with normal subjects and patients with coronary artery disease. Circulation 49: 1153–1159
69 Corya BC, Black MJ, McHenry PL (1976) Echocardiographic findings after acute carbon monoxide poisoning. Br Heart J 38: 712–717
70 Crawford MH, Karliner JS, O'Rourke RA (1976) Favorable effects of oral maintenance digoxin therapy on left ventricular performance in normal subjects: echocardiographic study. Am J Cardiol 38: 843–847
71 Curtiss EI, Reddy PS, O'Toole JD, Shaver JA (1976) Alterations of right ventricular systolic time intervals by chronic pressure and volume overloading. Circulation 53: 997–1003
72 Dashkoff N, Karacuschansky M, Come PC, Fortuin NJ (1977) Echocardiographic features of mitral annulus calcification. Am Heart J 94: 585–592

73 Davis RH, Feigenbaum H, Chang S, Konecke LL, Dillon JC (1974) Echocardiographic manifestations of discrete subaortic stenosis. Am J Cardiol 33: 227–280
74 D'Cruz IA, Cohen HC, Prabhu R, Bisla V, Glick G (1977) Clinical manifestations of mitral annulus calcification, with emphasis on its echocardiographic features. Am Heart J 94: 367–377
75 D'Cruz, Prabhu R, Cohen HC, Glick G (1977) Potential pitfalls in quantification of pericardial effusions by echocardiography. Br Heart J 39: 529–535
76 Delgado CE, Fortuin NJ, Rose RS (1975) Acute effects of low doses of alcohol on left ventricular function by echocardiography. Circulation 51: 535–540
77 Devereux RB, Perloff JK, Reichek N, Josephson ME (1976) Mitral valve prolapse. Circulation 54: 3–14
78 Diamond MA, Dillon JC, Haine CL, Chang S, Feigenbaum H (1971) Echocardiographic features of atrial septal defect. Circulation 43: 129–135
79 Dillon JC, Feigenbaum H, Konecke LL (1973) Echocardiographic manifestations of valvular vegetations. Am Heart J 86: 698–704
80 Dillon JC, Feigenbaum H, Konecke LL, Keutel J, Hurwitz RA, Davis RH, Chang S (1973) Echocardiographic manifestations of d-transposition of the great vessels. Am J Cardiol 32: 74–78
81 Dillon JC, Chang S, Feigenbaum H (1974) Echocardiographic manifestations of left bundle branch block. Circulation 49: 876–880
82 Dillon JC, Weyman AE, Feigenbaum H, Eggleton RC, Johnston K (1977) Cross-sectional echocardiographic examination of the interatrial septum. Circulation 55: 115–120
83 Dorp WG van, Spitaels S, Villeneuve VH de, Roelandt J (1976) Echocardiology II. Application to patients with congenital heart disease. Hart Bull 7: 189–200
84 Dorp WG van, TenCate FJ, Vletter WB, Dohmen H, Roelandt J (1976) Familial prevalence of asymmetric septal hypertrophy. Eur J Cardiol 4: 349–357
85 Dorp WG van, Vogel JA, Zwieten G van, Roelandt J (1976) Cardiac applications of ultrasound. Neth J Med 19: 103–110
86 Duchak JM, Chang S, Feigenbaum H (1972) Echocardiographic features of torn chordae tendineae. Am J Cardiol 29: 260 (Abstract)
87 Duff DF, Gutgesell HP (1977) The use of saline or blood for ultrasonic detection of a right-to-left intracardiac shunt in the early postoperative patient. Am Heart J 94: 402–406
88 Ehlers KH, Haystrom JWC, Lukas DS (1962) Glycogen storage of the myocardium with obstruction of the left ventricular outflow. Circulation 25: 96–109
89 Ehrich DA, Vieweg WVR, Alpert JS, Folkerth TL, Hagan AD (1977) Cor triatriatum: report of a case in a young adult with special reference to the echocardiographic features and etiology of the systolic murmur. Am Heart J 94: 217–221
90 Epstein ML, Goldberg SJ, Allen HD, Konecke L, Wood J (1975) Great vessel, cardiac chamber, and wall growth patters in normal children. Circulation 51: 1124–1129
91 Estevez CM, Weyman AE, Feigenbaum H (1976) Detection of left ventricular diverticulum by cross-sectional echocardiography. Chest 69: 544–546
92 Farooki ZQ, Henry JG, Arciniegas E, Green EW (1974) Ultrasonic pattern of ventricular rhabdomyoma in 2 infants. Am J Cardiol 34: 842–844
93 Farooki ZQ, Henry JG, Green EW (1975) Echocardiographic diagnosis of right atrial extension of Wilm's tumor. Am J Cardiol 36: 363–367
94 Farooki ZQ, Henry JG, Green EW (1976) Echocardiographic spectrum of Ebstein's anomaly of the tricuspid valve. Circulation 53: 63–68
95 Farooki ZQ, Henry JG, Green EW (1976) Echocardiographic spectrum of the hypoplastic left heart syndrome. A clinicopathologic correlation in 19 newborns. Am J Cardiol 38: 337–343
96 Farooki ZQ, Adelman S, Green EW (1977) Echocardiographic differentiation of a cystic and solid tumor of the heart. Am J Cardiol 39: 107–111
97 Feigenbaum H (1975) Echocardiographic diagnosis of pericardial effusion. Am J Cardiol 26: 475–479
98 Feigenbaum H (1976) Echocardiography. Lea and Febiger, Philadelphia
99 Felner JM, Brewer DB, Franch RH (1976) Echocardiographic manifestations of single ventricle. Am J Cardiol 38: 80–84
100 Finegan RE, Harrison DC (1970) Diagnosis of left atrial myxoma by echocardiography. N Engl J Med 282: 1022–1023
101 Fortuin NJ, Hood WP, Craige E (1972) Evaluation of left ventricular function by echocardiography. Circulation 46: 26–35

102 Francis GS, Theroux P, O'Rourke RA, Hagan AD, Johnson AD (1976) An echocardiographic study of interventricular septal motion in the WPW syndrome. Circulation 54: 174–178

103 French JW, Popp R (1975) Variability of echocardiographic discontinuity in double outlet right ventricle and truncus arteriosus. Circulation 51: 848–854

104 French JW, Baum D, Popp RI (1975) Echocardiographic findings in Uhl's anomaly. Demonstration of diastolic pulmonary valve opening. Am J Cardiol 36: 349–353

105 Garrard CL, Weissler AM, Dodge HT (1970) The relationship of alterations in systolic time intervals to ejection fraction in patients with cardiac disease. Circulation 42: 455–462

106 Ghose JC, Mitra SK, Chhetri MK (1976) Systolic time intervals in the differential diagnosis of constrictive pericarditis and cardiomyopathy. Br Heart J 38: 47–50

107 Gibson DG (1977) Detection of incoordinate left ventricular contraction by echocardiography In: Bom N (ed) Echocardiology. Nijhoff, The Hague

108 Gibson DG, Honey M, Lennox SC (1974) Cor triatriatum, diagnosed by echocardiography. Br Heart J 36: 835–838

109 Gibson DG, Grossman W, McLaurin LP, Moos S, Craige E (1976) An echocardiographic study of the interventricular septum in constrictive pericarditis. Br Heart J 38: 738–743

110 Gilbert BW, Schatz RA, Ramm OT von, Behar VS, Kisslo JA (1976) Mitral valve prolapse. Two-dimensional echocardiographic and angiocardiographic correlations. Circulation 54: 716–723

111 Gilbert BW, Haney RS, Crawford F, McClellan J, Gallis HA, Johnson ML, Kisslo JA (1977) Two-dimensional echocardiographic assessment of vegetative endocarditis. Circulation 55: 346–353

112 Girard DE (1977) Mitral valve prolapse-click syndrome in twins. Am Heart J 94: 813–815

113 Glanz S, Hellenbrand WR, Berman MA, Talner NS (1976) Echocardiographic assessment of the severity of aortic stenosis in children and adolescents. Am J Cardiol 38: 620–625

114 Glaser J, Whitman V, Liebman J (1972) The differential diagnosis of total anomalous pulmonary venous drainage in infancy by echocardiography. Circulation [Suppl II] 45/46: 38 (Abstract)

115 Glaser J, Bharati S, Whitman V, Liebman J (1973) Echocardiographic findings in patients with anomalous origin of the left coronary artery. Circulation [Suppl IV] 47/48: 63 (Abstract)

116 Glasser SP, Baucum RW (1977) Pulmonary valve fluttering in subpulmonic ventricular septal defect. Am Heart J 94: 3–5

117 Godman MJ, Tham P, Langford Kidd BS (1974) Echocardiography in the evaluation of the cyanotic newborn infant. Br Heart J 36: 154–166

118 Goldberg SJ, Allen HD, Sahn DJ (1975) Pediatric and adolescent echocardiography. Year Book Medical Publisher, Chicago

119 Goldschlager A, Popper R, Goldschlager N, Gerbode F, Prozan G (1972) Right atrial myxoma with right-to-left shunt and polycythemia presenting as congenital heart disease. Am J Cardiol 30: 82–86

120 Gomes JA, Calderon J, Zama Q (1975) Improvement in cardiac performance after maintenance digoxin in alcoholic cardiomyopathy: an echocardiographic study. Circulation [Suppl II] 51/52: 49 (Abstract)

121 Goodman DJ, Harrison DC, Popp RL (1974) Echocardiographic features of primary pulmonary hypertension. Am J Cardiol 33: 438–443

122 Gottlieb S, Khuddus SA, Balooki H, Dominguez AE, Meyerburg RJ (1974) Echocardiographic diagnosis of aortic valve vegetations in candida endocarditis. Circulation 50: 826–830

123 Graham TP, Jarmakani JM, Canent RV (1972) Left heart volume characteristics with a right ventricular volume overload. Circulation 45: 389–396

124 Gramiak R, Nanda NC (1972) Echocardiographic diagnosis of ostium primum septal defect. Circulation [Suppl II] 46: 137 (Abstract)

125 Gramiak S, Shah PM (1971) Cardiac ultrasonography. A review of current applications. Radiol Clin North Am 9: 469–490

126 Gramiak R, Shah PM (1971) Detection of intracardiac blood flow by pulsed echo-ranging ultrasound. Radiology 100: 415–418

127 Gramiak R, Chung KJ, Nanda N, Manning J (1973) Echocardiographic diagnosis of transposition of the great vessels. Radiology 106: 187–189

128 Greene DA, Kleid JJ, Naidu S (1977) Unusual echocardiographic manifestations of pericardial effusions. Am J Cardiol 39: 112–115

129 Greenwald J, Yap JF (1975) Echocardiographic mitral systolic motion in left ventricular aneurysm. Br Heart J 37: 684–690

130 Griffith JM, Henry WL (1974) A sector scanner for real time two-dimensional echocardiography. Circulation 49: 1147–1152

131 Guntheroth WG (1968) Tetralogy of Fallot. In: Moss AJ, Adams FH (eds) Heart disease in infants, children and adolescents. Williams and Wilkins, Baltimore

132 Gutgesell HP (1978) Echocardiographic estimation of pulmonary artery pressure in transposition of the great arteries. Circulation 57: 1151–1153

133 Gutgesell HP, Duff D, Adams J (1976) Left ventricular and right ventricular systolic time intervals in the neonate: comparison of transposition and respiratory distress in normal newborns. Circulation [Suppl II] 54: 47 (Abstract)

134 Gutgesell HP, Mullins CE, Gilette PC, Speer M, Rudolph AJ, McNamara DG (1976) Transient hypertrophic subaortic stenosis in infants of diabetic mothers. J Pediatr 89: 120–125

135 Gutgesell HP, Paquet M, Duff DF, McNamara DG (1977) Evaluation of left ventricular size and function by echocardiography. Results in normal children. Circulation 56: 457–462

136 Hagan AD (1973) Echocardiographic criteria for normal newborn infants. Circulation 48: 1221–1226

137 Hagan AD, Francis GS, Sahn DJ, Karliner JS, Friedman WF, O'Rourke RA (1974) Ultrasound evaluation of systolic anterior septal motion in patients with and without right ventricular volume overload. Circulation 50: 248–254

138 Hagemeijer F, Serruys PW, Dorp WG van (1977) Contrast echocardiology. In: Bom N (ed) Echocardiology. Nijhoff, The Hague

139 Hagler DJ (1976) Echocardiographic findings in atrioventricular canal defects In: Feldt RH (ed) Atrioventricular canal defect. Saunders, Philadelphia

140 Hagler DJ (1976) The utilization of echocardiography in the differential diagnosis of cyanosis in the neonate. Mayo Clin Proc 51: 143–154

141 Hagler DJ, Tajik AJ, Ritter DG (1975) Fluttering of the atrioventricular valves in patients with d-transposition of the great arteries after Mustard operation. Mayo Clin Proc 50: 69–75

142 Hall SW, Theologides A, From AHL, Gobel FL, Fortuny IE, Lawrence CJ, Edwards JE (1977) Hypereosinophilic syndrome with biventricular involvement. Circulation 55: 217–222

143 Halliday H, Hirschfeld S, Riggs T, Liebman J, Fanaroff A, Bormuth C (1977) Respiratory distress syndrome: echocardiographic assessment of cardiovascular function and pulmonary vascular resistance. Pediatrics 60: 444–449

144 Henning H, Roeske W, Karliner I, Crawford M, O'Rourke (1976) Inferior myocardial infarction: a common cause of asymmetric septal hypertrophy. Circulation [Suppl II] 53/54: 191 (Abstract)

145 Henry WL, Borer JS (1977) Echocardiographic assessment of cardiomyopathies. In: Bom N (ed) Echocardiology. Nijhoff, The Hague

146 Henry WL, Clark CE, Epstein SE (1973) Asymmetric septal hypertrophy. The unifying link in the IHSS disease spectrum: observations regarding its pathogenesis, pathophysiology, and course. Circulation 47: 827–832

147 Henry WL, Clark CE, Griffith JM, Epstein SE (1975) Mechanism of left ventricular outflow obstruction in patients with obstructive asymmetric septal hypertrophy (idiopathic hypertrophic subaortic stenosis). Am J Cardiol 35: 337–345

148 Henry WL, Maron BJ, Griffith JM, Redwood DR, Epstein SE (1975) Differential diagnosis of anomalies of the great arteries by real-time two-dimensional echocardiography. Circulation 51: 283–291

149 Henry WL, Morganroth J, Pearlman AS, Clark CE, Redwood DR, Itscoitz SB, Epstein SE (1976) Relation between echocardiographically detemined left atrial size and atrial fibrillation. Circulation 53: 273–279

150 Hess PG, Nanda NC, Weese JA de, Reeves WC, Gramiak R (1977) Echocardiographic features of combined membranous subaortic stenosis and acquired calcific aortic valvulopathy. Am Heart J 94: 349–352

151 Hess PG, Nanda NC, Thomson KR, Schwartz RG, Ross A, Gramiak R (1977) Systolic motion patterns of the aortic valve: clinico-echo correlates. Circulation [Suppl III] 55/56: 50 (Abstract)

152 Hirschfeld S, Meyer RA, Schwartz DC, Korfhagen J, Kaplan S (1975) Measurement of right and left ventricular systolic time intervals by echocardiography. Circulation 51: 304–309

153 Hirschfeld S, Meyer RA, Schwartz DC, Korfhagen J, Kaplan S (1975) The echocardiographic assessment of pulmonary artery pressure and pulmonary vascular resistance. Circulation 52: 642–650

154 Hirschfeld S, Meyer R, Korfhagen J, Kaplan S, Liebman J (1976) The isovolumic contraction time of the left ventricle. An echocardiographic study. Circulation 54: 751–756

155 Hirschfeld S, Meyer RA, Schwartz D, Korfhagen J, Kaplan S (1976) Echo assessment of pulmonary vascular resistance. (Letter to the editor). Circulation 54: 525–526

156 Hirschfeld DS, Schiller N (1976) Localisation of aortic valve vegetations by echocardiography. Circulation 53: 280–285

157 Hirschfeld DS, Rodriguez HJ, Schiller NB (1976) Duplication of aortic wall seen by echocardiography. Br Heart J 38: 943–950

158 Hishida H, Sobobata I, Koike Y, Okumura M, Mizuno Y (1976) Echocardiographic patterns of ventricular contraction in the Wolff-Parkinson-White syndrome. Circulation 54: 567–570

159 Horowitz MS, Schultz CS, Stinson EB (1974) Sensitivity and specificity of echocardiographic diagnosis of pericardial effusion. Circulation 50: 239–247

160 Houston AB, Gregory NL, Shaw A, Wheatley DJ, Coleman EN (1977) Two-dimensional echocardiography with a wide angle (60°) sector scanner. Br Heart J 39: 1071–1075

161 Houston AB, Gregory NL, Coleman EN (1978) Echocardiographic identification of aorta and main pulmonary artery in complete transposition. Br Heart J 40: 377–382

162 Houston AB, Gregory NL, Coleman EN (1978) Two-dimensional sector-scanner echocardiography in cyanotic congenital heart disease. Br Heart J 39: 1076–1081

163 Hunter S, Mortera C, Terry G, Goodwin A, Tynan M, Holden M (1977) Echocardiographic visualization of the interatrial baffle after Mustard's operation. Br Heart J 39: 954–957

164 Jacobs JJ, Feigenbaum H, Corya BC, Phillips JF (1973) Detection of left ventricular asynergy by echocardiography. Circulation 48: 263–271

165 Johnson GL, Meyer RA, Schwartz DC, Korfhagen J, Kaplan S (1976) Left ventricular function by echocardiography in children with fixed aortic stenosis. Am J Cardiol 38: 611–619

166 Johnson GL, Meyer RA, Schwartz DC, Korfhagen J, Kaplan S (1977) Echocardiographic evaluation of fixed left ventricular outlet obstruction in children. Pre- and postoperative assessment of ventricular systolic pressures. Circulation 56: 299–304

167 Johnson GL, Meyer RA, Korfhagen J, Schwartz DC, Kaplan S (1978) Echocardiographic assessment of pulmonary arterial pressure in children with complete right bundle branch block. Am J Cardiol 41: 1264–1269

168 Johnson ML, Warren CG, Waugh RA, Kisslo JA, Sabiston DC, Lesten R (1974) Echocardiography of the aortic valve in non-rheumatic left ventricular outflow tract lesions. Radiology 112: 677–684

169 Johnson SL, Baker DW, Lute RA, Murray JA (1974) Detection of mitral regurgitation by Doppler echocardiography. Am J Cardiol 33: 147 (Abstract)

170 Jones WB, Hefner LL, Bancroft WH, Klip W (1959) Velocity of blood flow and stroke volume obtained from the pressure pulse. J Clin Invest 38: 2087–2090

171 Joyner CR, Hey ED, Johnson J, Reid JM (1967) Reflected ultrasound in the diagnosis of tricuspid stenosis. Am J Cardiol 19: 66–73

172 Kamigaki M, Goldschlager N (1972) Echocardiographic analysis of mitral valve motion in atrial septal defect. Am J Cardiol 30: 343–348

172b Katz NM, Buckley MJ, Liberthson RR (1977) Discrete membranous subaortic stenosis: report of 31 patients. Review of the literature and delineation of management. Circulation 56: 1034–1041

173 Kaye HH, Tynan M, Hunter S (1975) Validity of echocardiographic estimates of left ventricular size and performance in infants and children. Br Heart J 37: 371–375

174 Kerber RE, Payvandi MN (1977) Echocardiography in acute hemopericardium: production of false negative echocardiograms by pericardial clots. Circulation [Suppl III] 55/56: 24 (Abstract)

175 Kerber RE, Dippel WF, Abboud FM (1973) Abnormal motion of the interventricular septum in right ventricular volume overload: experimental and clinical echocardiographic studies. Circulation 48: 86–96

176 Kerber RE, Kioschos JM, Lauer RM (1974) Use of an ultrasonic contrast method in the diagnosis of valvular regurgitation and intracardiac shunts. Am J Cardiol 34: 722–727

177 King DL, Steeg CN, Ellis K (1973) Visualization of ventricular septal defects by cardiac ultrasonography. Circulation 48: 1215–1220

178 King JF, Maria AN de (1974) Marked abnormal mitral valve motion without simultaneous intraventricular pressure gradient due to uneven mitral septal contact in idiopathic hypertrophic subaortic stenosis. Am J Cardiol 34: 360–366

179 Kirklin JW, Pacifico AD, Bargeron LM, Soto B (1973) Cardiac repair in anatomically corrected malposition of the great arteries. Circulation 48: 153–159

180 Kisslo J, Ramm OT von, Haney R, Jones R, Juk SS, Behar VS (1976) Echocardiographic evaluation of tricuspid valve endocarditis. An M-mode and twodimensional study. Am J Cardiol 38: 502–507
181 Kisslo J, Ramm OT von, Thurstone FL (1976) Cardiac imaging using a phased array altrasound system, II: clinical technique and application. Circulation 53: 262–267
182 Komatsu Y, Nagai Y, Shibuya M, Takao A, Hirosawa K (1976) Echocardiographic analysis of intracardiac anatomy in endocardial cushion defect. Am Heart J 91: 210–218
183 Konecke LL, Feigenbaum H, Chang S, Corya BS, Fischer JC (1973) Abnormal mitral valve motion in patients with elevated left ventricular diastolic pressures. Circulation 47: 989–996
184 Kotler MN, Segal BL, Mintz C, Parry WR (1977) Pitfalls and limitations of M-mode echocardiography. Am Heart J 94: 227–249
185 Kovick RB, Fogelman AM, Abbasi AS, Peter JB, Pearce ML (1975) Echocardiographic evaluation of posterior left ventricular wall motion in muscular dystrophy. Circulation 52: 447–454
186 Krajcer Z, Orzan F, Pechacek LW, Garcia E, Leachman RD (1978) Early systolic closure of the aortic valve in patients with hypertrophic subaortic stenosis and discrete subaortic stenosis. Correlation with preoperative and postoperative hemodynamics. Am J Cardiol 41: 823–829
187 Kramer NE, Gill SS, Patel R, Towne WD (1977) Pulmonary valve vegetations detected with echocardiography. Am J Cardiol 39: 1064–1067
188 Kronzon I, Schloss M, Danilowicz D, Singh A (1975) Fixed membranous subaortic stenosis. Chest 67: 473–474
189 Krovetz LJ, Gessner IH, Schiebler GL (1967) Truncus arteriosus. In Handbook of pediatric cardiology. Harper and Row, New York
190 Krueger SK, Starke H, Forker AD, Eliot RS (1975) Echocardiographic mimics of aortic root dissection Chest 67: 441–441
191 Lacorte MA, Fellows KE, Williams RG (1976) Overriding tricuspid valve: echocardiographic and angiocardiographic features. Am J Cardiol 37: 911–919
192 Lacorte M, Harada K, Williams R (1976) Echocardiographic features of congenital left ventricular inflow obstruction. Circulation 54: 562–566
193 Larter WE, Allen HD, Sahn DJ, Goldberg SJ (1976) The asymmetrically hypertrophied septum. Further differentiation of its causes. Circulation 53: 19–27
194 Laurenceau JL, Guay JM, Gagné S (1973) Echocardiography in the diagnosis of subaortic membranous stenosis. Circulation [Suppl IV]: 47/48: 46 (Abstract)
195 Lee CC, Das G, Weissler AM (1974) Characteristic echocardiographic manifestations in ruptured aortic valve leaflet. Circulation [Suppl III] 49/50: 144 (Abstract)
196 Leech GJ (1977) Right-sided heart valves. In: Bom N (ed) Echocardiology. Nijhoff, The Hague
197 Lemire F, Tajik AJ, Hagler DJ (1976) Asymmetric left atrial enlargement. An echocardiographic observation. Chest 69: 779–781
198 Lev M, Bharati S, Meng L (1972) A concept of double outlet right ventricle. J Thorac Cardiovasc Surg 64: 271–281
199 Levisman JA (1977) Echocardiographic diagnosis of mitral regurgitation in congestive cardiomyopathy. Am Heart J 93: 33–39
200 Levisman JA, Abbasi AS (1976) Abnormal motion of the mitral valve with pericardial effusion: pseudo prolapse of the mitral valve. Am Heart J 91: 18–20
201 Levisman JA, Abbasi AS, Pearce ML (1975) Posterior mitral leaflet motion in mitral stenosis. Circulation 51: 511–514
202 Levisman JA, MacAlpin RN, Abbasi AS, Ellis N, Eber LM (1975) Echocardiographic diagnosis of a mobile, pedunculated tumor in the left ventricular cavity. Am J Cardiol 36: 957–959
203 Lewis AB, Takahashi M (1976) Echocardiographic assessment of left-to-right shunt volume in children with ventricular septal defect. Circulation 54: 78–82
204 Liberthson RR, Paul MH, Muster AJ (1971) Straddling and displaced atrioventricular orifices and valves with primitive ventricles. Circulation 43: 213–226
205 Liberthson RR, Buckley MJ, Boucher CA (1976) Pulmonary regurgitation in large atrial shunt without pulmonary hypertension. Circulation 54: 966–968
206 Lieppe W, Scallion R, Behar VS, Kisslo J (1977) Two-dimensional echocardiographic findings in atrial septal defect. Circulation 56: 447–456
207 Lieppe W, Behar VS, Scallion R, Kisslo JA (1978) Detection of tricuspid regurgitation with two-dimensional echocardiography and peripheral vein injection. Circulation 57: 128–132

208 Lintermans JP, Dorp WG van (1977) Le diagnostique échocardiographique de la d-transposition des gros vaisseaux par analyse déductive. Arch Mal Coeur 70: 1337–1343

209 Lintermans JP, Roberts DB, Guntheroth WG, Figley MM (1968) Two-chambered right ventricle without outflow obstruction in ventricular septal defect. Am J Cardiol 21: 582–587

210 Lundström NR (1972) Ultrasound-cardiographic studies of the mitral valve region in young infants with mitral atresia, mitral stenosis, hypoplasia of the left ventricle and cor triatriatum. Circulation 45: 324–334

211 Lundström NR (1973) Echocardiography in the diagnosis of Ebstein's anomaly of the tricuspid valve. Circulation 47: 597–605

212 Maria AN de, King JF, Bogren HG, Lies JE, Mason DT (1974) The variable spectrum of echocardiographic manifestations of the mitral valve prolapse syndrome. Circulation 50: 33–41

213 Maria AN de, Vismara LA, Miller RR, Neumann A, Mason DT (1975) Unusual echographic manifestations of right and left heart myxomas. Am J Med 59: 713–720

214 Maria AN de, Miller RR, Amsterdam EA, Markson W, Mason DT (1976) Mitral valve early diastolic closing velocity in the echocardiogram: relation to sequential diastolic flow and ventricular compliance. Am J Cardiol 37: 693–700

215 Maria AN de, Neumann A, Lee G, Fowler W, Mason DT (1978) Alterations in ventricular mass and performance induced by exercise training in man evaluated by echocardiography. Circulation 57: 237–244

215 a Marin-Garcia J, Tandon R, Moller JH (1974) Common (single) ventricle with normally related great vessels. Circulation 49: 565–573

215 b Markiewicz W, Stoner J, London E, Hunt S, Popp RL (1976) Mitral valve prolapse in one hundred presumably healthy young females. Circulation 53: 464–473

216 Maron BJ, Edwards JE, Henry WL, Clark CE, Bingle GJ, Epstein SE (1974) Asymmetric septal hypertrophy (ASH) in infancy. Circulation 50: 809–820

217 Maron BJ, Henry WL, Griffith JM, Freedom RM, Kelly DT, Epstein SE (1975) Identification of congenital malformations of the great arteries in infants by real-time two-dimension echocardiography. Circulation 52: 671–677

218 Maron BJ, Henry WL, Clark CE, Redwood DR, Roberts WC, Epstein SE (1976) Asymmetric septal hypertrophy in childhood. Circulation 53: 9–19

219 Maron BJ, Redwood DR, Roberts WC, Henry WL, Morrow AG, Epstein SE (1976) Tunnel subaortic stenosis. Left ventricular outflow tract obstruction produced by fibromuscular tubular narrowing. Circulation 54: 404–416

220 Maron B, Clark C, Henry W, Fukuda T, Edwards J (1976) Is the disproportionately thickened ventricular septum always genetically transmitted asymmetric septal hypertrophy? Circulation [Suppl II] 53/54: 80 (Abstract)

221 Maron BJ, Clark CE, Henry WL Fukuda T, Edwards JE, Matthews EC, Redwood DR, Epstein SE (1977) Prevalence and characteristics of disproportionate ventricular septal thickening in patients with acquired or congenital heart diseases. Echocardiographic and morphologic findings. Circulation 55: 489–496

222 Maron BJ, Gottdiener JS, Roberts WC, Henry WL, Sause DD, Epstein SE (1978) Left ventricular outflow tract obstruction due to systolic anterior motion of the anterior mitral valve leaflet in patients with concentric left ventricular hypertrophy. Circulation 57: 527–533

223 Maron BJ, Savage DD, Clark CE, Henry WL, Vlodaver. Z, Edwards JE, Epstein SE (1978) Prevalence and characteristics of disproportionate ventricular septal thickening in patients with coronary artery disease. Circulation 57: 250–256

224 Martinez EC, Burch GE, Giles TD (1974) Echocardiographic diagnosis of vegetative aortic bacterial endocarditis. Am J Cardiol 34: 645–651

225 Mathey DG, Decoodt PR, Allen HN, Swan HJC (1975) The determinants of mitral valve prolapse in the systolic click – late systolic murmur syndrome. Circulation [Suppl II] 52: 77 (Abstract)

226 Matsumoto M, Matsuo H, Beppu S, Yoshioka Y, Kawashima Y, Nimura Y, Abe H (1976) Echocardiographic diagnosis of ruptured aneurysm of sinus of Valsalva. Circulation 53: 382–389

227 Matsumoto M, Matsuo H, Nagata S, Hamanaka Y, Fujita T, Kawashima Y, Nimura Y, Abe H (1976) Visualization of Ebstein's anomaly of the tricuspid valve by two-dimensional and standard echocardiography. Circulation 53: 69–79

228 McCann WD, Harbold NB, Guilliania ER (1972) The echocardiogram in right ventricular overload. JAMA 221: 1243–1245

229 McDonald IG (1976) Echocardiographic assessment of left ventricular function in aortic valve disease. Circulation 53: 860–864
230 McDonald IG (1976) Echocardiographic assessment of left ventricular function in mitral valve disease. Circulation 53: 865–871
231 McLaurin LP, Gibson TC, Waider W, Grossman W, Craige E (1973) An appraisal of mitral valve echograms mimicking mitral stenosis in conditions with right ventricular pressure overload. Circulation 48: 801–809
232 Meurs van-Woezik H van, Klein HW, Krediet P (1977) Normal internal calibres of ostia of great arteries and of aortic isthmus in infants and children. Br Heart J 39: 860–865
233 Meyer JF, Frank MJ, Goldberg S, Cheng TO (1977) Systolic mitral flutter, An echocardiographic clue to the diagnosis of ruptured chordae tendineae. Am Heart J 93: 3–8
234 Meyer RA (1977) Pediatric echocardiography. Lea and Febiger, Philadelphia
235 Meyer RA, Kaplan S (1972) Echocardiography in the diagnosis of hypoplasia of the left and right ventricle in the neonate. Circulation 46: 55–64
236 Meyer RA, Kaplan S (1973) Noninvasive techniques in pediatric cardiovascular disease. Prog Cardiovasc Dis 14: 341–367
237 Meyer RA, Schwartz DC, Benzing G, Kaplan S (1972) Ventricular septum in right ventricular volume overload. Am J Cardiol 30: 349–353
238 Meyer R, Bloom K, Schwartz D, Kaplan S (1973) Mitral flutter without aortic incompetence. Circulation [Suppl IV] 47/48: 81 (Abstract)
239 Meyer RA, Schwartz DC, Covitz W, Kaplan S (1974) Echocardiographic assessment of cardiac malposition. Am J Cardiol 33: 896–903
240 Meyer RA, Stockert J, Kaplan S (1975) Echocardiographic determination of left ventricular volumes in pediatric patients. Circulation 51: 297–303
241 Mierop LHS van, Eisen S, Schiebler GL (1970) The radiographic appearance of the tracheobronchial tree as an indicator of visceral situs. Am J Cardiol 26: 432–435
242 Mills PG, Leech GJ, Leatham A, Ginks WR (1975) Noninvasive estimation of pulmonary artery end-diastolic pressure. Circulation [Suppl II] 50: 190 (Abstract)
243 Mills P, Amara I, Fujii J, McLaurin L, Koch G, Craige E (1977) Dual echocardiographic right ventricular isovolumic contraction in estimation of pulmonary artery pressures. Circulation [Suppl III] 55/56: 67 (Abstract)
244 Mills P, McLaurin L, Smith C, Murray G, Craige E (1977) Echocardiographic findings in left ventricular to right atrial shunts. Br Heart J 39: 594–597
245 Miller GAH, Gibson DG, Kerr IH (1977) Discrete subaortic stenosis with abnormal left ventricular function In: Proceedings of the 15th Annual General Meeting of the Association of European Pediatric Cardiologists. Belgium, 1977. Akademisch Ziekenhuis, Gent
246 Millward DK, Robinson NJ, Craige E (1972) Dissecting aortic aneurysm diagnosed by echocardiography in a patient with rupture of the aneurysm into the right atrium. Am J Cardiol 30: 427–431
247 Milner S, Meyer RA, Venables AW, Korfhagen J, Kaplan S (1976) Mitral and tricuspid valve closure in congenital heart disease. Circulation 53: 513–518
248 Mintz GS, Kotler MN, Segal BL, Parry WR (1978) Systolic anterior motion of the mitral valve in the absence of asymmetric septal hypertrophy. Circulation 57: 256–263
249 Mintz GS, Kotler MN, Segal BL, Parry WR (1978) Two-dimensional echocardiographic recognition of ruptured chordae tendineae. Circulation 57: 244–250
250 Moodie DS, Hagler DJ, Ritter DG (1976) Cor triatriatum. Echocardiographic findings. Mayo Clin Proc 51: 289–295
251 Moothart RW, Spangler RD, Blount SG (1975) Echocardiography in aortic root dissection and dilatation. Am J Cardiol 36: 11–16
252 Morganroth J, Maron BJ, Krovetz LJ, Henry WL, Epstein SE (1975) Electrocardiographic evidence of left ventricular hypertrophy in otherwise normal children. Clarification by echocardiography. Am J Cardiol 35: 278–281
253 Morris DC, Felner JM, Schlant RC, Franch RH (1975) Echocardiographic diagnosis of tetralogy of Fallot. Am J Cardiol 36: 908–913
254 Mortera C, Hunter S, Terry G, Tynan M (1977) Echocardiography of primitive ventricle. Br Heart J 39: 847–855
255 Mortera C, Hunter S, Tynan M (1977) Diagnosis of ventriculo-arterial discordance (transposition of the great arteries) by contrast echocardiography. Br Heart J 39: 844–846

256 Moulaert A, Bruins C, Buis-Liem T, Oppenheimer-Dekker A (1977) Different types of ventricular septal defects with subaortic stenosis In: Proceedings of the 15 th Annual General Meeting of the Association of European Pediatric Cardiologists. Belgium, 1977. Akademisch Ziekenhuis, Gent

257 Murphy KF, Kotler MN, Reichek N, Perloff JK (1975) Ultrasound in the diagnosis of congenital heart disease. Am Heart J 89: 638–656

258 Nanda NC, Gramiak R, Shah PM (1973) Diagnosis of aortic root dissection by echocardiography. Circulation 48: 506–513

259 Nanda NC, Gramiak R, Manning JA (1974) Echocardiographic studies of the tricuspid valve in atrial septal defect. Circulation [Suppl III] 49/50: 236 (Abstract)

260 Nanda NC, Gramiak R, Manning JA, Mahoney EB, Lipchik EO, Weese JA de (1974) Echocardiographic recognition of the congenital bicuspid aortic valve. Circulation 49: 870–875

261 Nanda NC, Gramiak R, Robinson TI, Shah PM (1974) Echocardiographic evaluation of pulmonary hypertension. Circulation 50: 575–581

262 Nanda NC, Gramiak R, Shah PM, Stewart S, Weese JA de (1974) Echocardiography in the diagnosis of hypertrophic subaortic stenosis co-existing with aortic valve disease. Circulation 50: 752–757

263 Nanda NC, Gramiak R, Manning JA (1975) Echocardiography of the tricuspid valve in congenital left ventricular-right atrial communication. Circulation 51: 268–272

264 Nanda NC, Stewart S, Gramiak R, Manning JA (1975) Echocardiography of the intra-atrial baffle in dextro-transposition of the great vessels. Circulation 51: 1130–1135

265 Nanda NC, Gramiak R, Manning JA, Lipchik EO (1975) Echocardiographic features of subpulmonic obstruction in dextrotransposition of the great vessels. Circulation 51: 515–521

266 Nanda NC, Gramiak R, Gross CM (1976) Echocardiography of cardiac valves in pericardial effusion. Circulation 54: 500–504

267 Nanda NC, Lever H, Gramiak R, Ross A, Reeves W, Hess P, Zesk J, Combs R (1977) Reliability of echocardiography in the diagnosis of aortic root dilatation. Circulation [Suppl III] 55/56: 68 (Abstract)

268 Nasrallah AT, Nihill M (1975) Supravalvular aortic stenosis. Echocardiographic features. Br Heart J 37: 662–667

269 Nasser WK, Davis RH, Dillon JC, Tavel ME, Helman CH, Feigenbaum H, Fisch C (1972) Atrial myxoma. Part II: phonocardiographic, echocardiographic, hemodynamic and angiocardiographic features in 9 cases. Am Heart J 83: 810–824

269a Neufeld HN, Dushane JW, Edwards JE (1961) Origin of both great vessels from the right ventricle. II With pulmonary stenosis. Circulation 23: 603–612

270 Neumann A, Maria AD de, Miller RR, Mason DT (1976) Noninvasive quantification of valvular aortic stenosis by echographic mitral valve early diastolic closing velocity. Circulation [Suppl II] 53/54: 83 (Abstract)

271 Nichol PM, Gilbert BW, Kisslo JA (1977) Two-dimensional echocardiographic assessment of mitral stenosis. Circulation 55: 120–128

272 Nimura Y, Matsumoto M, Beppu S, Matsuo H, Sakakibara H, Abe HL (1974) Noninvasive preoperative diagnosis of cor triatriatum with ultrasonocardiotomogram and conventional echocardiogram. Am Heart J 88: 240–250

273 Nimura Y, Nagata S, Matsumoto M, Beppu S, Tamal M, Yamada Y, Matsuo H, Sakakibara H, Abe H (1975) An unusual pattern of the mitral echocardiogram observed in cases of congestive cardiomyopathy and other myocardial diseases. Jpn Heart J 16: 500–511

274 Nishimura K, Hibi N, Kato T, Fukui Y, Arakawa T, Tatematsu H, Miwa A, Tada H, Kambe T, Sakamoto N (1976) Real-time observation of ruptured right sinus of Valsalva aneurysm by high speed ultrasono-cardiotomography. Report of a case. Circulation 53: 732–735

275 Orsmond GS, Knight L, Dehner LP, Nicoloff DM, Nesbitt M, Bessinger FB (1976) Alveolar rhabdomyosarcoma involving the heart: an echocardiographic, angiographic and pathologic study. Circulation 54: 837–843

276 Orsmond GS, Ruttenberg HD, Bessinger FB, Moller JH (1978) Echocardiographic features of total anomalous pulmonary venous connection to the coronary sinus. Am J Cardiol 41: 597–601

277 Owens JP, Williams RG, Fellows KE (1974) Prolapsing mitral leaflet associated with secundum atrial defect. Circulation [Suppl III] 50: 263 (Abstract)

277 a Paquet M, Gutgesell H (1975) Echocardiographic features of total anomalous pulmonary venous connection. Circulation 51: 599–605

277 b Parisi AF, Tow DE, Felix RW, Sasahara AA (1977) Noninvasive cardiac diagnosis. N Engl J Med 296: 316–320, 368–374, 427–432

278 Park SC, Neches WH, Zuberbuhler JR, Matthews RA, Lenox CC, Fricker FJ (1978) Echocardiographic and hemodynamic correlates in transposition of the great arteries. Circulation 57: 291–298

279 Patton R, Dragatakis L, Marpole D, Sniderman A (1978) The posterior left atrial echocardiogram of mitral regurgitation. Circulation 57: 1134–1139

280 Payvandi MN, Kerber RE (1976) Echocardiography in congenital and acquired absence of the pericardium. An echocardiographic mimic of right ventricular volume overload. Circulation 53: 86–92

281 Payvandi MN, Kerber RE, Phelps CD, Judisch GE, El-Khoury G, Schrott HG (1977) Cardiac, skeletal and opthalmologic abnormalities in relatives of patients with the Marfan syndrome. Circulation 55: 797–802

282 Pearlman AS, Clark CE, Henry WL, Morganroth J, Itscoitz SB, Epstein SE (1976) Determinants of ventricular septal motion. Influence of relative right and left ventricular size. Circulation 54: 83–91

283 Pearlman AS, Borer JS, Clark CE, Henry WL, Redwood DR, Morrow AG, Epstein SE (1978) Abnormal right ventricular size and ventricular septal motion after atrial septal defect closure. Etiology and functional significance. Am J Cardiol 41: 295–301

284 Perloff JK (1970) The clinical recognition of congenital heart disease. Saunders, Philadelphia

285 Pernod J, Piwnica A, Duret JC (1978) Right atrial myxoma: an echocardiographic study. Br Heart J 40: 201–203

286 Pieroni DR, Park SC, Holbrook PR, Houghton PB (1973) Echocardiographic diagnosis of septic pericarditis in infancy. J Pediatr 82: 689–691

287 Pieroni DR, Homcy E, Freedom RM (1975) Echocardiography in atrioventricular canal defect. Am J Cardiol 35: 54–58

288 Popio KA, Gorlin R, Teichholz LE, Cohn PF, Bechtel D, Herman MV (1975) Abnormalities of left ventricular function and geometry in adults with an atrial septal defect. Ventriculographic, hemodynamic and echocardiographic studies. Am J Cardiol 36: 302–308

289 Popp RL (1976) Echocardiographic assessment of cardiac disease. Circulation 54: 538–552

290 Popp RL, Carmichael BM (1971) Cardiac echography in the diagnosis of prosthetic mitral valve malfunction. Circulation [Suppl II] 44: 33 (Abstract)

291 Popp RL, Harrison DC (1969) Ultrasound in the diagnosis and evaluation of therapy of idiopathic hypertrophic subaortic stenosis. Circulation 40: 905–914

292 Popp RL, Wolfe SB, Hirata T, Feigenbaum H (1969) Estimation of right and left ventricular size by ultrasound: a study of the echoes from the interventricular septum. Am J Cardiol 24: 523–530

293 Popp RL, Silverman JF, French JW, Stinson EB, Harrison DC (1974) Echocardiographic findings in discrete subvalvular aortic stenosis. Circulation 49: 226–231

293 a Popp RL, Brown OR, Silverman JF, Harrison DC (1974) Echocardiographic abnormalities in mitral valve prolapse syndrome. Circulation 49: 428–433

294 Ports TA, Schiller NB, Strunk BL (1977) Echocardiography of right ventricular tumors. Circulation 56: 439–447

294 a Ports TA, Silverman NH, Schiller NB (1978) Two-dimensional echocardiographic assessment of Ebstein's anomaly. Circulation 58: 336–343

295 Praagh R van (1977) Terminology of congenital heart disease. Glossary and commentary. Circulation 56: 139–143

295 a Praagh R van, Durnin RE, Jockin H (1975) Anatomically corrected malposition of the great arteries (S.D.L.). Circulation 51: 20–31

296 Praagh R van, Praagh S van (1965) The anatomy of common aorticopulmonary trunk (truncus arteriosus communis) and its embryologic implications. Am J Cardiol 16: 406–425

296 a Praagh R van, Praagh S van (1966) Isolated ventricular inversion. A consideration of the morphogenesis, definition and diagnosis of nontransposed and transposed great arteries. Am J Cardiol 17: 395–406

297 Procacci PM, Savran SV, Schreiter SL, Bryson AL (1975) Clinical frequency and implications of mitral valve prolapse in the female population. Circulation [Suppl II] 52: 78 (Abstract)

298 Quinones MA, Gaasch WH, Waisser E (1974) Reduction in the rate of diastolic descent of the mitral vale echogram in patients with altered left ventricular diastolic pressure-volume relations. Circulation 49: 246–254

299 Radford DJ, Bloom KR, Izukawa T, Moes CAF, Rowe RD (1976) Echocardiographic assessment of bicuspid aortic valves. Angiographic and pathological correlates. Circulation 53: 80–85
300 Radtke WE, Tajik AJ, Gau GT, Schattenberg TT, Guiliani ER, Tancredi RG (1976) Atrial septal defect: Echocardiographic observations. Studies in 120 patients. Ann Intern Med 84: 246–253
301 Raizada V, Benchimol A, Desser KB, Reich FD, Sheasby C, Graves C (1977) Mitral valve prolapse in patients with coronary artery disease. Br Heart J 39: 53–60
302 Ray WVJ, Bennett DH, Stovin PGI, Evans DW (1976) Echocardiographic assessment of mitral valve calcification. Br Heart J 38: 81–84
303 Rees A, Elbl, F, Minhas K, Solinger R (1976) Echocardiographic evidence of outflow tract obstruction in Pompe's disease (glycogen storage disease of the heart). Am J. Cardiol 37: 1103–1106
304 Rees AH, Rao PS, Rigby JJ, Miller MD (1978) Echocardiographic estimation of a left-to-right shunt in isolated ventricular septal defects. Eur J Cardiol 7: 25
305 Reeves W, Grigges R, Nanda NC, Gramiak R (1976) Echocardiographic demonstration of mitral valve prolapse in muscular dystrophy. Circulation [Suppl II] 53/54: 97
306 Reinhold J, Rudhe U (1957) Relation of the first and second heart sounds to events in the cardiac cycle. Br Heart J 19: 473
307 Reitman M, Goldberg H, Boris G, Bakst A, Gluck R (1978) Echocardiographic assessment of a Blalock-Taussig shunt. J Clin U 6: 55
308 Riggs T, Hirschfeld S, Bormuth C, Fanaroff A, Liebman J (1977) Neonatal circulatory changes: an echocardiographic study. Pediatrics 59: 338–344
309 Riggs T, Hirscheld S, Borkat G, Knoke J, Liebman J (1978) Assessment of the pulmonary vascular bed by echocardiographic right ventricular systolic time intervals. Circulation 57: 939–947
310 Rizzon P, Biasco G, Brindicci G, Mauro F (1973) Familial syndrome of midsystolic click and late systolic murmur. Br Heart J 35: 245–259
311 Robertson D, Stevens RM, Friesinger GC, Oates JA (1977) The effect of the valsalva manoever on echocardiographic dimension in man. Circulation 55: 596–602
312 Rocchini AP, Rosenthal A, Castaneda AR, Keane JF, Jeresaty R (1976) Subaortic obstruction after the use of an intracardiac baffle to tunnel the left ventricle to the aorta. Circulation 54: 957–960
313 Rodger JC (1976) Motion of mitral apparatus in hypertrophic cardiomyopathy with obstruction. Br Heart J 38: 732–737
314 Roelandt J (1975) Echocardiology. Current applications of echotechniques in cardiology. Hart Bull 6: 9–20
315 Roelandt J (1977) Practical echocardiology. Research Studies Press, Forest Grove
316 Roelandt J, Brand M van den, Vletter WB, Nauta J, Hugenholtz PG (1975) Echocardiographic diagnosis of pseudoaneurysm of the left ventricle. Circulation 52: 466–472
317 Roelandt J, Dorp WG van, Bom N, Laird JD, Hugenholtz PG (1976) Resolution problems in echocardiology: a source of interpretation errors. Am J Cardiol 37: 256–262
318 Roeske WR, O'Rourke RA, Klein A, Leopold G, Karliner JS (1976) Noninvasive evaluation of ventricular hypertrophy in professional athletes. Circulation 53: 286–292
319 Rogé CLL, Silverman NH, Hart PA, Ray RM (1978) Cardiac structure growth pattern determined by echocardiography. Circulation 57: 285–290
320 Ross J (1976) Afterload mismatch and preload reserve: a conceptual framework for the analysis of ventricular function. Prog Cardiovasc Dis 18: 255–264
321 Rossen RM, Goodman DJ, Ingham RE, Popp RL (1974) Ventricular systolic septal thickening and excursion in idiopathic hypertrophic subaortic stenosis. N Engl J Med 291: 1317–1319
322 Rothbaum DA, Dillon JC, Chang S, Feigenbaum H (1974) Echocardiographic manifestation of right sinus of Valsalva aneurysm. Circulation 49: 768–771
323 Rudolp AM (1970) The changes in the circulation after birth. Their importance in congenital heart disease. Circulation 41: 342
324 Ruttenberg HD, Neufeld HN, Lucas RV (1964) Syndrome of congenital cardiac defects with asplenia: distinction from other forms of congenital cyanotic cardiac disease. Am J Cardiol 13: 387–406
325 Sahn DJ, Allen HD (1978) Real-time cross-sectional echocardiographic imaging and measurement of the patent ductus arteriosus in infants and children. Circulation 58: 343–354
326 Sahn DJ, Deely WJ, Hagan AD, Froedman WF (1974) Echocardiographic assessment of left ventricular performances in normal newborns. Circulation 49: 232–236

327 Sahn DJ, Terry R, O'Rourke R, Leopold G, Friedman WF (1974) Multiple crystal cross-sectional echocardiography in the diagnosis of cyanotic congenital heart disease. Circulation 50: 230–238

328 Sahn DJ, Terry RW, O'Rourke R, Leopold G, Friedman WF (1974) Multiple crystal echocardiographic evaluation of endocardial cushion defect. Circulation 50: 25–32

329 Sahn DJ, Vaucher Y, Williams DE, Allen HD, Goldberg SJ, Friedman WF (1976) Echocardiographic detection of large left-to-right shunts and cardiomyopathies in infants and children. Am J Cardiol 38: 73–79

330 Sahn DJ, Allen HD, Goldberg SJ (1976) Echocardiographic vs anatomical "discontinuity". (Letter to the editor). Circulation 53: 201–204

331 Sahn DJ, Allen HD, Goldberg SJ, Friedman WF (1976) Mitral valve prolapse in children. A problem defined by real-time cross-sectional echocardiography. Circulation 53: 651–657

332 Sahn DJ, Allen HD, George W, Mason M, Goldberg SJ (1977) The utility of contrast echocardiographic techniques in the care of critically ill infants with cardiac and pulmonary disease. Circulation 56: 959–968

333 Sahn DJ, Allen HD, McDonald G, Goldberg SJ (1977) Real-time cross-sectional echocardiographic diagnosis of coarctation of the aorta. A prospective study of echocardiographic-angiographic correlation. Circulation 56: 762–769

334 Sahn DJ, Bom N, Lancée CT, Egmond FC van, Roelandt J (1977) A dual M-mode system for simultaneous time motion analysis of cardiac structures and evaluation of cardiac function: initial clinical applications. In: Bom N (ed) Echocardiology. Nijhoff, The Hague

335 Sahn DJ, Wood J, Allen HD, Peoples W, Goldberg SJ (1977) Echocardiographic spectrum of mitral valve motion in children with and without mitral valve prolapse: the nature of false positive diagnosis. Am J Cardiol 39: 422–431

336 Sakamoto T, Matsuhisa M, Hayashi T (1975) Echocardiogram and phonocardiogram related to the movement of the pulmonary valve. Jpn Heart J 16: 107–117

337 Salomon J, Shah PM, Heinle RA (1975) Thoracic skeletal abnormalities in idiopathic mitral valve prolapse. Am J Cardiol 36: 32–36

338 Sapire DW, Black FS (1975) Echocardiographic detection of aneurysm of the interventricular septum associated with ventricular septal defect. Am J Cardiol 36: 797–801

339 Schieken RM, Kerber RE (1976) Echocardiographic abnormalities in acute rheumatic fever. Am J Cardiol 38: 458–462

340 Schiller NB, Botvinick EH (1977) Right ventricular compression as a sign of cardiac tamponade. An analysis of echocardiographic ventricular dimensions and their clinical implications. Circulation 56: 774–779

341 Schmaltz AA, Ibrahim ZI, Apitz J (1978) Clinical and angio- and echocardiographic findings in 45 children with mitral valve prolapse syndrome. Eur J Cardiol 7: 49–58

342 Scovil JA, Nanda NC, Gramiak R, Lipchik EO (1976) Echocardiographic assessment of aortic valve morphology. Circulation [Suppl II] 53/54: 112 (Abstract)

343 Scovil JA, Nanda NC, Gross CM, Lombardi AC, Gramiak R, Lipchik EO, Manning JA (1976) Echocardiographic studies of abnormalities associated with coarcation of the aorta. Circulation 53: 953–956

344 Seides SF, Joseph RL de, Brown AE, Damato AN (1975) Echocardiographic findings in isolated, surgically created tricuspid insufficiency. Am J Cardiol 35: 679–682

345 Serwer GA, Armstrong BE, Anderson PAW, Sherman D, Benson DW, Edwards SB (1978) Use of contrast echocardiography for evaluation of right ventricular hemodynamics in the presence of ventricular septal defects. Circulation 58: 327–336

346 Settle HP, Adloph RJ, Fowler NO, Engel P, Agruss Ns, Levenson NI (1977) Echocardiographic study of cardiac tamponade. Circulation 56: 951–959

347 Seward JB, Tajik AJ, Guiliana ER, Mair DD (1976) Aneurysm of the membranous ventricular septum in TGA. Echo features (letter to the editor). Circulation 54: 161–162

348 Seward JB, Tajik AJ, Hagler DJ, Guiliani ER, Gau GT, Ritter DG (1977) Echocardiogram in common (single) ventricle: angiographic-anatomic correlation. Am J Cardiol 39: 217–225

349 Seward JB, Tajik AJ, Hagler DJ, Ritter DG (1977) Contrast echocardiography in single or common ventricle. Circulation 55: 513–519

350 Seward JB, Tajik AJ, Hagler DJ, Ritter DG (1978) Echocardiographic spectrum of tricuspid atresia. Mayo Clin Proc 53: 100–112

351 Shah PM, Gramiak R, Kramer DH (1969) Ultrasound localization of left ventricular outflow obstruction in hypertrophic obstructive cardiomyopathy. Circulation 40: 3–11

352 Shapiro J, Boxer R, Krongrad F (1976) Echocardiographic observations in patients with postoperative right bundle branch block pattern. Circulation [Suppl II] 53/54: 46 (Abstract)

353 Shinebourne EA, Anderson RH, Bowyer JJ (1975) Variations in clinical presentation of Fallot's tetralogy in infancy. Angiographic and pathologic implications. Br Heart J 37: 946–955

354 Shinebourne EA, Macartney FJ, Anderson RH (1976) Sequential chamber localization – logical approach to diagnosis in congenital heart disease. Br Heart J 38: 327–340

355 Shiu MF, Jenkins BS, Webb-Peploe MM (1978) Echocardiographic analysis of posterior mitral leaflet movement in mitral stenosis. Br Heart J 40: 372–376

356 Shrivastava S, Tadavarthy SM, Fukuda T, Edwards JE (1976) Anatomic causes of pulmonary stenosis in complete transposition. Circulation 54: 154–159

357 Silverman NH, Schiller NB (1978) Apex echocardiography. A two-dimensional technique for evaluating congenital heart disease. Circulation 57: 503–511

358 Silverman NH, Lewis AB, Heymann MA, Rudolph AM (1974) Echocardiographic assessment of ductus arteriosus shunt in premature infants. Circulation 50: 821–825

359 Smith ER, Sangalang VE, Hefferman LP, Welch JP, Flemington ES (1977) Hypertrophic cardiomyopathy: the heart disease of Friedreich's ataxia. Am Heart J 94: 428–434

360 Solinger R, Elbl F, Minhas K (1973) Echocardiography in the normal neonate. Circulation 47: 108–118

361 Solinger R, Elbl F, Minhas K (1974) Deductive echocardiographic analysis in infants with congenital heart disease. Circulation 50: 1072–1096

362 Sommerville J, Ross D (1977) Atypical aortic valve stenosis causing diffuse left ventricular obstruction. Diagnosis and management (Abstract). In: Proceedings of the 15th Annual Meeting of the Association of European Pediatric Cardiologists. Belgium, 1977. Akademisch Ziekenhuis, Gent

363 Spangler RD, Okin JT (1975) Echocardiographic demonstration of a left atrial thrombus. Chest 67: 716–718

364 Spangler RD, Nord JJ, Lortscher RW, Wolfe RR, Okin JT (1976) Echocardiography in Marfan's syndrome. Chest 69: 72–78

365 Spitaels S, Arbogast R, Fouron JC, Davignon A (1974) The influence of heart rate and age on the systolic and diastolic time intervals in children. Circulation 49: 1107–1115

366 Sridaromont S, Feldt RH, Ritter DG, Davis GD, Edwards JE (1976) Double outlet right ventricle: hemodynamic and anatomic correlations. Am J Cardiol 38: 85–94

367 Stanger P, Rudolph AM, Edwards JE (1977) Cardiac malpositions. An overview based on study of 65 necropsy specimens. Circulation 56: 159–172

368 Stefadouros MA, Witham AC (1975) Systolic time intervals by echocardiography. Circulation 51: 114–117

369 Stevenson JG, Kawabori I, Dooley T, Guntheroth WG (1978) Diagnosis of ventricular septal defect by pulsed Doppler echocardiography. Circulation 58: 322–326

370 Story WE, Felner JM, Schlant R (1977) Echocardiographic criteria for the diagnosis of mitral-semilunar continuity. Am Heart J 93: 575–580

371 Strunk BL, Guss SB, Hicks RE, Kotler MN (1975) Echocardiographic recognition of the mitral valve – posterior aortic wall relationship. Circulation 51: 594–598

372 Strunk BL, Fitzgerald JW, Lipton M, Popp RL, Barry WH (1976) The posterior aortic wall echocardiogram. Its relationship to left atrial volume change. Circulation 54: 744–750

373 Sutton MGSJ, Hagler DJ, Tajik AJ, Giuliani ER, Seward JB (1978) Cardiac function in the normal newborn. Additional information by complete analysis of the M-mode echocardiogram. Circulation 57: 1198–1204

374 Sweatman T, Selzer A, Kamagaki M, Cohn K (1972) Echocardiographic diagnosis of mitral regurgitation due to ruptured chordae tendineae. Circulation 46: 580–586

375 Tajik AJ, Giuliani ER (1974) Echocardiographic observations in idiopathic hypertrophic subaortic stenosis. Mayo Clin Proc 49: 89–97

376 Tajik AJ, Giuliani ER (1977) Diastolic opening of the aortic valve. An echocardiographic observation. Mayo Clin Proc 52: 112–116

377 Tajik AJ, Gau GT, Schattenberg TT, Ritter DG (1972) Normal ventricular septal motion in atrial septal defect. An echocardiographic observation. Mayo Clin Proc 47: 635–638

378 Tajik AJ, Gau GT, Ritter DG, Schattenberg TT (1972) Echocardiographic pattern of right ventricular diastolic volume overload in children. Circulation 46: 36–43

379 Tajik AJ, Gau GT, Schattenberg TT (1972) Echocardiogram in atrial septal defect. Chest 62: 213–214

380 Tajik AJ, Gau GT, Schattenberg TT (1972) Echocardiogram in total anomalous pulmonary venous drainage. Mayo Clin Proc 47: 247–250

381 Tajik AJ, Gau GT, Schattenberg TT (1972) Echocardiographic "pseudo IHSS" pattern in atrial septal defect. Chest 62: 324–325

382 Tajik AJ, Gau GT, Giuliani ER, Ritter DG, Schattenberg TT (1973) Echocardiogram in Ebstein's anomaly with Wolff-Parkinson-White preexicitation syndrome, type B. Circulation 47: 813–818

383 Tajik AJ, Gau GT, Ritter DG, Schattenberg TT (1973) Echocardiogram in tetralogy of Fallot. Chest 64: 107–108

384 Tamer DM, Watson DD, Kenny PJ, Janowitz WR, Gelband H, Gilson AJ (1977) Noninvasive detection and quantification of left-to-right shunts in children using oxygen-15 labeled carbon dioxide. Circulation 56: 626–631

385 Ten Cate FJ (1977) Echocardiologic assessment in asymmetric septal hypertrophy In: Bom N (ed) Echocardiology. Nijhoff, The Hague

386 Ten Cate FJ, Hugenholtz PG, Roelandt J (1977) Ultrasound study of dynamic behaviour of the left ventricle in genetic asymmetric septal hypertrophy. Br Heart J 39: 627–633

387 Termini BA, Jackson PA, Williams CD (1977) Systolic anterior motion of the mitral valve following annuloplasty. Vasc Surg 11: 55–60

388 Thomson K, Nanda N, Gramiak R (1976) Reliability of echocardiography in the diagnosis of infective endocarditis. Circulation [Suppl II] 53/54: 112 (Abstract)

389 Ticzon AR, Damato AN, Caracta AR, Russo G, Foster JR, Lau SH (1976) Interventricular septal motion during preexcitation and normal conduction in Wolff-Parkinson-White syndrome. Echocardiographic and electrophysiologic correlation. Am J Cardiol 37: 840–847

390 Tingelstad JB, Robertson LW (1976) Fluttering of the interventricular septum. Chest 69: 119–120

391 Traill T, Sutton M, Sanderson J, Brown D, Gibson D, Goodwin J (1976) Echocardiographic study of left ventricular filling in hypertrophic cardiomyopathy Circulation [Suppl II] 53/54: 190 (Abstract)

392 Traill TA, Gibson DG, Brown DJ (1978) Study of left ventricular wall thickness and dimension changes using echocardiography. Br Heart J 40: 162–169

393 Ultan LB, Segal BL, Likoff W (1967) Echocardiography in congenital heart disease. Preliminary observation. Am J Cardiol 19: 74–83

394 Upton MT, Gibson DG, Brown DJ (1976) Echocardiographic assessment of abnormal left ventricular relaxation in man. Br Heart J 38: 1001–1009

395 Usher BW, Goulden D, Murgo JP (1974) Echocardiographic detection of supravalvular aortic stenosis. Circulation 48: 1257–1259

396 Valdes-Cruz LM, Pieroni DR, Roland JMA, Varghese PJ (1976) Echocardiographic detection of intracardiac right-to-left shunts following peripheral vein injections. Circulation 54, 558–562

397 Valdes-Cruz LM, Pieroni DR, Roland JMA, Shematek JP (1977) Recognition of residual postoperative shunts by contrast echocardiographic techniques. Circulation 55: 148–152

398 Verani MS, Lauer RM (1975) Echocardiographic findings in right coronary arterial – right ventricular fistula. Report of a neonate with fatal congestive heart failure. Am J Cardiol 35: 444–447

399 Vidne BA, Subramanian S, Wagner HR (1976) Aneurysm of the membranous ventricular septum in transposition of the great arteries. Circulation 53: 157–161

400 Vignola P, Boucher C, Gurfman G, Walker H, Pohost G, Dinsmore R, Shea W (1977) Postoperative echocardiographic abnormal septal motion: clinical, hemodynamic and surgical correlates. Circulation [Suppl III] 55/56: 24 (Abstract)

401 Vignola PA, Walker HJ, Gold HK, Leinbach RC (1977) Alteration of the left ventricular pressure-volume relationship in man and its effect on the mitral echocardiographic early diastolic closure slope. Circulation 56: 586–592

402 Waggoner AD, Adyanthaya AV, Quinones MA, Alexander JK (1976) Left atrial enlargement. Echocardiographic assessment of electrocardiographic criteria. Circulation 54: 553–557

403 Wanderman KL, Goldberg MJ, Stack RS, Weissler AM (1976) Left ventricular performance in mitral regurgitation assessed with systolic time intervals and echocardiography. Am J Cardiol 38: 831–835

404 Wanderman KL, Ovsyshcher I, Gueron M (1978) Left ventricular performance in patients with atrial septal defect: evaluation with noninvasive methods. Am J Cardiol 41: 487–493

405 Wann LS, Dillon JC, Weyman AE, Feigenbaum H (1976) Echocardiography in bacterial endocarditis. N Engl J Med 295: 135–139

406 Wann LS, Weyman AE, Dillon JC, Feigenbaum H (1977) Premature pulmonary valve opening. Circulation 55: 128–133

407 Wann LS, Feigenbaum H, Weyman AE, Dillon JC (1978) Cross-sectional echocardiographic detection of rheumatic mitral regurgitation. Am J Cardiol 41: 1258–1263

408 Warren SG, Waugh RA, Kisslo J, Johnson ML (1974) Echocardiographic abnormalities in ruptured right coronary sinus of Valsalva aneurysm. Circulation [Suppl III] 49/50: 249 (Abstract)

409 Waxler EB, Kawai N, Kasparian H (1972) Right atrial myxoma, echocardiographic, phonocardiographic and hemodynamic signs. Am Heart J 83: 251–257

410 Weaver WF, Wilson CS, Rourke T, Caudill CC (1977) Mid-diastolic aortic valve opening in severe acute aortic regurgitation. Circulation 55: 145–148

411 Weinnert L, Bommer W, Neumann A, George L, Mason DT, Maria AN de (1977) Evaluation of right atrial and right ventricular size by cross-sectional echocardiography: comparison of normals and right ventricular overload. Circulation [Suppl III] 55/56: 24 (Abstract)

412 Weiss AN, Chaval S, Ludbrook PA (1974) Echocardiographic recognition of paradoxical interventricular septal motion associated with right ventricular premature beats. Circulation [Suppl III] 49/50: 250 (Abstract)

413 Weiss AN, Nimbs JW, Ludbrook PA, Sobel BE (1975) Echocardiographic detection of mitral valve prolapse. Circulation 52: 1091–1096

414 Weissler AM (1977) Current concepts in cardiology. Systolic time intervals. N Engl J Med 296: 321–324

415 Weissler AM, Lewis RP, Leighton RF (1972) The systolic time intervals as a measure of left ventricular performance in man. In: Yu PN (ed) Progress in cardiology, vol I. Lea and Febiger, Philadelphia

416 Werner JA, Schiller NB, Prasquier R (1976) Occurence and significance of echographically demonstrated tricuspid valve prolapse. Circulation [Suppl II] 53/54: 232 (Abstract)

417 Weyman AE, Dillon JC, Feigenbaum H, Chang S (1974) Echocardiographic patterns of pulmonic valve motion in pulmonic stenosis. Am J Cardiol 33: 178 (Abstract)

418 Weyman AE, Dillon JC, Feigenbaum H, Chang S (1974) Echocardiographic patterns of pulmonic valve motion with pulmonary hypertension. Circulation 50: 905–910

419 Weyman AE, Dillon JC, Feigenbaum H, Chang S (1975) Echocardiographic differentiation of infundibular from valvular pulmonary stenosis. Am J Cardiol 36: 21–26

420 Weyman AE, Dillon JC, Feigenbaum H, Chang S (1975) Premature pulmonic valve opening following sinus of Valsalva aneurysm rupture into the right atrium. Circulation 51: 556–560

421 Weyman AE, Dillon JC, Feigenbaum H, Chang S (1975) Pulmonary valve echo motion in pulmonary regurgitation. Br Heart J 37: 1184–1190

422 Weyman AE, Feigenbaum H (1976) Echocardiography. Where are we now and where are we going. Am J Med 60: 315–320

423 Weyman AE, Wann S, Feigenbaum H, Dillon JC (1976) Mechanism of abnormal septal motion in patients with right ventricular volume overload. Circulation 54: 179–186

424 Weyman AE, Feigenbaum H, Hurwitz RA, Girod DA, Dillon JC, Chang S (1976) Cross-sectional echocardiography in evaluating patients with discrete subaortic stenois. Am J Cardiol 37: 358–365

425 Weyman AE, Feigenbaum H, Hurwitz RA, Girod DA, Dillon JC, Chang S (1976) Localization of left ventricular outflow obstruction by cross-sectional echocardiography. Am J Med 60: 33–38

426 Weyman AE, Hurwitz RA, Girod DA, Dillon JC, Feigenbaum H, Green D (1977) Cross-sectional echocardiographic visualization of the stenotic pulmonary valve. Circulation 56: 769–774

427 Weyman AE, Caldwell RL, Hurwitz RA, Girod DA, Dillon JC, Feigenbaum H, Green D (1978) Cross-sectional echocardiographic characterization of aortic obstruction. 1 Supravalvular aortic stenosis and aortic hypoplasia. Circulation 57: 491–497

428 Weyman AE, Caldwell RL, Hurwitz RA, Girod DA, Dillon JC, Feigenbaum H, Green D (1978) Cross-sectional echocardiographic detection of aortic obstruction. 2. Coarctation of the aorta. Circulation 57: 498–502

429 Weyman AE, Feigenbaum H, Hurwitz RA, Girod DA, Dillon JC (1977) Cross-sectional echocardiographic assessment of the severity of aortic stenosis in children. Circulation 55: 773–778

430 Williams R, Rudd M (1974) Echocardiographic features of endocardial cushion defect. Circulation 49: 418–422

431 Williams RG, Tucker CR (1977) Echocardiographic diagnosis of congenital heart disease. Little Brown, Boston

432 Williams DE, Sahn DJ, Friedman WF (1976) Cross-section echocardiographic localization of sites of left ventricular outflow tract obstruction. Am J Cardiol 37: 250–255
433 Wing JP, Findlay WA, Sahn DJ, McDonald G, Allen AD, Goldberg SJ (1978) Serial echocardiographic profiles in infants and children with coarctation of the aorta. Am J Cardiol 41: 1270–1277
434 Wolfe SB, Popp RL, Feigenbaum H (1969) Diagnosis of atrial tumors by ultrasound. Circulation 39: 615–622
435 Wray TM (1975) The variable echocardiographic features in aortic valve endocarditis. Circulation 52: 658–662
436 Yabek SM, Isabel-Jones J, Bhatt DR, Nakazawa M, Marks RA, Jarmakani JM (1972) Echocardiographic determination of left atrial volumes in children with congenital heart disease. Circulation 53: 268–272
437 Yoshikawa J, Tanaka K, Owaki T, Kato H (1976) Cord-like aortic valve vegetation in bacterial endocarditis. Demonstration by cardiac ultrasonography. Report of a case. Circulation 53: 911–914
438 Zoneraich S, Zoneraich O, Rhee JJ (1977) Echocardiographic evaluation of septal motion in patients with artificial pacemakers: vectorcardiographic correlations. Am Heart J 93: 596–602

Subject Index

Page nummers in *italics* refer to chapter index.

GPSR Compliance
The European Union's (EU) General Product Safety Regulation (GPSR) is a set of rules that requires consumer products to be safe and our obligations to ensure this.

If you have any concerns about our products, you can contact us on

ProductSafety@springernature.com

In case Publisher is established outside the EU, the EU authorized representative is:

Springer Nature Customer Service Center GmbH
Europaplatz 3
69115 Heidelberg, Germany

www.ingramcontent.com/pod-product-compliance
Lightning Source LLC
Chambersburg PA
CBHW061206240926
51846CB00006B/1126
* 9 7 8 3 6 4 2 6 7 5 1 7 1 *